RHEUMATOID ARTHRITIS – ETIOLOGY, CONSEQUENCES AND CO-MORBIDITIES

Edited by **Andrew B. Lemmey**

Rheumatoid Arthritis – Etiology, Consequences and Co-Morbidities
Edited by Andrew B. Lemmey

Published by InTech

Janeza Trdine 9, 51000 Rijeka, Croatia

Publishing Process Manager Anja Filipovic

Technical Editor Teodora Smiljanic

Cover Designer InTech Design Team

Additional hard copies can be obtained from orders@intechopen.com

Rheumatoid Arthritis – Etiology, Consequences and Co-Morbidities,
Edited by Andrew B. Lemmey
p. cm.
ISBN 978-953-307-847-2

For EU product safety concerns:
IN TECH d.o.o., Prolaz Marije Krucifikse Kozulić 3, 51000 Rijeka, Croatia,
info@intechopen.com or visit our website at intechopen.com.

Meet the editor

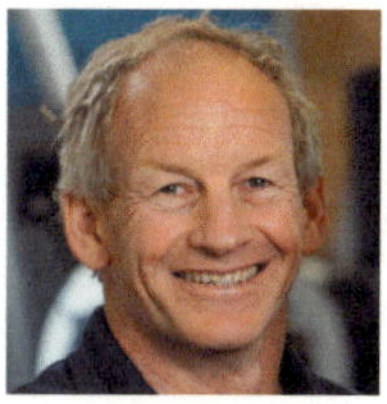

Dr. Andrew B. Lemmey, BSc (Hons), MA, PhD, is a clinical exercise physiologist in the School of Sport, Health and Exercise Sciences at Bangor University in the UK He has a 14 year background in leading groundbreaking research into restoring physical function and attenuating disabilities in patients with rheumatoid arthritis (RA). His expertise in this field was recognized by the American College of Sports Medicine, who invited him to author the chapter on arthritis in their influential text "Clinical Exercise Physiology (3rd Ed.)" (Human Kinetics). Dr. Lemmey has over 50 peer-reviewed publications, is a regular speaker at international conferences, and is a member of the British Society for Rheumatology. After gaining his PhD from the University of Adelaide, Dr. Lemmey was a post-doctoral research fellow at Cambridge and Bristol prior to accepting his current academic post at Bangor.

Contents

Preface

Rheumatoid arthritis (RA) is a chronic, autoimmune, inflammatory arthritis, which features destruction of synovial joints, systemic inflammation, functional disability, reduced quality of life, and increased morbidity and mortality. It is relatively common, having a world-wide prevalence of between 0.5-2%, and is associated with huge social and economic costs. Consequently, it is the most important of the inflammatory arthritides.

The aim of *Rheumatoid Arthritis – Etiology, Consequences and Co-Morbidities* is not to provide a comprehensive commentary on RA (several of these are already in publication), but rather to provide interesting, thought-provoking, and up-to-date perspectives on a variety of aspects of current research into this condition. In taking this approach, *Rheumatoid Arthritis – Etiology, Consequences and Co-Morbidities* includes topics not usually covered by conventional publications. As such, it is an ideal reference and source of inspiration and direction for investigators, whatever their level, in the challenging and exciting field of rheumatology research.

This book is broadly divided into: "Etiology" (chapters 1-10), and "Consequences and Co-Morbidities" (chapters 11-16).

The editor would like to thank the chapter authors for their excellent contributions, and extend to them the wish that their current and future research endeavors are fruitful. Special thanks are also given to Anja Filipovic and other InTech staff for their expert editorial assistance in publishing this book.

RA is an exciting condition to investigate. Hopefully, this book will help to advance research into the mechanisms and treatment of the disease.

Dr. Andrew B. Lemmey
School of Sport, Health & Exercise Sciences,
College of Health & Behavioral Sciences,
Bangor University,
UK

Part 1

Etiology

1

Cytokine Profile of T Cells in the Joints of Rheumatoid Arthritis and Its Murine Models

Takashi Usui
Center for Innovation in Immunoregulative Technology and Therapeutics, Graduate School of Medicine, Kyoto University
Japan

1. Introduction

Rheumatoid arthritis (RA) is a chronic autoimmune disease that results in the destruction of cartilage and bone in joints. The murine Collagen-Induced Arthritis (CIA) model has been used to investigate the pathogenesis of RA representatively, because it shares many features with RA (Courtenay, et al., 1980; Luross & Williams, 2001). Susceptibility to arthritis of both CIA and RA is associated with the specific major histocompatibility complex class II allele (Gregersen, et al., 1987; Wooley, et al., 1989). In addition, autoantibodies to type II collagen (CII) have been detected from the synovial fluid of RA patients and it has an aggravating effect in both CIA mice and RA (Clague & Moore, 1984; Cook, et al., 1996; Mullazehi, et al., 2007; Tarkowski, et al., 1989). Finally, pathogenic contributions of $CD4^+$ helper T (Th) cells have been reported in both CIA mice and RA (Weyand & Goronzy, 1999; Weyand, et al., 1998). More recently, the SKG mouse which carries a point mutation of the gene encoding zeta-chain-associated protein kinase 70 (ZAP-70) has been reported as a new model of RA. However, there is little information available about the similarities and differences in the pathogenesis of arthritis among these murine models and RA.

Interleukin-17 (IL-17) is a cytokine secreted by T cells, natural killer (NK) cells, and neutrophils (Ferretti, et al., 2003), and it induces IL-6, IL-8, chemokine, and metalloproteinase production by target cells (Weaver, et al., 2007). Central pathogenic roles of IL-17 in CIA have also been reported recently. For example, systemic or local IL-17 gene transfer aggravated CIA, whereas administration of an IL-17-blocking antibody ameliorated CIA even after the onset of arthritis (Lubberts, et al., 2001; Lubberts, et al., 2004) and IL-17 deficient mice also showed reduced severity of CIA (Nakae, et al., 2003). Furthermore, IL-23 deficient mice, which show impaired Th17 response, do not exhibit CIA because IL-23 is an essential factor for the maintenance of Th17 cells (Murphy, et al., 2003). Consequently, although the pathological contribution of IL-17 to CIA is evident, it remains unclear with RA.

In the present study, we analyzed the phenotypes and cytokine profiles of T cells in the joints of CIA mice kinetically, for the first time, and then analyzed those of SKG mice and RA.

2. Most of the IL-17-producing T cells in the swollen joints of CIA were gamma/delta T cells

To analyze the phenotype and cytokine profile of T cells in the joints of CIA mice, we choose foot pad injection for CII-CFA (complete Freund's adjuvant) instead of tail base injection to distinguish the inflammatory effect of adjuvant itself from real CIA. Each joint was thus designated as immunized joint (CII-CFA injected site), swollen joint (real CIA), or non-swollen joint (Figure 1A). First, the phenotypes and cytokine profiles of T cells in swollen joints of CIA mice were analyzed using intra-cellular cytokine staining by FACS at the peak of CIA (Figure 1B). Surprisingly, most of the IL-17-producing T cells were gamma/delta TCR+ T cells, and did not express CD4, CD8, and DX5. The remainder of the IL-17-producing cells were Th17 cells which express alpha/beta TCR+ (data not shown) and CD4, and neither $CD8^+$ cells nor $DX5^+$ NK cells produced IL-17.

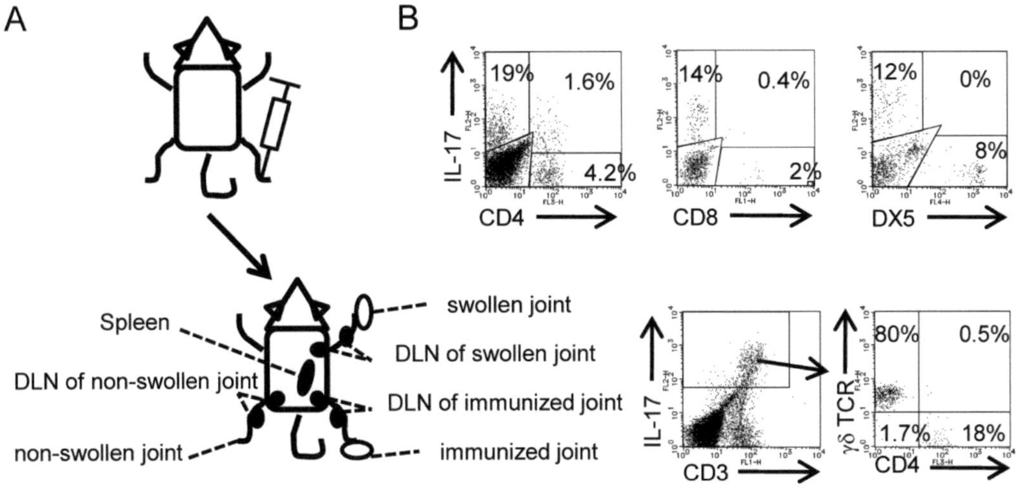

Fig. 1. Phenotypes of IL-17 producing T cells in the swollen joints of CIA

A, Schema of analyzed joints and their DLNs of mice with CIA. **B**, Infiltrated cells of swollen joint of CIA mice were obtained by collagenase digestion, and stained with antibodies against CD3, CD4, CD8, DX5, and gamma/delta TCR. IL-17-producing cells were detected by intracellular cytokine staining. The percentage of cells in each region or quadrant is noted.

3. Distribution and kinetics of IL-17- and IFN-gamma-producing T cells in the joints of CIA

We next analyzed the kinetics of phenotypes and cytokine profiles of infiltrated T cells in the joints of CIA mice at six distinct phases: before immunization (naïve mice), one day after immunization (day 1), before onset (day 10), onset (day 32), peak (day 42), and ankylosing phase (day 70) of arthritis. At each phase, cells were collected from the swollen joint, immunized joint and non-swollen joint, as well as the DLN and spleen (Fig. 1A).

In the swollen joints, absolute numbers of IL-17-producing gamma/delta T cells were larger than those of Th17 cells (CD4+, alpha/beta TCR+ T cells) with the maximal counts at the peak of arthritis (Fig. 2A and B). Surprisingly, neither IFN-gamma-producing $CD4^+$ (Th1) cells nor IFN-gamma-producing gamma/delta T cells were detected at any phase analyzed in the swollen joints. In contrast, IFN-gamma-producing T cells were detected in their DLNs (Fig. 2A). In the immunized joints, IL-17-producing gamma/delta T cells and Th17 cells were already observed on Day 1, reached the first peak on day 10 after immunization, and then reached their highest counts with the peak of arthritis. The absolute numbers of IL-17-producing gamma/delta T cells were consistently larger than those of Th17 cells at most time points analyzed. In contrast to the swollen joints, IFN-gamma-producing T cells were detected in the immunized joints after immunization (Fig. 2A and B). For both swollen and immunized joints, the percentages of IL-17-producing gamma/delta T cells among IL-17-producing cells were larger than those in their DLNs (Fig. 2A). In the non-swollen joints, both IL-17-producing T cells and IFN-gamma-producing T cells were rarely observed. In addition, IFN-gamma-producing gamma/delta T cells were a minor population in the joints of CIA (Fig. 2A). These data suggest that CIA is an IL-17-driven arthritis that is produced mainly by gamma/delta T cells, while IFN-gamma-producing T cells are probably dispensable.

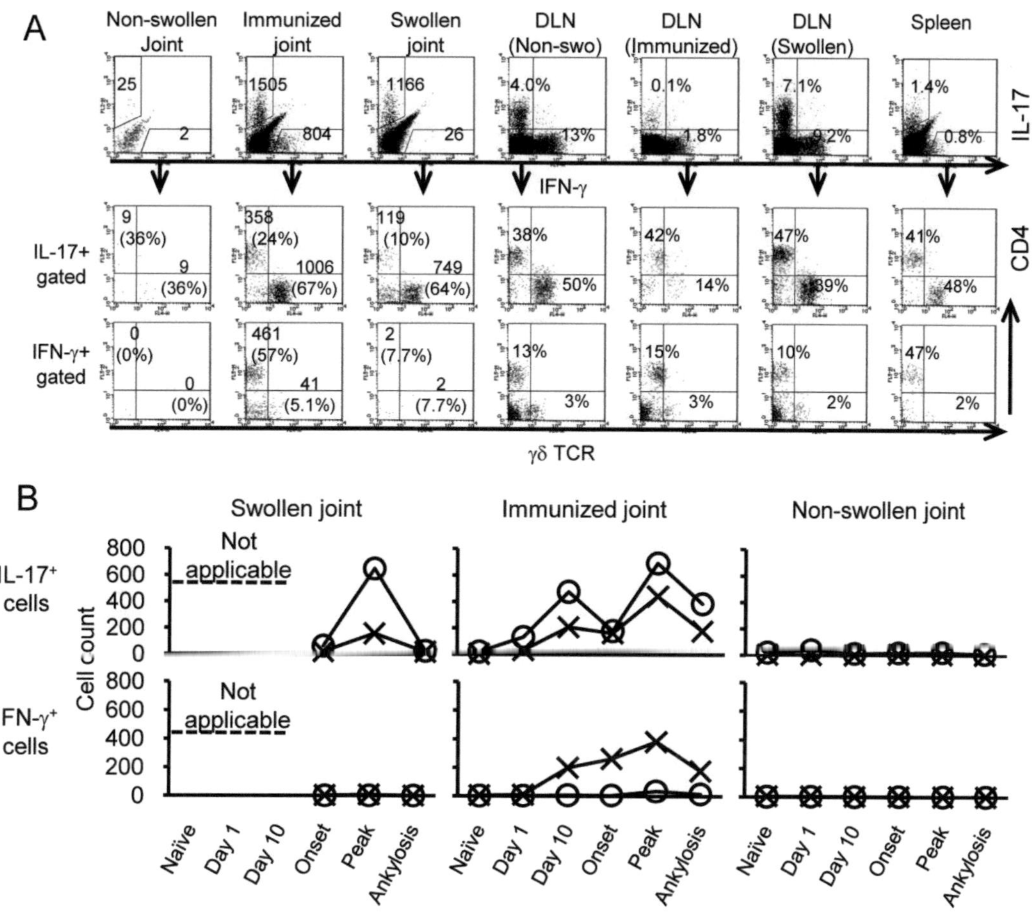

Fig. 2. Distribution and kinetics of IL-17- and IFN-gamma-producing T cells in the CIA joints

A, Cells were obtained from joints, their DLNs, and the spleens of mice with CIA at the peak of arthritis. IL-17-producing T cells and IFN-gamma-producing T cells were detected by intracellular cytokine staining (top row). IL-17-producing T cells (second row) or IFN-gamma-producing T cells (bottom row) were gated and plotted by their expression of gamma/delta TCR and CD4. The absolute number and the percentage of T cells among them are indicated in the joint panels. In panels of DLNs and spleens, the percentages of cells in each quadrant are noted. **B**, Cells were recovered from swollen joints, immunized joints, and non-swollen joints of CIA mice at the six distinct phases of arthritis. IL-17-producing T cells and IFN-gamma-producing T cells were detected by intracellular cytokine staining, and their absolute numbers were counted (open circle; gamma/delta T cell, cross; $CD4^+$ T cells).

4. IL-23 and IL-1 beta efficiently stimulate IL-17 production by gamma/delta T cells

It is known that a subset of gamma/delta T cells already differentiate to acquire the IL-17-producing function in the thymus (Jensen, et al., 2008), and CCR6 is suggested as a specific marker of Th17 cells (Acosta-Rodriguez, et al., 2007; Annunziato, et al., 2007; Hirota, et al., 2007; Singh, et al., 2008). Therefore, the expression of CCR6 on IL-17-producing gamma/delta T cells in the thymus of naïve DBA1/J mice was evaluated. IL-17-producing, but not IFN-gamma-producing gamma/delta T cells preferentially expressed CCR6 (Fig. 3A). As it has also been reported that small numbers of gamma/delta T cells are present in the normal joints of mice (Arai, et al., 1996), we next examined whether de novo $CCR6^+$ IL-17-producing gamma/delta T cells are present in the normal joints of naïve DBA1/J mice. Cells were collected from the normal joints of naïve mice and intracellular cytokine staining was performed. By analyzing cells from two normal paws and ankles at a time, $CCR6^+$ IL-17-producing gamma/delta T cells could be detected (data not shown). In addition, in CIA mice, 92% of $CCR6^+$ gamma/delta T cells produced IL-17 (Fig. 3B). Next, the signal requirements of IL-17-producing gamma/delta T cells were analyzed. Gamma/delta T cells from naïve DBA1/J mice were stimulated with cytokines in the presence or absence of anti-gamma/delta TCR activating mAb (Fig. 3C). Although small numbers of IL-17-producing gamma/delta T cells were detected by stimulations with anti- gamma/delta TCR mAb, IL-23, or IL-1 beta alone, IL-23 plus IL-1 beta induced IL-17-producing gamma/delta T cells quite efficiently without anti- gamma/delta TCR stimulation. These observations indicated that TCR signaling was not necessary to stimulate IL-17-producing gamma/delta T cells. Furthermore, a combination of IL-23 and IL-1 beta was a much more potent stimulator than TCR signaling. Similar results were obtained with gamma/delta T cells sorted from DLNs of swollen joints at the peak of CIA (Fig. 3C, right panel).

A, Thymocytes from naïve mice were stimulated with PMA and ionomycin for 4 h. Gamma/delta TCR^+ cells were gated and $CCR6^+$ cells among IL-17-producing or IFN-gamma-producing gamma/delta T cells were detected. The percentages of cells in each quadrant are indicated. **B**, Cells were collected from DLNs of swollen joints of CIA mice. IL-17-producing cells were detected by intracellular cytokine staining. $CCR6^+$ cells were gated and IL-17-producing cells were analyzed. The percentage of IL-17-producing cells among $CCR6^+$ gamma/delta T cells is noted. **C**, Gamma/delta T cells were sorted from peripheral lymph nodes of naïve DBA1/J mice (upper panel) or DLNs of swollen joints of CIA mice at the peak of arthritis (lower panel) and stimulated with cytokines, activating anti-gamma/delta TCR antibodies, and anti-CD28 antibodies for 24 h. By intracellular cytokine staining, the percentages of IL-17-producing cells among gamma/delta T cells were determined. Mean ± SEM is shown from three different mice.

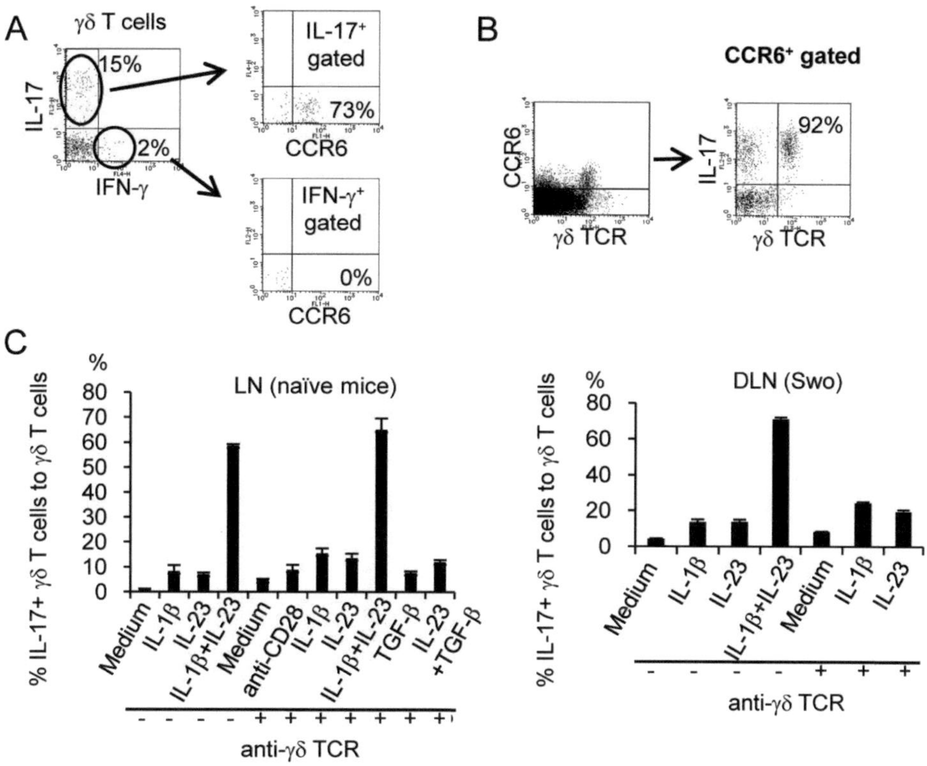

Fig. 3. IL-23 and IL-1 beta efficiently stimulate IL-17-producing gamma/delta t cells without TCR stimulation

5. IL-17-producing gamma/delta T cells were maintained by IL-23 but not by CII in vitro and induced by IFA in vivo

Since IL-23 plays important roles in the maintenance of Th17 cells (Bettelli, et al., 2006; Harrington, et al., 2005; Infante-Duarte, et al., 2000; Mangan, et al., 2006; Park, et al., 2005; Veldhoen, et al., 2006), we next analyzed the maintaining effect of IL-23 or CII on IL-17-producing gamma/delta T cells. To test this, cells from DLNs of swollen joints of CIA mice were cultured with IL-23, CII, or medium alone (Fig. 4A). Both IL-17-producing gamma/delta T cells and Th17 cells were maintained by the presence of IL-23. However, IL-17-producing gamma/delta T cells were not maintained by the presence of CII, and Th17 cells showed CII-dependency. To further investigate the factors that enhance the accumulation of IL-17-producing gamma/delta T cells in the inflamed joints, the numbers of IL-17-producing gamma/delta T cells were counted in the joints of differently-immunized mice on day 10. Mice were immunized with PBS, IFA+solution (0.05 mM of acetic acid for CII solvent), IFA+CII, or CFA+CII (Fig. 4B). The numbers of IL-17-producing gamma/delta T cells were not significantly different between mice immunized with IFA+solution, IFA+CII, or CFA+CII. In contrast, the numbers of IL-17-producing gamma/delta T cells were significantly smaller in mice immunized with PBS than in the other three conditions, while the numbers of Th17 cells were significantly larger in mice immunized with IFA+CII than those in mice treated with IFA+solution. These data suggested that IL-17-producing gamma/delta T cells do not specifically respond to CII and may just respond to adjuvant (IFA+solution) or adjuvant-induced IL-23.

6. IL-17-producing gamma/delta T cells did not induce but amplified CIA

Next, the pathogenic roles of IL-17-producing gamma/delta T cells in CIA were evaluated. Because we found that CCR6 is an exclusive marker for IL-17-producing T cell even in the case of gamma/delta T cells, CCR6⁺ gamma/delta T cells were sorted from DLN of the swollen joints of CIA mice as the source of IL-17-producing gamma/delta T cells (data not shown). When CCR6⁺ gamma/delta T cells were transferred to the joints of naïve mice, arthritis was not indiced. However, when it was transferred to the joints of mice immunized with CII+CFA, it significantly worsened the arthritis score compared with PBS (Fig. 4C). The arthritis-exacerbating effect of CCR6⁺ gamma/delta T cells from swollen joints was equivalent to CCR6⁺ gamma/delta T cells from DLNs of swollen joints (data not shown).

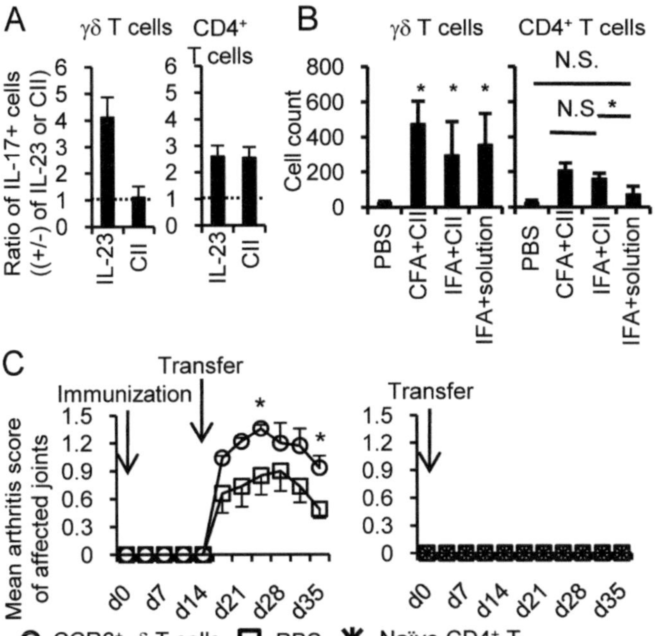

Fig. 4. IL-17-producing gamma/delta T cells were maintained by IL-23, and did not induce but amplified CIA

A, Cells were prepared from the DLNs of swollen joints and cultured for 7 days in the presence of IL-23, CII, or medium alone. IL-17-producing T cells were detected using FACS analysis. The ratio of the numbers of IL-17-producing T cells in the presence of IL-23 or CII to those in medium alone was calculated. Mean ± SEM is shown from at least three different experiments. **B**, Various combinations of substances were administered into the footpads of DBA1/J mice. Ten days later, the absolute numbers of IL-17-producing cells were counted by FACS analysis. Mean ± SEM is shown from at least three different mice. * = $P < 0.05$. **C**, CCR6⁺ gamma/delta T cells were sorted from DLNs of swollen joints of CIA mice, then those cells or PBS alone were injected to unimmunized wrists or ankles of mice immunized with CII+CFA two weeks before. For naïve mice, CCR6+ gamma/delta T cells, naïve CD4+ T cells, or PBS alone were injected. Mean ± SEM of the arthritis score of affected joints is shown. * = $P < 0.05$.

7. IL-17-producing gamma/delta T cells were not detected in the swollen joints of SKG mice

To elucidate the pathological differences from other murine arthritis models, the same analysis was performed using SKG mice (Sakaguchi, et al., 2003). SKG mice carry a point mutation of the gene encoding zeta-chain-associated protein kinase 70 (ZAP-70), and homozygous mice show IL-17-dependent arthritis resembling RA. Although the present study could detect only a few IL-17-producing gamma/delta T cells in the DLNs of swollen joints, surprisingly almost all of the IL-17-producing cells were Th17 cells and the numbers of IL-17-producing gamma/delta T cells were negligible in the swollen joints of SKG mice (Fig. 5A). As SKG is a BALB/c-background strain, and SKG arthritis is induced by zymosan as an adjuvant (Sakaguchi, et al., 2003; Yoshitomi, et al., 2005), the possibility that IL-17-producing gamma/delta T cells are absent in the joints of SKG arthritis should be excluded because of the differences in strain or adjuvant from CIA. Thus we counted the absolute numbers of cell subsets from joints immunized with CFA+CII of SKG or BALB/c mice. Even in this condition, IL-17-producing gamma/delta T cells were not detected in SKG mice, whereas IL-17-producing gamma/delta T cells were more abundant than Th17 cells in BALB/c (Fig. 5B). These data suggested that SKG mice have some impairment of development or maintenance in IL-17-producing gamma/delta T cells.

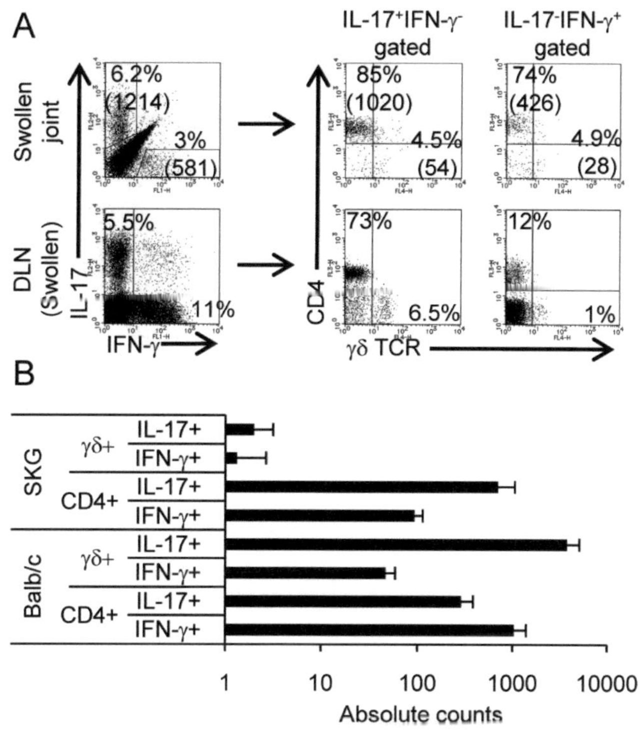

Fig. 5. IL-17-producing gamma/delta T cells were not detected in swollen joints of SKG mice

A, Cells were collected from an ankle with maximum arthritis and its DLNs of SKG mice treated with zymosan 7 weeks previously. IL-17-producing cells and IFN-gamma-producing cells were detected by intracellular cytokine staining (left column). IL-17-producing IFN-gamma-negative cells (middle column) or IFN-gamma-producing IL-17-negative cells (right column) were gated and plotted by their expressions of gamma/delta TCR and CD4. The absolute numbers and percentages of $CD4^+$ cells and gamma/delta TCR^+ cells are indicated. **B**, SKG or BALB/c mice were immunized with CFA+CII and cells in their immunized joints were collected 10 days later. Absolute numbers of cells were counted by FACS analysis. Mean ± SEM is shown from three different mice.

8. In RA affected joints, IL-17-producing gamma/delta T cells were not detected, and IFN-gamma-producing T cells were dominant

Finally, cells in synovial tissues or fluids with RA patients were analyzed to determine the presence of IL-17-producing gamma/delta T cells, Th17 and Th1 cells. In contrast to CIA, IL-17-producing gamma/delta T cells could not be detected in either synovial tissues or synovial fluids of the affected joints with RA, whereas a small number of IFN-gamma-producing gamma/delta T cells were present in synovial tissues (Fig. 6A). Among the $CD4^+$ T cells in both synovial tissues and synovial fluids, IL-17-producing cells were rarely present, and IFN-gamma-producing T cells were clearly dominant in the affected joints of RA patients (Fig. 6A and B). Although this finding is consistent with a previous report (Yamada, et al., 2007), we confirmed it in both synovial tissues and fluids of RA patients.

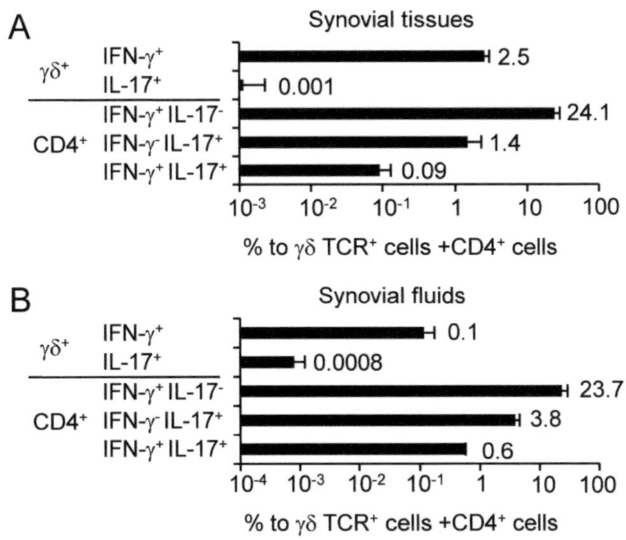

Fig. 6. IL-17-producing gamma/delta T cells were not detected, and IFN-gamma-producing T cells were dominant in the affected joints of RA

Cells in synovial tissues (n=4) or synovial fluids (n=7) of RA were isolated and stained with antibodies against CD4, gamma/delta TCR, IL-17, and IFN-gamma after stimulation by PMA/ionomycin for 6 hours. The percentages of cells out of the total of gamma/delta T cells plus $CD4^+$ T cells were determined. Mean ± SEM is shown.

9. Conclusion

This study initially focused on IL-17-producing T cells in the swollen joints of CIA. We found that gamma/delta T cells were the predominant source of IL-17 and were more abundant than Th17 cells, and DX5+ NK cells did not secrete IL-17 in swollen joints of CIA mice. Although it is known that gamma/delta T cells are dispensable for the induction of CIA, because gamma/delta TCR deficient mice can mount CIA (Corthay, et al., 1999), the present findings in the kinetic study and adoptive transfer experiments, together with previous reports (Arai, et al., 1996; Peterman, et al., 1993; Roark, et al., 2007), suggest that not only Th17 cells but also IL-17-producing gamma/delta T cells contribute to the exacerbation of CIA. On the other hand, alpha/beta T cells, especially Th17 cells, are essential for the induction of CIA because alpha/beta TCR deficient mice cannot mount CIA (Corthay, et al., 1999). In addition, IL-17-producing iNKT cells in CIA have been reported recently (Yoshiga, et al., 2008), but these cells were not analyzed in this study.

The origin and functions of IL-17-producing gamma/delta T cells in physiological and pathological conditions have been elucidated recently. It was reported that a subset of gamma/delta T cells acquired IL-17-produing function in the thymus (Jensen, et al., 2008) and produced cytokines immediately responding to the initial stimulation. In various murine infectious disease models, these gamma/delta T cells predominantly produce IL-17 and eradicate pathogens (Lockhart, et al., 2006; Romani, et al., 2008; Shibata, et al., 2007; Umemura, et al., 2007). Although IL-23 is known to be a sufficient stimulant of IL-17-production by gamma/delta T cells in naïve mice (Shibata, et al., 2007), the precise requirements of IL-17 production by gamma/delta T cells especially in CIA are unknown. We herein demonstrated that the combination of IL-23 and IL-1 beta synergistically stimulated IL-17 production, but stimulation via gamma/delta TCR had a limited effect. Given the enhanced expression of IL-1 beta and IL-23 in inflamed joints of CIA (Kim, et al., 2007; Weiss, et al., 2005), these findings suggest that IL-17-production by gamma/delta T cells in CIA might mainly be an inflammatory cytokine-driven, and not a TCR-signal-driven process.

The present study showed that IL-17-producing gamma/delta T cells were CCR6 positive, and CCR6 was already expressed on IL-17-producing gamma/delta T cells in the thymus of naive mice. CC chemokine ligand 20 (CCL20), the only chemokine known to interact with CCR6, is physiologically expressed at epithelial surfaces (Schutyser, et al., 2003) and fibroblast-like synoviocytes (Hirota, et al., 2007), and is upregulated in inflammatory conditions (Hirota, et al., 2007; Schutyser, et al., 2003). These findings suggest that CCR6 might have some role in determining the physiological distribution of IL-17-producing gamma/delta T cells. In fact, it was found that a small number of CCR6+ IL-17-producing gamma/delta T cells were present in the joints of naïve mice.

Next, the differences between IL-17-producing gamma/delta T cells and Th17 cells were focused upon. IL-17-producing gamma/delta T cells are maintained by IL-23 but not by a specific antigen (CII, in this case). In contrast, Th17 cells responded to both CII and IL-23. Furthermore, IL-17-producing gamma/delta T cells were induced equivalently in response to stimulation by IFA+solution in the absence of CII. Together with the previous study demonstrating that IL-17-producing gamma/delta T cells are induced equally by CFA+CII and CFA (Roark, et al., 2007), the present data suggest that IL-17-producing gamma/delta T cells do not recognize the specific antigen (CII) but rather proliferate in response to IL-23, which may be produced locally by synovial cells (Kim, et al., 2007). The ligands of gamma/delta T cells are largely unknown and further analysis of possible antigens of IL-17-producing gamma/delta T cells in CIA could be difficult (Konigshofer & Chien, 2006). However, we confirmed the diverse usage of gamma/delta TCR in IL-17-producing gamma/delta T cells in CIA (Ito, et al., 2009), which supported the present conclusion that IL-17-producing gamma/delta T cells are antigen-independently induced by inflammatory cytokines.

In summary, the sequence of pathology of CIA is speculated to be as follows. First, CII-specific Th17 cells are induced by CII+CFA, which then infiltrate into the joints and cause primary inflammation. Although antigen-independent IL-17-producing gamma/delta T cells could be induced simultaneously by CFA, they are dispensable for the induction of arthritis. Next, primary inflammation induces local production of IL-23 from synoviocytes and increases the expression of IL-1 beta in the joint cartilage and pannus (Weiss, et al., 2005). Locally-produced IL-23 induces the proliferation of resident IL-17-producing gamma/delta T cells. These gamma/delta T cells, stimulated by IL-1 beta and IL-23, produce enhanced amounts of IL-17 and exacerbate the arthritis of CIA. Another, but not mutually exclusive, possibility is that primary inflammation enhances CCL20 expression in vascular endothelial cells and fibroblast-like synoviocytes (Hirota, et al., 2007) in inflamed joints, and recruits $CCR6^+$ IL-17-producing cells. In the ankylosing phase, the burned out tissue does not produce inflammatory cytokines, and then the activities and the number of IL-17-producing gamma/delta T cells decrease to the basal level.

The cytokine profiles of T cells were compared in the inflamed joints of SKG mice and RA with those of CIA mice. In contrast to CIA, IL-17-producing gamma/delta T cells were not detected in the swollen joints of SKG mice. A lack of IL-17-producing gamma/delta T cells in SKG mice was not caused by the differences in strain or adjuvant. It was also found that IL-17-producing gamma/delta T cells are hardly induced, not only in immunized joints but also in their DLNs and the spleens of SKG mice by immunization with CFA+CII (data not shown). Given that the TCR signals in SKG mice are attenuated because of a point mutation in ZAP-70 (Sakaguchi, et al., 2003) and differentiation of gamma/delta T cells requires a strong signal via TCR (Haks, et al., 2005; Hayes, et al., 2005), there may be some defects in the gamma/delta T cell differentiation in SKG mice. This speculation was supported by the data of impaired development of specific subsets of gamma/delta T cells in ZAP-70 knockout mice (Kadlecek, et al., 1998). Therefore, it is true that both murine RA models share the property of IL-17-driven arthritis, and IFN-gamma-producing Th1 cells seem dispensable in these models. However, there is also a significant dissimilarity in their pathogeneses. CIA mice appear to be an arthritis model that is driven by innate factor, because the major population of swollen joints was antigen-independent gamma/delta T cell. In contrast, SKG arthritis seems to be a pure Th17-driven arthritis (Fig 7). However, the target antigen of Th17 cells in the affected joint of SKG mice is still unknown.

Contrary to the findings of murine RA models, there are big differences in the phenotypes and the cytokine profiles in the affected joints of RA patients. IL-17-production from gamma/delta T cells in synovial tissues of RA was negligible, and a small number of IFN-gamma-producing gamma/delta T cells were present in RA synovium. Furthermore, the most notable difference was predominance of Th1 cells (IFN-gamma-producing Th cell) rather than Th17 cells in the jointd of RA, and this observation is consistent with a previous report (Yamada, et al., 2007). This discrepancy could be explained by some artifacts. For example, the synovium samples of RA available are not from an early phase but a relatively late phase. In fact, Leipe et al. (2011) reported recently that the percentages of Th17 cells correlate strongly with the activity of RA using very early active and naïve RA patients, and concluded that Th17 cells play an important role in human RA. However, their data also indicated that IFN-gamma-producing T cells were dominant even in those cases. This discrepancy may also be explained by the differences between mice and humans. Alternatively, IL-17-producing T cells may play important roles in RA as well, but are suppressed by the effects of medicines. In conclusion, we have to wait for the results of clinical trials of IL-17 blocking agents in RA patients to further understand the true roles of Th17 cells in RA.

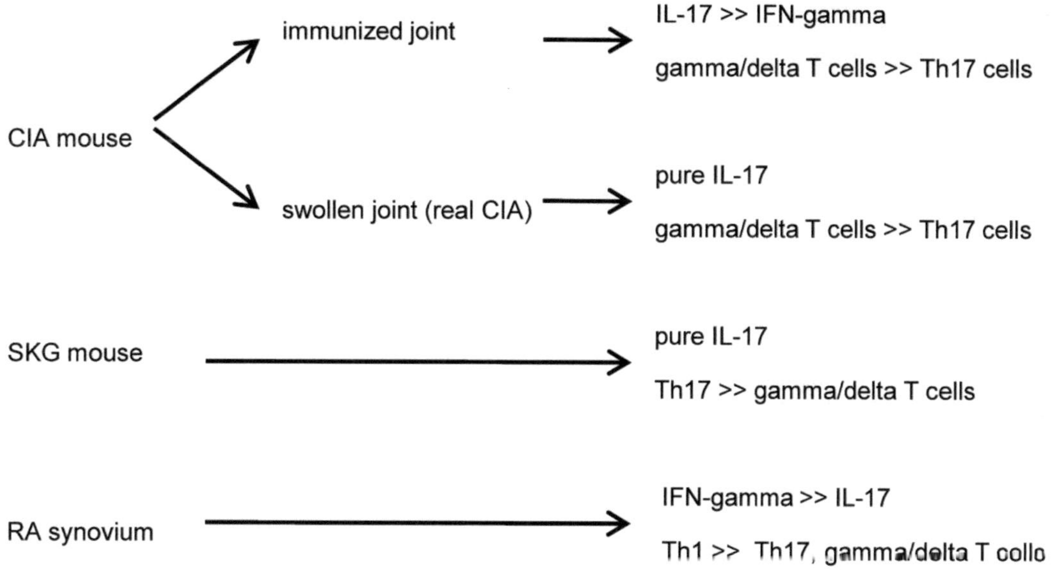

Fig. 7. A schema of cytokine profiles and T cell phenotype of two murine arthritis models and RA

10. Acknowledgment

This work was mainly conducted by Dr. Ito Yoshinaga (Ito, et al., 2009).

11. References

Acosta-Rodriguez, E. V., Rivino, L., Geginat, J., Jarrossay, D., Gattorno, M., Lanzavecchia, A., Sallusto, F. & Napolitani, G. (2007). Surface phenotype and antigenic specificity of human interleukin 17-producing T helper memory cells. *Nat Immunol*, Vol.8, No.6, pp.639-646, ISSN 1529-2908

Annunziato, F., Cosmi, L., Santarlasci, V., Maggi, L., Liotta, F., Mazzinghi, B., Parente, E., Fili, L., Ferri, S., Frosali, F., Giudici, F., Romagnani, P., Parronchi, P., Tonelli, F., Maggi, E. & Romagnani, S. (2007). Phenotypic and functional features of human Th17 cells. *J Exp Med*, Vol.204, No.8, pp.1849-1861, ISSN 0022-1007

Arai, K., Yamamura, S., Hanyu, T., Takahashi, H. E., Umezu, H., Watanabe, H. & Abo, T. (1996). Extrathymic differentiation of resident T cells in the joints of mice with collagen-induced arthritis. *J Immunol*, Vol.157, No.11, pp.5170-5177, ISSN 0022-1767

Bettelli, E., Carrier, Y., Gao, W., Korn, T., Strom, T. B., Oukka, M., Weiner, H. L. & Kuchroo, V. K. (2006). Reciprocal developmental pathways for the generation of pathogenic effector TH17 and regulatory T cells. *Nature*, Vol.441, No.7090, pp.235-238, ISSN 1476-4687

Clague, R. B. & Moore, L. J. (1984). IgG and IgM antibody to native type II collagen in rheumatoid arthritis serum and synovial fluid. Evidence for the presence of collagen-anticollagen immune complexes in synovial fluid. *Arthritis Rheum*, Vol.27, No.12, pp.1370-1377, ISSN 0004-3591

Cook, A. D., Rowley, M. J., Mackay, I. R., Gough, A. & Emery, P. (1996). Antibodies to type II collagen in early rheumatoid arthritis. Correlation with disease progression. *Arthritis Rheum*, Vol.39, No.10, pp.1720-1727, ISSN 0004-3591

Corthay, A., Johansson, A., Vestberg, M. & Holmdahl, R. (1999). Collagen-induced arthritis development requires alpha beta T cells but not gamma delta T cells: studies with T cell-deficient (TCR mutant) mice. *Int Immunol*, Vol.11, No.7, pp.1065-1073, ISSN 0953-8178

Courtenay, J. S., Dallman, M. J., Dayan, A. D., Martin, A. & Mosedale, B. (1980). Immunisation against heterologous type II collagen induces arthritis in mice. *Nature*, Vol.283, No.5748, pp.666-668, ISSN 0028-0836

Ferretti, S., Bonneau, O., Dubois, G. R., Jones, C. E. & Trifilieff, A. (2003). IL-17, produced by lymphocytes and neutrophils, is necessary for lipopolysaccharide-induced airway neutrophilia: IL-15 as a possible trigger. *J Immunol*, Vol.170, No.4, pp.2106-2112, ISSN 0022-1767

Gregersen, P. K., Silver, J. & Winchester, R. J. (1987). The shared epitope hypothesis. An approach to understanding the molecular genetics of susceptibility to rheumatoid arthritis. *Arthritis Rheum*, Vol.30, No.11, pp.1205-1213, ISSN 0004-3591

Haks, M. C., Lefebvre, J. M., Lauritsen, J. P., Carleton, M., Rhodes, M., Miyazaki, T., Kappes, D. J. & Wiest, D. L. (2005). Attenuation of gammadeltaTCR signaling efficiently diverts thymocytes to the alphabeta lineage. *Immunity*, Vol.22, No.5, pp.595-606, ISSN 1074-7613

Harrington, L. E., Hatton, R. D., Mangan, P. R., Turner, H., Murphy, T. L., Murphy, K. M. & Weaver, C. T. (2005). Interleukin 17-producing CD4+ effector T cells develop via a lineage distinct from the T helper type 1 and 2 lineages. *Nat Immunol*, Vol.6, No.11, pp.1123-1132, ISSN 1529-2908

Hayes, S. M., Li, L. & Love, P. E. (2005). TCR signal strength influences alphabeta/gammadelta lineage fate. *Immunity*, Vol.22, No.5, pp.583-593, ISSN 1074-7613

Hirota, K., Yoshitomi, H., Hashimoto, M., Maeda, S., Teradaira, S., Sugimoto, N., Yamaguchi, T., Nomura, T., Ito, H., Nakamura, T., Sakaguchi, N. & Sakaguchi, S. (2007). Preferential recruitment of CCR6-expressing Th17 cells to inflamed joints via CCL20 in rheumatoid arthritis and its animal model. *J Exp Med*, Vol.204, No.12, pp.2803-2812, ISSN 1540-9538

Infante-Duarte, C., Horton, H. F., Byrne, M. C. & Kamradt, T. (2000). Microbial lipopeptides induce the production of IL-17 in Th cells. *J Immunol*, Vol.165, No.11, pp.6107-6115, ISSN 0022-1767

Ito, Y., Usui, T., Kobayashi, S., Iguchi-Hashimoto, M., Ito, H., Yoshitomi, H., Nakamura, T., Shimizu, M., Kawabata, D., Yukawa, N., Hashimoto, M., Sakaguchi, N., Sakaguchi, S., Yoshifuji, H., Nojima, T., Ohmura, K., Fujii, T. & Mimori, T. (2009). Gamma/delta T cells are the predominant source of interleukin-17 in affected joints in collagen-induced arthritis, but not in rheumatoid arthritis. *Arthritis Rheum*, Vol.60, No.8, pp.2294-2303, ISSN 0004-3591

Jensen, K. D., Su, X., Shin, S., Li, L., Youssef, S., Yamasaki, S., Steinman, L., Saito, T., Locksley, R. M., Davis, M. M., Baumgarth, N. & Chien, Y. H. (2008). Thymic selection determines gammadelta T cell effector fate: antigen-naive cells make interleukin-17 and antigen-experienced cells make interferon gamma. *Immunity*, Vol.29, No.1, pp.90-100, ISSN 1074-7613

Kadlecek, T. A., van Oers, N. S., Lefrancois, L., Olson, S., Finlay, D., Chu, D. H., Connolly, K., Killeen, N. & Weiss, A. (1998). Differential requirements for ZAP-70 in TCR signaling and T cell development. *J Immunol*, Vol.161, No.9, pp.4688-4694, ISSN 0022-1767

Kim, H. R., Cho, M. L., Kim, K. W., Juhn, J. Y., Hwang, S. Y., Yoon, C. H., Park, S. H., Lee, S. H. & Kim, H. Y. (2007). Up-regulation of IL-23p19 expression in rheumatoid arthritis synovial fibroblasts by IL-17 through PI3-kinase-, NF-kappaB- and p38 MAPK-dependent signalling pathways. *Rheumatology (Oxford)*, Vol.46, No.1, pp.57-64, ISSN 1462-0324

Konigshofer, Y. & Chien, Y. H. (2006). Gammadelta T cells - innate immune lymphocytes? *Curr Opin Immunol*, Vol.18, No.5, pp.527-533, ISSN 0952-7915

Leipe, J., Grunke, M., Dechant, C., Reindl, C., Kerzendorf, U., Schulze-Koops, H. & Skapenko, A. (2011). Role of Th17 cells in human autoimmune arthritis. *Arthritis Rheum*, Vol.62, No.10, pp.2876-2885, ISSN 1529-0131

Lockhart, E., Green, A. M. & Flynn, J. L. (2006). IL-17 production is dominated by gammadelta T cells rather than CD4 T cells during Mycobacterium tuberculosis infection. *J Immunol*, Vol.177, No.7, pp.4662-4669, ISSN 0022-1767

Lubberts, E., Joosten, L. A., Oppers, B., van den Bersselaar, L., Coenen-de Roo, C. J., Kolls, J. K., Schwarzenberger, P., van de Loo, F. A. & van den Berg, W. B. (2001). IL-1-independent role of IL-17 in synovial inflammation and joint destruction during collagen-induced arthritis. *J Immunol*, Vol.167, No.2, pp.1004-1013, ISSN 0022-1767

Lubberts, E., Koenders, M. I., Oppers-Walgreen, B., van den Bersselaar, L., Coenen-de Roo, C. J., Joosten, L. A. & van den Berg, W. B. (2004). Treatment with a neutralizing anti-murine interleukin-17 antibody after the onset of collagen-induced arthritis reduces joint inflammation, cartilage destruction, and bone erosion. *Arthritis Rheum*, Vol.50, No.2, pp.650-659, ISSN 0004-3591

Luross, J. A. & Williams, N. A. (2001). The genetic and immunopathological processes underlying collagen-induced arthritis. *Immunology*, Vol.103, No.4, pp.407-416, ISSN 0019-2805

Mangan, P. R., Harrington, L. E., O'Quinn, D. B., Helms, W. S., Bullard, D. C., Elson, C. O., Hatton, R. D., Wahl, S. M., Schoeb, T. R. & Weaver, C. T. (2006). Transforming growth factor-beta induces development of the T(H)17 lineage. *Nature*, Vol.441, No.7090, pp.231-234, ISSN 1476-4687

Mullazehi, M., Mathsson, L., Lampa, J. & Ronnelid, J. (2007). High anti-collagen type-II antibody levels and induction of proinflammatory cytokines by anti-collagen antibody-containing immune complexes in vitro characterise a distinct rheumatoid arthritis phenotype associated with acute inflammation at the time of disease onset. *Ann Rheum Dis*, Vol.66, No.4, pp.537-541, ISSN 0003-4967

Murphy, C. A., Langrish, C. L., Chen, Y., Blumenschein, W., McClanahan, T., Kastelein, R. A., Sedgwick, J. D. & Cua, D. J. (2003). Divergent pro- and antiinflammatory roles for IL-23 and IL-12 in joint autoimmune inflammation. *J Exp Med*, Vol.198, No.12, pp.1951-1957, ISSN 0022-1007

Nakae, S., Nambu, A., Sudo, K. & Iwakura, Y. (2003). Suppression of immune induction of collagen-induced arthritis in IL-17-deficient mice. *J Immunol*, Vol.171, No.11, pp.6173-6177, ISSN 0022-1767

Park, H., Li, Z., Yang, X. O., Chang, S. H., Nurieva, R., Wang, Y. H., Wang, Y., Hood, L., Zhu, Z., Tian, Q. & Dong, C. (2005). A distinct lineage of CD4 T cells regulates tissue inflammation by producing interleukin 17. *Nat Immunol*, Vol.6, No.11, pp.1133-1141, ISSN 1529-2908

Peterman, G. M., Spencer, C., Sperling, A. I. & Bluestone, J. A. (1993). Role of gamma delta T cells in murine collagen-induced arthritis. *J Immunol*, Vol.151, No.11, pp.6546-6558, ISSN 0022-1767

Roark, C. L., French, J. D., Taylor, M. A., Bendele, A. M., Born, W. K. & O'Brien, R. L. (2007). Exacerbation of collagen-induced arthritis by oligoclonal, IL-17-producing gamma delta T cells. *J Immunol*, Vol.179, No.8, pp.5576-5583, ISSN 0022-1767

Romani, L., Fallarino, F., De Luca, A., Montagnoli, C., D'Angelo, C., Zelante, T., Vacca, C., Bistoni, F., Fioretti, M. C., Grohmann, U., Segal, B. H. & Puccetti, P. (2008). Defective tryptophan catabolism underlies inflammation in mouse chronic granulomatous disease. *Nature*, Vol.451, No.7175, pp.211-215, ISSN 1476-4687

Sakaguchi, N., Takahashi, T., Hata, H., Nomura, T., Tagami, T., Yamazaki, S., Sakihama, T., Matsutani, T., Negishi, I., Nakatsuru, S. & Sakaguchi, S. (2003). Altered thymic T-cell selection due to a mutation of the ZAP-70 gene causes autoimmune arthritis in mice. *Nature*, Vol.426, No.6965, pp.454-460, ISSN 1476-4687

Schutyser, E., Struyf, S. & Van Damme, J. (2003). The CC chemokine CCL20 and its receptor CCR6. *Cytokine Growth Factor Rev*, Vol.14, No.5, pp.409-426, ISSN 1359-6101

Shibata, K., Yamada, H., Hara, H., Kishihara, K. & Yoshikai, Y. (2007). Resident Vdelta1+ gammadelta T cells control early infiltration of neutrophils after Escherichia coli infection via IL-17 production. *J Immunol*, Vol.178, No.7, pp.4466-4472, ISSN 0022-1767

Singh, S. P., Zhang, H. H., Foley, J. F., Hedrick, M. N. & Farber, J. M. (2008). Human T cells that are able to produce IL-17 express the chemokine receptor CCR6. *J Immunol*, Vol.180, No.1, pp.214-221, ISSN 0022-1767

Tarkowski, A., Klareskog, L., Carlsten, H., Herberts, P. & Koopman, W. J. (1989). Secretion of antibodies to types I and II collagen by synovial tissue cells in patients with rheumatoid arthritis. *Arthritis Rheum*, Vol.32, No.9, pp.1087-1092, ISSN 0004-3591

Umemura, M., Yahagi, A., Hamada, S., Begum, M. D., Watanabe, H., Kawakami, K., Suda, T., Sudo, K., Nakae, S., Iwakura, Y. & Matsuzaki, G. (2007). IL-17-mediated regulation of innate and acquired immune response against pulmonary Mycobacterium bovis bacille Calmette-Guerin infection. *J Immunol*, Vol.178, No.6, pp.3786-3796, ISSN 0022-1767

Veldhoen, M., Hocking, R. J., Atkins, C. J., Locksley, R. M. & Stockinger, B. (2006). TGFbeta in the context of an inflammatory cytokine milieu supports de novo differentiation of IL-17-producing T cells. *Immunity*, Vol.24, No.2, pp.179-189, ISSN 1074-7613

Weaver, C. T., Hatton, R. D., Mangan, P. R. & Harrington, L. E. (2007). IL-17 family cytokines and the expanding diversity of effector T cell lineages. *Annu Rev Immunol*, Vol.25, pp.821-852, ISSN 0732-0582

Weiss, R. J., Erlandsson Harris, H., Wick, M. C., Wretenberg, P., Stark, A. & Palmblad, K. (2005). Morphological characterization of receptor activator of NFkappaB ligand (RANKL) and IL-1beta expression in rodent collagen-induced arthritis. *Scand J Immunol*, Vol.62, No.1, pp.55-62, ISSN

Weyand, C. M. & Goronzy, J. J. (1999). T-cell responses in rheumatoid arthritis: systemic abnormalities-local disease. *Curr Opin Rheumatol*, Vol.11, No.3, pp.210-217, ISSN 1040-8711

Weyand, C. M., Klimiuk, P. A. & Goronzy, J. J. (1998). Heterogeneity of rheumatoid arthritis: from phenotypes to genotypes. *Springer Semin Immunopathol*, Vol.20, No.1-2, pp.5-22, ISSN 0344-4325

Wooley, P. H., Whalen, J. D. & Chapdelaine, J. M. (1989). Collagen-induced arthritis in mice. VI. Synovial cells from collagen arthritic mice activate autologous lymphocytes in vitro. *Cell Immunol*, Vol.124, No.2, pp.227-238, ISSN 0008-8749

Yamada, H., Nakashima, Y., Okazaki, K., Mawatari, T., Fukushi, J. I., Kaibara, N., Hori, A., Iwamoto, Y. & Yoshikai, Y. (2007). Th1 but not Th17 cells predominate in the joints of patients with rheumatoid arthritis. *Ann Rheum Dis*, ISSN 1468-2060

Yoshiga, Y., Goto, D., Segawa, S., Ohnishi, Y., Matsumoto, I., Ito, S., Tsutsumi, A., Taniguchi, M. & Sumida, T. (2008). Invariant NKT cells produce IL-17 through IL-23-dependent and -independent pathways with potential modulation of Th17 response in collagen-induced arthritis. *Int J Mol Med*, Vol.22, No.3, pp.369-374, ISSN 1107-3756

Yoshitomi, H., Sakaguchi, N., Kobayashi, K., Brown, G. D., Tagami, T., Sakihama, T., Hirota, K., Tanaka, S., Nomura, T., Miki, I., Gordon, S., Akira, S., Nakamura, T. &

Sakaguchi, S. (2005). A role for fungal {beta}-glucans and their receptor Dectin-1 in the induction of autoimmune arthritis in genetically susceptible mice. *J Exp Med*, Vol.201, No.6, pp.949-960, ISSN 0022-1007

2

Invariant Natural Killer T Cells in Rheumatoid Arthritis and Other Inflammatory Arthritides

Evin Sowden and Wan-Fai Ng
Newcastle University
United Kingdom

1. Introduction

Like cells of the adaptive immune system, natural killer T (NKT) cells possess immune recognition receptors formed by germline DNA rearrangement. However, in common with cells of the innate immune system, the repertoire of NKT cell receptors is limited and NKT cells can mount a robust effector response with little capacity for immunological memory, sharing some of the characteristics of other innate-like lymphocytes such as γδ T cells, marginal zone B cells, B1 B cells and NK cells. NKT cells have been shown to play a staggering array of roles in infection, cancer and autoimmunity. Autoimmune diseases in which NKT cells have been implicated include type I diabetes, multiple sclerosis, systemic lupus erythematosus and graft-versus-host disease. In rheumatoid arthritis, much work has been done to characterise the frequency and phenotype of NKT cells. Animal models such as collagen-induced arthritis or the antibody-mediated arthritis in the K/BxN serum transfer model have provided valuable insight into the multi-faceted potential of these remarkable cells and in time, pharmacological manipulation of their immune function may provide us with the prospect of novel therapeutic tools.

2. Biology of natural killer T cells

Natural killer T cells were first recognised in 1990 as $CD4^-CD8^-$ double negative (DN) thymocytes bearing the murine natural killer (NK) cell marker NK1.1 or the orthologous CD161 in humans (Ballas & Rasmussen, 1990). Since their discovery, the unexpected ontological complexity, development, function and pathophysiological roles of NKT cells have begun to unravel. Here, we briefly review the biology of NKT cells and focus on a subset known as invariant NKT (iNKT) cells by virtue of their CD1d-restricted, semi-invariant T cell receptor in order to better understand their significance in autoimmune diseases such as rheumatoid arthritis.

2.1 CD1 molecules & the ontogeny of the NKT cell

The first mouse anti-human monoclonal antibody recognised an antigen found on human thymocytes and certain B cell lymphoma lines subsequently termed the first cluster of differentiation or CD1. Five CD1 protein isoforms encoded on chromosome 1 bear resemblance to the α chains of MHC class I encoded on chromosome 6. CD1 molecules associate non-covalently with β_2-microglobulin, but unlike MHC class I molecules they show very limited polymorphism. Human CD1a, -1b and -1c (CD1 group 1) are widely expressed on dendritic cells and other professional antigen presenting cells (APC). CD1d (CD1 group 2) expression appears to be independent of group 1 isoforms and can be found on lymph node mantle zone B cells, cortical thymocytes, activated T cells, gut and liver tissues. CD1b was first shown to present microbial antigen in 1992 which was later identified as lipid antigen. Since then it has become clear that CD1 molecules bind diverse hydrophobic ligands, with the exception of CD1e which remains intracellular and is thought to be involved in lipid antigen processing and loading (Brigl & Brenner, 2004; Strominger, 2010).

After the discovery of NK1.1$^+$ CD4$^-$CD8$^-$ double negative (DN) thymocytes, further work led to iNKT cells bearing a TCR consisting of an invariant Vα14-Jα18 rearrangement and a limited repertoire of Vβ8.2, -7 or -2 chains in mice or the homologous Vα24-Vα18 and Vβ11 chains in humans. Later, the TCR of iNKT cells was shown to be CD1d-restricted and these cells were coined the type I NKT cells (Godfrey et al., 2004). Like iNKT cells, type II NKT cells are CD1d-restricted but possess a more diverse TCR repertoire that also displays bias. They have been shown to possess regulatory and pathogenic functions but have been less well studied than iNKT cells. Non-CD1d restricted T cells that possess NK cell markers also exist and are referred to as NKT-like or type III NKT cells. In mice, 20-80% of CD3$^+$NK1.1$^+$ T cells stain with α-GalCer/CD1d-tetramer. In humans, while 20-25% of T cells are CD161$^+$, less than 1% are α-GalCer/CD1d-tetramer$^+$ and many staining cells are CD161$^-$. These cells comprise CD1 group 1-restricted NKT cells that can be αβ$^+$, γδ$^+$, CD4$^+$, CD8$^+$, or CD4$^-$CD8$^-$ T cells, and may also include mucosa associated invariant T cells (MAIT) that express an invariant TCRα chain restricted to the MHC class I-like molecule MR1 (Godfrey et al., 2010).

2.2 iNKT cell development and homeostasis

iNKT cells develop in the thymus when invariant TCRα rearrangement and CD1d recognition initiate positive and negative selection, but unlike conventional T cells positive selection of iNKT cells involves double-positive CD4$^+$CD8$^+$ cortical thymocytes rather than cortical epithelial cells. TCR, SLAM and other co-stimulatory signals (CD28, ICOS, TGF-β) are required for maturation, expression of activation (CD44, CD69, CD122) and NK (KLRG1 and NK1.1) markers, and acquisition of innate effector functions dependent on the transcriptional regulator promyelocytic leukaemia zinc finger protein (PZLF). Maturation to NK1.1$^+$ or CD161$^+$ occurs in the periphery in mice and humans, or in the thymus in mice where a long lived population of thymic mature iNKT cells may contribute to fine-tuning the negative selection of conventional T cells (D'Cruz et al., 2010).

Similar to naïve conventional T cells, peripheral iNKT cell are not expanded in unchallenged mice, with an average clonal size of 5-10 cells that do not require interaction with CD1d for homeostasis. Nevertheless, iNKT cell frequency is orders of magnitude higher than that of naïve MHC class I and II restricted T cells. Humans have fewer iNKT cells than mice although there is wide variation amongst individuals, varying between undetectable and 3% of peripheral lymphocytes. It is not known whether this is related to thymic development and migration, or peripheral proliferation and maintenance differences but the phenomenon appears to be a stable, genetically determined phenotype in both mice and humans (Van Kaer et al., 2011).

iNKT cells are most abundant in the liver and spleen in mice but exceed the number of antigen-specific T cells in the lymph nodes by 500-5000 fold. In keeping with their innate function, NKT cells also accumulate in inflammatory lesions where they can rapidly become activated to release a diverse range of cytokines, proliferate and influence the subsequent adaptive immune response (Fox et al., 2010).

2.3 Antigen and antigen-independent activation pathways

Unlike conventional T cells, iNKT cells appear to be selected in the thymus for their ability to recognise both microbial lipid antigen and self-antigen. The direct pathway of activation involves recognition of microbial lipid antigen presented on CD1d. In the case of the lipoglycan α-GalCer, CD1d-restricted antigen presentation is sufficient for iNKT cell activation although co-stimulatory signalling mediated by constitutive CD28 expression can further augment the iNKT response. Alternatively, the indirect pathway activates iNKT cells in response to microbial organisms lacking cognate glycolipid antigens by recognition of self-antigen, together with co-stimulatory cytokine signals (IL-12, IL-18) from toll-like receptor (TLR) ligand-activated APCs. Finally, cytokine-mediated iNKT cell activation independently of CD1d involvement has also been observed in response to lipopolysaccharide (LPS) or viral CpG-activated APCs (Reilly et al., 2010).

By virtue of their semi-invariant TCR, all iNKT cells can recognise glycolipids consisting of a galactose or glucose moiety α-linked to the polar head of a lipid. The prototypical extrinsic iNKT antigen is the α-linked galactosylceramide α-GalCer, a glycosphingolipid extracted from the non-sterile marine sponge *Agelas mauritianus*. α-GalCer and related glycosphingolipids are not present in mammalian cells but can be found in the cell walls of *Novosphingobium*, previously known as *Sphingomonas* bacteria that colonise the marine sponge. Glycosylated diacylglycerol lipids in *Borrelia burgdorferi* are also recognised by a sub-population of murine iNKT cells and iNKT cell deficiency is associated with reduced spirochete clearance and chronic inflammation. Other microbial CD1d-restricted lipids are thought to be present in *Plasmodium falciparum*, *Trypanosoma* spp, *Leishmania* spp, *Ehrlichia* spp, *Streptococcus pneumoniae*, *Helicobacter pylori* and *M bovis*. The importance of these other microbial lipid antigens is however unclear as they are not strong TCR agonists (Brigl & Brenner, 2010).

The nature of relevant lipid self-antigen(s) has remained a matter of considerable debate. Phospholipids such as phosphatidylinositol, phosphatidylethanolamine, and phosphatidylglycerol can be eluted from CD1d but most however are not stimulatory or stimulate only a small fraction of iNKT cells. In contrast, sphingolipids such as the tumour-derived ganglioside GD3 or the lysosomal β-linked glycosphingolipid isoglobotrihexosylceramide (iGb3) have been shown to be recognised by iNKT cells (Gapin, 2010). Lysophosphatidylcholine (LPC) is produced from membrane phosphatidylcholine by phospholipase-A2, an enzyme produced by myeloid APC and activated during the inflammatory response. Thus increased presentation of LPC to iNKT cells during inflammation has been proposed to lead to their enhanced activation and cytokine production (Fox et al., 2010). In addition to constitutive stimulatory self-antigens, neo-self-antigens have been proposed to arise following exposure of APC to microbial or viral danger signals resulting in increased iNKT cell sensitivity to existing self-lipids, generation of novel lipid entities that are not constitutively expressed or increased antigen presentation and co-stimulation (Reilly et al., 2010).

2.4 iNKT cell activation and effector functions

Stimulatory antigens such as α-GalCer rapidly activate iNKT cells within hours, up-regulating surface markers such as CD25 and CD69 and producing cytokines through constitutive expression of mRNA for IL-4 and IFN-γ. iNKT cells proliferate and expand up to 10-fold in the spleen, 5-fold in blood, bone marrow and lymph nodes, and 2- to 3-fold in liver with a peak at 3-4 days after antigen exposure. Unlike conventional T cells, iNKT cells show not only a lack of secondary memory response but a hyporesponsive state of immunological anergy lasting up to 2 months (Van Kaer et al., 2011).

Upon activation, iNKT cells have been reported to be capable of producing a wide variety of both Th1 and Th2 cytokines (IL-2, IL-3, IL-4, IL-5, IL-6, IL-9, IL-10, IL-13, IL-17, IL-21, IFN-γ, TNF-α, GM-CSF) (Coquet, 2008). The precise pattern of cytokines produced may depend on factors such as tissue distribution, iNKT cell subset, antigen processing, activation pathway, TCR signal strength and cytokine milieu. In addition, chemokines and chemokine receptors allow homing to inflammatory sites where iNKT cells form a bridge between the innate and adaptive immune systems by jump starting antigen-specific responses (Salio et al., 2010).

Activated iNKT cells can stimulate inflammatory myeloid APC, NK and B cell function by the production of CD40L and pro-inflammatory cytokines such as IFN-γ and TNF-α which can induce maturation with up-regulation of co-stimulatory molecules, perpetuation of cytokine and chemokine production, thus enhancing MHC-restricted T cell stimulation and ensuing adaptive immune responses. In contrast, iNKT cells have also been shown to potentiate antigen-specific immune tolerance in a number of animal models of autoimmunity, organ transplantation and therapeutic mucosal immune tolerance induction. The mechanisms by which iNKT cells induce or maintain tolerance may be mediated by a shift in secretion toward regulatory cytokines such as IL-10 and IL-4 although experimental data have not been consistent and cytokine-independent mechanisms such as generation of regulatory DCs may play a role (Hegde et al., 2010).

2.5 Pathophysiological roles of iNKT cells

In summary, iNKT cells are a unique subset of T cells that can help orchestrate both pro-inflammatory and regulatory immune responses. Despite their small population size, they can simultaneously promote resistance against microbial infection, participate in tumour immunosurveillance, maintain peripheral tolerance and prevent autoimmunity.

iNKT cells have long been known to react to self. Such autoreactivity is TCR and CD1d dependent in both mice and human iNKT cells. It has been suggested that the antigens responsible for autoreactivity are the same as those involved in thymic selection so that iNKT cells are autoreactive by design (Gapin, 2010). An immunosuppressive role for iNKT cells has now been shown in a number of animal models of autoimmunity including type I diabetes in non-obese diabetic (NOD) mice, experimental autoimmune encephalomyelitis as a model of multiple sclerosis in C57BL/6 and NOD mice, models of systemic lupus erythematosus (SLE) and graft-versus-host disease (GvHD). In some cases, iNKT cells have been shown to play a pathogenic rather than protective role. Despite such apparently conflicting results, iNKT function can be harnessed for tolerance induction, as demonstrated most notably in the prevention of GvHD. In this chapter, we will focus our discussion on the possible roles of iNKT cells in rheumatoid arthritis (RA) and other inflammatory arthritis.

3. iNKT cells in rheumatoid arthritis

RA is an inflammatory arthritis affecting small and large synovial joints, mediated by a destructive interplay between T cells, B cells, macrophage-like synoviocytes and fibroblast-like synoviocytes, ending with synovial cartilage invasion and ultimately joint destruction

(Scott et al., 2010). Given the dual pro-inflammatory and regulatory potential of iNKT cells, the study of their frequency and phenotype in RA, and their role in animal models of inflammatory arthritis, have been of significant interest to researchers in the field.

3.1 iNKT cell frequency

Until the advent of α-GalCer/CD1d-tetramers and invariant TCR chain-specific monoclonal antibodies, much of the earlier work on iNKT cells had been muddied by the lack of specific reagents for reliable iNKT cell identification. However, despite the limitations posed by older identification methods, most studies have consistently shown that NKT or iNKT cell absolute and relative frequencies are reduced in RA. Here we review studies examining the peripheral and synovial compartments, individual iNKT cell subsets and the relationship between iNKT cell frequency, disease activity and treatment response.

3.1.1 Peripheral blood compartment

In the earliest published study on NKT cells in RA, Yanagihara et al. (1999) looked at $CD3^+NKR\text{-}P1A^+(CD161^+)$ NKT cells in 60 patients with established RA compared with 36 healthy controls. They found a 5.8 fold difference in NKT cells but no difference in NK cells. Although patients and controls were mismatched for age, no correlation with age was found in either group. There was no apparent correlation with disease duration, clinical disease activity, inflammatory markers, RF status or drug treatment.

Recent studies of iNKT cell frequency using more specific detection reagents have confirmed results from earlier studies. Parietti et al. (2010) detected iNKT cells with a monoclonal antibody (mAb) against the canonical Vα24Jα18 invariant TCR chain in 36 RA, 43 SLE and 31 healthy subjects. The investigators confirmed the lower frequencies and percentages of iNKT in RA and SLE vs controls (0.09% and 0.01% vs 0.26%, respectively). They found no effect of age, gender or treatment on iNKT cell frequency.

Our own group analysed the frequency of $V\alpha24^+V\beta11^+$ NKT cells among 46 RA and 22 healthy controls, taking care to use a statistically robust minimum number of lymphocyte-gated events set at 500,000 in order to reliably measure the infrequent iNKT cells. Our results showed that RA patients have a 15-fold lower iNKT cell relative frequency compared to healthy controls (0.001% vs 0.21%, respectively), either before or after commencing immunosuppressive treatment (Tudhope et al., 2010).

3.1.2 Synovial compartment

In a comparative analysis of NKT cell frequency in different compartments, Spadaro et al. (2004) studied 29 patients with psoriasis and psoriatic arthritis (PsA), 27 patients with RA and 27 healthy controls. Blood and synovial fluid (SF) lymphocyte subsets, including $CD3^+CD16^+CD56^+$ NKT cells, were measured and compared. In peripheral blood, there was no statistically significant difference in NKT cell absolute or relative numbers between PsA, RA and healthy control subjects (61 cells/μL or 3.6%, 93 cells/μL or 5% and 89 cells/μL or 3.9%, respectively). SF NKT cells however were significantly reduced in both absolute and relative numbers as compared to peripheral blood in PsA and RA (2% vs 3.2% and 1.6% vs 4.1%, respectively) (Spadaro et al., 2004).

Linsen et al. (2005) studied 23 RA and 22 healthy control patients using peripheral blood and, when available, synovial fluid and tissue specimens. They found that $V\alpha24^+V\beta11^+CD3^+$ NKT cells were significantly reduced in relative frequency in RA as compared to control peripheral blood (0.03% vs 0.11%, respectively) but unlike Spadaro et al. (2004), their synovial fluid samples showed an inconsistent trend toward higher percentage of NKT cells in SF from seven patients as compared to matched peripheral blood (0.08% vs 0.05%, respectively).

3.1.3 iNKT cell subsets

iNKT cell subsets include $CD4^-$ (DN), $CD4^+$ and $CD8^+$ cells. iNKT cells from these subsets have been shown to be functionally distinct and therefore individual subset frequency may be immunologically more relevant than global iNKT cell numbers.

In a study of patients with a range of autoimmune diseases including 20 patients with RA, $V\alpha24J\alpha18^+$ DN T cells were found to express polymorphic Vб11 and CD161 almost universally, suggesting that these were likely to be true iNKT cells. The frequency of these DN NKT cells was markedly reduced in RA patients who had a mean of 48.8 cells/ml as compared to 290 cells/ml in healthy controls. Similar findings applied to patients with SLE, systemic sclerosis (SSc) and Sjogren's syndrome (SS) but not Behcet's disease (BD), and $CD4^+$ NKT cells were similarly reduced in frequency (Kojo et al., 2001).

$V\alpha24^+CD8^+$ NKT cells have been shown to consist mainly of $CD161^+$, CD1d-restricted NKT cells that have an immunoregulatory phenotype (Ho et al. 2004; Takahashi 2002). Mitsuo et al. (2006) examined the frequency of this NKT cell subset in patient with RA (n=24), SLE (n=54), SSc (n=14), mixed connective tissue disease (MCTD) (n=15) and polymyositis/dermatomyositis (PM/DM) (n=13) compared to healthy controls (n=18). The absolute frequency of $CD161^+CD8^+$ T cells was reduced in all patients compared to healthy donors, although in RA patients the relative frequency was not statistically significantly lower. No correlation with age, gender or treatment was noted (Mitsuo et al., 2006).

3.1.4 Correlation with disease activity and treatment response

Whilst Yanagihara et al. (1999) found no correlation between iNKT cell frequency and clinical disease activity, Parietti et al. (2010) noted a trend toward lower iNKT cell numbers with higher disease activity (DAS28), ESR and CRP. Our group also found no correlation with disease activity although a moderate but statistically significant inverse relationship with CRP could be demonstrated (Tudhope et al., 2010).

Parietti et al. (2010) measured iNKT cell frequencies in seven patients before and after treatment with rituximab, an anti-CD20 monoclonal antibody targeting B cells. They found a significant increase in NKT frequency and percentage from baseline at days 45 and 120 post-infusion (1.7, 3.4 and 4.1 cells/µL, or 0.1%, 0.32% and 0.3%, respectively). There was also a clear correlation between clinical outcome and NKT cell frequency change with non-responders showing no change whilst responders saw a 600% increase in frequency. In our study, we measured iNKT cell frequencies in seven patients before and after initiating methotrexate therapy and found that iNKT frequency increased as early as two weeks after the start of treatment. Unlike Parietti et al.'s results however, we found no obvious link to clinical response (Tudhope et al., 2010).

3.2 iNKT cell phenotype

3.2.1 Response to α-GalCer

Kojo et al. (2001) examined the functional phenotype of $V\alpha24J\alpha18^+$ DN iNKT cells in patients with RA and other autoimmune diseases. Peripheral blood mononuclear cells

(PBMC) stimulated with α-GalCer for 10 days resulted in expansion of iNKT cells in just 3 out of 10 RA patients (from 0-10 to 61-1480 cells/10^5 lymphocytes) as compared to all 7 healthy controls (from 6-123 to 350-3169 cells/10^5 lymphocytes). The proportion of responders was 50% in patients with SLE (n=10) and SSc (n=8). No clear relationship was noted to disease activity.

In further experiments, Linsen et al. (2005) also characterised the phenotype of $V\alpha24^+V\beta11^+CD3^+$ iNKT cells in RA compared to healthy controls. The capacity of NKT cells to respond to α-GalCer was tested in peripheral blood of 7 healthy and 13 RA patients as well as the SF from 5 RA patients. PBMC or synovial mononuclear cells (SFMC) were stimulated with α-GalCer and re-stimulated at day 7 with pulsed, irradiated PBMCs then analysed by flow cytometry at day 14. The number of NKT cells from RA peripheral blood (PB) and SF remained lower than that of healthy controls (8.4 and 4.4 vs 15.8%, respectively). Like Kojo et al. (2001), the investigators noted two separate RA populations comprised of non-responders (6/13 patients) and responders (7/13 patients). In fact, RA responders showed stronger responses than healthy controls (294 vs 149 fold, respectively). They too did not find any correlation between response and clinical or treatment phenotype. SF iNKT cells however responded in all tested patients.

In keeping with these earlier results, our own experiments showed that peripheral iNKT cells stimulated with α-GalCer for 12 days display impaired expansion in RA patients compared to controls (31 vs 121 fold, respectively). Using the 25th percentile of fold-expansion in healthy controls, 75% of RA vs 20% of healthy controls are non-responders with no detectable differences between early and late RA (Tudhope et al., 2010).

While investigating the mechanism underlying non-response to α-GalCer in RA patients, Kojo et al. (2001) found that non-responder APCs could expand responder iNKT cells in the presence of α-GalCer and IL-2, albeit with a lower response than responder APCs. In contrast, non-responder iNKT cells failed to expand in the presence of responder APCs under the same culture conditions. This suggested that in non-responders, the defect lay within iNKT cells rather than APCs.

3.2.2 Cytokine production

In keeping with iNKT cell frequency as measured by flow cytometry, linsen et al. performed ELISPOT analysis of cytokine production by isolated PBMC stimulated with α-GalCer and found a decreased frequency of reactive cells producing IFN-γ (2.3 vs 24.3, respectively) and IL-4 (0.2 vs 3.9, respectively) in RA patients compared to healthy controls. The IL-4/IFN-γ ratio was also reduced (0.07 vs 0.30, respectively), suggesting a Th1-like phenotypic bias in RA which could not be explained by any differences in $CD4^+$ and $CD4^-$ subsets, or selective clonal expansion as shown by Vα24 and Vβ11 TCR CDR3 fragment length spectra analysis (Linsen et al., 2005).

Intracellular cytokine staining of iNKT cells in PB revealed marked differences between RA patients and healthy controls for IFN-γ^+ (92.5 vs 64.5%, respectively), IL-4^+ (1.4 vs 15.7%, respectively) and IFN-γ^+IL-4^+ iNKT cells (6.1 vs 19.7%, respectively), confirming the Th1 bias in PBMC-derived iNKT cells. In contrast, cytokine profiles for SF iNKT cells were more similar to that of healthy control PB iNKT cells, with smaller proportion of IL-4^+ and higher proportion of IFN-γ^+IL-4^+ iNKT cells (5.3 and 28.4%, respectively), suggesting a Th0-profile in SF-derived iNKT cells. No correlation with response to α-GalCer, or disease and treatment parameters was noted (Linsen et al., 2005).

3.2.3 Clonal heterogeneity

Linsen et al. (2005) also examined clonal heterogeneity by TCR CDR3 region fragment length analysis using primers for Vα24 and the TCR-α constant region on PBMC from 5 healthy controls and 7 paired PB-SF or PB-ST samples from RA patients. In PB, whilst healthy controls exhibited a polyclonal peak profile corresponding to the invariant NKT TCR α chain at 350 base pairs, RA patients exhibited a more restricted monoclonal (1 peak) or oligoclonal (2-4 peaks) pattern which included the invariant TCR-α chain in all patients. In SF or ST, Vα24 TCR usage was more variably skewed or polyclonal although all samples peaked corresponding to the invariant TCR-α chain thus confirming iNKT cells are present in SF and ST.

3.3 Why are iNKT cells defective in RA?

The above studies suggest that cross-subset iNKT cell frequency is reduced in RA as compared to healthy controls in peripheral blood, with conflicting reports on the synovial fluid compartment. This reduction is not specific for RA and at best would appear to correlate weakly with disease activity or systemic inflammation. Notably, iNKT cell frequency deficiency is reversible as shown by the response to treatment with methotrexate or rituximab. This is associated with a functional defect in a majority of RA patients, as shown by impaired proliferative and altered cytokine responses to α-GalCer.

So why are iNKT cells reduced in frequency and defective in peripheral blood of RA patients? Peripheral blood iNKT cell homeostasis depends on both thymic output, cell turnover and migration into extra-vascular compartments. It has previously been shown that recent thymic emigrants of conventional T cells, identified by the presence of T-cell receptor excision circles (TRECs), are reduced in number compared to age-matched controls (Koetz et al., 2000; Ponchel et al., 2002). Whether similar thymic dysregulation applies to iNKT cells remains yet to be investigated. Whether the survival of iNKT cells in the periphery is abnormally shortened in RA patients also remains undetermined, although it seems unlikely that the reduced frequency is due to a selective loss of a limited number of iNKT clones as shown by the polyclonal Vб11 profile of expanded peripheral RA iNKT cells. In non-responders, impaired iNKT cell response to α-GalCer and potentially to self-lipid ligands could be a sign of an intrinsic defect that might lead to reduced physiological expansion or a shortened cellular lifespan, but this phenomenon was restricted to the PB compartment only. Abnormal CD1d-mediated ligand presentation by APCs could similarly also impact on iNKT cell homeostasis but experimental data do not support a major defect in APC function. In fact, CD1d expression on PBMC from RA patients is similar to that of healthy controls (Kojo et al., 2003). Intriguingly, a soluble form of CD1d with capacity to bind α-GalCer and stimulate iNKT cells is significantly reduced in RA as compared to healthy controls, and correlates with $V\alpha24^{+}V\delta11^{+}$ NKT cell frequency (Segawa et al., 2009).

It has been suggested by Kojo et al. (2001) that low iNKT cell number and functional defect could be due to chronic activation and overstimulation as has been shown for anti-CD3ε or IL-12 stimulated NKT cells (Eberl & MacDonald, 1998). In this respect, it would be interesting to analyse markers of iNKT cell activation to support or refute this theory. In the same vein, Linsen et al. (2005) proposed that the measured deficiency in iNKT cell numbers is in fact artefactual, stemming from down-regulation of the TCR as a result of chronic activation (Wilson et al., 2003). Further studies are also required to examine this latter proposition.

Finally, migration of iNKT cells into secondary lymphoid, liver or joint compartments might account for some of the apparent reduction in iNKT cell numbers in RA. Selective migration into joint synovial tissue or synovial fluid however is not supported by analysis of cell frequency and clonality in these compartments, but we cannot exclude migration into secondary lymphoid organs or liver as a possible factor. As most iNKT cells are found in the spleen or liver tissues, with relatively significantly fewer iNKT cells in peripheral blood, assessing the iNKT cell population size from peripheral blood frequency alone is therefore potentially misleading (Eberl et al., 1999; Matsuda et al., 2000).

3.4 Animal models of rheumatoid arthritis

Given the distribution of iNKT cells to organs which are not easily amenable to investigation in human subjects, animal models of RA-like inflammatory arthritis have provided invaluable insight into the possible pathogenic or protective roles played by iNKT cells, particularly with the help of CD1d$^{-/-}$ or invariant Jα281$^{-/-}$ knockout mice deficient in iNKT cells. Furthermore, these models have given investigators an opportunity to explore interventions to either harness or subdue iNKT cell functions for therapeutic benefit. In this section, we review the findings and attempt to make sense of the occasionally puzzling and conflicting data arising from experimental animal studies.

3.4.1 Collagen-induced arthritis

Collagen-induced arthritis (CIA) in mice was first demonstrated in 1981 by Wooley et al. as a promising animal model of inflammatory arthritis. The parenteral administration of heterologous chicken or bovine-derived type II collagen (CII) in complete Freund's adjuvant (CFA) containing heat-killed *Mycobacterium tuberculosis*, followed by a booster 21 days later to genetically susceptible mice results in a persistent inflammatory arthritis sharing many of the features of RA, including mononuclear synovial infiltrate, presence of rheumatoid factor and pannus formation, leading to cartilage destruction and bone erosion. CD4^{+} T cells are thought to be the primary mediators of disease induction characterised by early Th1 polarisation, whilst complement-fixing anti-CII autoantibody are responsible for the chronic inflammation during the effector phase of the immune response (Luross & Williams, 2001). CIA has been extensively characterised and has proved useful not only in furthering our understanding of basic pathophysiological mechanisms involved in inflammatory arthritis, but also in testing the therapeutic efficacy of potential new treatments for RA (Hegen et al., 2008).

3.4.1.1 C57BL/6 mice

Unlike the susceptible DBA/1 mice normally used in collagen-induced arthritis models, C57BL/6 mice NKT cells express the NK1.1 marker but are also susceptible to CIA with a 70% arthritis incidence. Prior to the widespread availability of more specific detection reagents, Wang et al. (2003) first noted that C57BL/6 mice with higher clinical arthritis scores had lower NK1.1^{+}CD3^{+} T cell spleen and LN frequency but greater synovial membrane infiltration in more severely affected joints. NK1.1^{+} cell depletion before CIA induction however did not lead to disease amelioration.

In a further C57BL/6 model of CIA, Ohnishi et al. (2005) found significantly reduced arthritis incidence and severity in Jα281 and CD1d knockout mice. Serum anti-CII autoantibody levels were also significantly reduced. Splenocyte proliferation assays to CII at day 9 post-primary immunisation however revealed no significant difference and neither did IL-4 and IFN-γ cytokine responses differ between Jα281 knockout and wild-type C57BL/6 mice. At 5 days after booster immunisation on day 21, and therefore during the disease development phase, there were fewer activated CD69^{+} T and B cells in Jα281 knockout mice. This was associated with lower splenocyte mRNA for IL-4 and IL-1β, and higher IFN-γ expression.

Using more specific detection reagents, Chiba et al. (2005) analysed the frequency of Vα24^{+} iNKT cells stained with α-GalCer-loaded CD1d dimers in C57BL/6 murine models of CIA. Unlike human and earlier murine studies using less specific detection reagents, they found increased liver and peripheral blood, but not lymph node or spleen iNKT cell numbers which peaked with clinical disease severity in CIA compared with control mice. Anti-CD1d blocking antibody administered bi-weekly from day 21 resulted in disease amelioration but not susceptibility. Furthermore, Jα281 knockout mice showed an increased IgG1/IgG2a ratio of anti-CII antibodies in keeping with a Th2 deviation in iNKT cell deficient mice. Accordingly, draining lymph node (DLN) lymphoid cells stimulated with CII 10 days post-secondary immunisation produced much more IL-10 in Jα281 knockout mice than wild-type C57BL/6 mice, but less IL-2 and IFN-γ although levels of these two cytokines were already low in wild-type mice.

IL-17 produced by Th17 lymphocytes has been shown to mediate an IL-1-independent role in synovial inflammation and joint destruction in CIA (Lubberts et al., 2001). Studies of IL17^{-}/$^{-}$ mice have shown a role in T cell priming, collagen-specific IgG2a production and a markedly suppressed CIA severity in the absence of this cytokine (Nakae et al., 2003). TGF-β and IL-6 promote Th17 cell development (Bettelli et al., 2006; Mangan et al., 2006; Veldhoen et al., 2006) whilst IL-23 has been shown to be essential to Th17 cell maintenance (Aggarwal et al., 2003; Langrish et al., 2005). Thus IL-23^{-}/$^{-}$ knockout mice lack Th17 cells, and similarly fail to develop clinical or histological disease in CIA (Murphy et al., 2003). Neutralisation with anti-IL-17 after the onset of arthritis results in suppression of disease in keeping with a role in both induction and effector phases of CIA (Lubberts et al., 2004). Interestingly, IFN-γ suppresses IL-17 production by CII-specific T cells and may be relevant to the suppressive role of IFN-γ during the effector stage of CIA (Chu et al., 2007). This was subsequently demonstrated in experiments showing that the neutralisation of IFN-γ after day 10 post-primary immunisation results in IL-17 dependent exacerbation of CIA (Sarkar et al., 2009).

Yoshiga et al. (2008) confirmed the pathogenic role of iNKT cells in C57BL/6 CIA by noting the reduced disease incidence and severity in Jα281 knockout mice compared to wild-type mice. DLN cells from Jα281^{-}/$^{-}$ mice stimulated with CII at day 11 post-primary immunisation produced similar amounts of IFN-γ and minimal IL-4, with increased IL-10 (not significantly) and significantly less IL-17. This was associated with a marked reduction in the percentage of IL-17 producing CD4^{+} cells. Administration of α-GalCer in C57BL/6 but not Jα281^{-}/$^{-}$ mice resulted in IL-17 production by splenocytes with detectable IL-17^{+} iNKT cells distinct from the IFN-γ^{+} and IL-4^{+} population, as well as increased IL-17 production by non-iNKT cells as compared to Jα281^{-}/$^{-}$ mice. Splenic naïve and stimulated iNKT cells were found to express IL-23R and RORγt mRNA similarly to Th17 cells, but only stimulated cells expressed IL-17. NK1.1^{+} and NK1.1^{-} iNKT cells splenocytes were incubated with mitomycin-C-treated CD11c^{+} DCs with either IL-23 or α-GalCer. Results showed that IL-17 is only produced by the NK1.1^{-} subset in response to α-GalCer and more weakly after IL-23 stimulation. Furthermore, α-GalCer-induced IL-17 could not be abrogated with IL-23 and IL-23 was not detectable in culture supernatant, suggesting that NK1.1^{-} iNKT cells can produce IL-17 is both IL-23-dependent and independent (Yoshiga et al., 2008).

3.4.1.2 DBA1/J mice

The DBA/1 mouse model of CIA is more susceptible to CIA than C57BL/6 mice despite similar CD1d/α-GalCer-dimer$^+$ NKT cell frequency and in vivo or in vitro function. In a DBA/1 model of CIA, Jung et al. (2009) showed that CD1d$^{-/-}$ knockout mice display a reduced incidence and severity of CIA, IgG2a and IgG1 CII-specific antibody levels, CII-stimulated production of IFN-γ, IL-17, IL-1β and IL-6, and increased production of IL-10 by splenocytes on day 35, as compared to CD1d$^{+/-}$ mice. In wild-type mice, iNKT cells producing IFN-γ were maintained throughout all disease stages whilst IL-17 producing iNKT cells steadily increased in frequency and number until the late stages of disease (Jung et al., 2009).
In a further DBA/1 model of CIA, Miellot-Gafsou et al. (2010) found that hepatic iNKT cells released IFN-γ, IL-4 and IL-17A in response to intra-peritoneal (i.p.) α-GalCer 2hr before euthanasia at day 6, i.e. early during the course of CIA. This was associated with increased expression of CD69 on CD1d/α-GalCer-tetramer+ hepatic iNKT cells without any difference in the proportion of iNKT cells as compared to non-immunized mice. In keeping with an early role in disease development, anti-CD1d administered early (days 0, 3 and 6 post-induction) but not late (days 27-39) delayed onset, reduced disease incidence and ameliorated clinical and histological severity. No difference in FoxP3$^+$ Treg frequency in spleen and lymph nodes or their suppressor function was noted. Splenic dendritic and macrophage APCs however showed reduced expression of CD40, CD80 and CD86 co-stimulatory molecules (Miellot-Gafsou et al., 2010).
In addition, Jung et al. (2010) have demonstrated a more subtle late regulatory role for NKT cells in tolerogenic DC (Tol-DC) mediated suppression of CIA. Thus TGF-β induced, peritoneal exudate cell (PEC)-derived Tol-DC from CD1d$^{+/-}$ but not CD1d$^{-/-}$ mice could suppress the incidence, onset and severity of CIA when administered on day 28. This was associated with suppressed serum and joint tissue IFN-γ and IL-17 cytokine and mRNA production, respectively. Anti-CII specific IgG2a was reduced whilst IgG1 was higher in CD1d$^{+/-}$ compared to CD1d$^{-/-}$ Tol-DC. Similarly, CII-stimulated splenocytes from CD1d$^{+/-}$ but not CD1d$^{-/-}$ Tol-DC produced lower levels of IFN-γ and IL-17, and higher levels of IL-4 and IL-10 .

3.4.2 Antibody mediated arthritis

Although the initating event and processes involved in RA and animal models of autoimmune arthritis may differ, the final inflammatory pathways leading to joint damage are more likely to be common to both (Nandakumar & Holmdahl 2006). Antibody-mediated models of autoimmune arthritis give us a unique opportunity to study these terminal events independently of the initation processes involved, and thereby to evaluate more clearly the role of iNKT cells during the terminal effector stage of disease.

3.4.2.1 K/BxN serum transfer model

The K/BxN mouse model of spontaneous autoimmune arthritis is a cross between the KRN TCR C57BL/6 transgenic mouse that is specific for an I-A^k restricted peptide of bovine ribonuclease (RNase), and the non-obese diabetic (NOD) mouse (Kouskoff et al., 1996). The K/BxN mouse T cells recognise an I-Ag7-restricted peptide from glucose-6-phosphate isomerase (G6PI) and B cells produce G6PI-specific antibodies (Matsumoto et al., 1999). Serum transfer alone into C57BL/6 mice can also mediate disease after just several days (Ji et al. 2001). Complement, neutrophils and mast cells play an essential role, and it is also apparent that Fcγ receptors (FcγRs) and IL-1 are also required in mediating joint inflammation and destruction (Ditzel, 2004).

In an earlier study of the K/BxN serum transfer model of inflammatory arthritis, Chiba et al. (2005) found an increased percentage of Vα24^{+}α-GalCer/CD1d-dimer^{+} iNKT cells in liver, peripheral blood, spleen and lymph nodes as compared to control mice given BxN serum. CD1d$^{-/-}$ and Jα281$^{-/-}$ knockout mice deficient in iNKT cells exhibited milder disease and reduced histological severity but not susceptibility, supporting a role for iNKT cells during the inflammatory effector phase of arthritis.

Subsequently, Kim et al. (2006) showed using in the K/BxN serum transfer model that CD1d$^{-/-}$ and Jα281$^{-/-}$ knockout mice have reduced clinical disease severity and neutrophil inflammatory infiltration, while transfer of liver NK1.1^{+}TCR-β^{+} NKT cells from normal B6 mice into CD1d$^{-/-}$ knockout mice restored wild-type disease severity. Furthermore, splenocytes from Vα14Jα281 TCR transgenic (Tg) RAG$^{-/-}$ mice but not Jα281$^{-/-}$ knockout mice restored disease severity in CD1d$^{-/-}$ mice, confirming the specific role of iNKT cells and in addition, the injection of α-GalCer as an in vivo activator of iNKT cells resulted in exacerbation of disease in B6 but not CD1d$^{-/-}$ mice. These investigators went on to dissect the mechanisms by which iNKT cells play a pro-inflammatory role in the KxB/N mouse model. Joint tissue Vα24Jα281 TCR mRNA measured by RT-PCR was observed at days 3, 5 and 7 in wild-type B6 (C57BL/6) mice, but not on day 0 or in CD1d$^{-/-}$ knockout mice, suggesting *de novo* iNKT cell infiltration during the inflammatory response. Joint tissue mRNA level of TGF-β1 was increased but IL-4 and IFN-γ were reduced in CD1d$^{-/-}$ mice compared to B6 mice, although similar levels were noted in splenocytes. Adoptive transfer of NKT cells reduced TGF-β1 and restored IL-4 and IFN-γ mRNA in joint tissue without changing splenic transcript levels. Postulating a role for TGF-β1 in resistance to joint inflammation, anti-TGF-β mAb was administered i.p. three times a week before and after serum transfer in CD1d$^{-/-}$ and wild-type mice. Anti-TGF-β increased disease severity to wild-type levels in CD1d$^{-/-}$ but had no effect in wild-type mice. Administration of recombinant TGF-β1 to wild-type mice in turn reduced disease severity, suggesting that iNKT cells mediate their pathogenic role in a TGF-β1-dependent fashion. But how do iNKT cells regulate TGF-β1 production? To answer this, synovial cells from B6 mice were stimulated with concanavalin A (ConA) to induce TGF-β1 production. This was suppressed by α-GalCer or anti-CD1d mAb in keeping with iNKT cell-mediated regulation. Similarly, injection of α-GalCer into treated B6 mice resulted in suppressed TGF-β1 production in joint tissues, indicating the capacity of NKT cells to specifically suppress TGF-β1 production. Blocking IL-4 and IFN-γ could restore TGF-β1 production, while IL-4$^{-/-}$ or IFN-γ$^{-/-}$ mice NKT cells transferred into CD1d$^{-/-}$ serum-treated mice resulted in minimal joint swelling and TGF-β1 transcriptional expression remained elevated. In contrast, transfer of NKT cells from B6 mice restored wild-type disease severity and TGF-β1 suppression. Finally, anti-IL-4 or anti-IFN-γ resulted in resistance to joint inflammation and enhanced TGF-β1 production in Vα14Jα281 TCR Tg RAG$^{-/-}$ mice (Kim, 2005).

Speculating that the observed NKT-mediated aggravation K/BxN serum transfer model of autoimmune arthritis may not be due to TCR-mediated recognition of CD1d-restricted self-lipid but instead could be due to Fcγ receptor engagement by immune complexes providing activating signals to NKT cells independently of TCR, Kim et al. (2006) showed that hepatic, splenic and thymic NK1.1^{+}TCR-β^{+} NKT cells in B6 mice selectively expressed FcγRIII, mainly on CD4+ or CD4- cells. Of these, 62% stained with α-GalCer/CD1d tetramer, indicating a mixed invariant and non-invariant NKT cell population. Furthermore, TCR stimulation of liver mononuclear cells (LMNCs) by α-GalCer/CD1d upregulated FcγRIII expression. Aggregated IgG but not soluble IgG, could activate NKT cells from B6 mice but not T or NK cells or NKT cells from Fcγ-/- mice, and upregulate activation markers CD25 and CD69. NKT cell FcγRIII engagement by aggregated IgG could upregulate expression of T-bet and GATA-3, and induce production of IL-4, IL-10, IL-13 and IFN-γ independently of simultaneous TCR stimulation. Simultaneous TCR and FcγRIII engagement resulted in cytokine output greater than either signal alone. In mice treated with K/BxN serum, joint swelling was detected at 4-5 days and maximal at 8-9 days. CD1d-/- mice administered NKT cells from B6 mice showed similar disease severity to wild-type mice, but administration of NKT from FcγR-/- B6 mice showed minimal joint swelling and only mild inflammatory infiltrate. Joint tissue Vα14Jα281 TCR mRNA was similar in CD1d-/- administered B6 NKT cells and CD1d-/- administered FcγR-/- B6 NKT cells. Furthermore, there was no difference in hepatic NKT, NK, CD4 and CD8 T cell numbers in Fcγ-/- B6 mice and α-GalCer/CD1d complex-stimulated LMNC cells from FcγR-/- mice produced IL-4, IL-10, IL-13 and IFN-γ similarly to wild-type B6 mice. These findings suggested that FcγR engagement rather than TCR engagement mediated NKT activation in the serum transfer model. RT-PCR analysis confirmed elevated joint tissue but not liver levels of TGFβ-1 and reduced levels of IL-4 and IFN-γ in CD1d-/- mice administered FcγR-/- NKT cells as compared to B6 NKT cells, indicating that FcγRIII engagement by joint tissue –deposited IgG enhances IL-4 and IFN-γ production and results in suppressed TFG-β1 (Kim et al., 2006).

IL-12 has previously been shown both to attenuate and to exacerbate CIA in C57BL/6 (Murphy et al., 2003) and DBA/1 mice (Butler et al., 1999; Malfait et al., 1998; Matthys et al., 1998), respectively. To elucidate the role of IL-12 in the terminal effector stages of arthritis, Park et al. (2010) studied the K/BxN mice serum transfer model in IL-12p35-/- and IL-12Rβ2-/- mice. Knockout mice had slower onset and less severe disease associated with milder inflammatory synovial infiltrate as compared to B6 mice. IL-12 mRNA was detected in joint tissues in B6 mice and recombinant (rm) IL-12 could restore arthritis severity in knockout mice. Serum transfer resulted in infiltration of large numbers of CD11b+ and Gr1+ granulocytes and smaller numbers of B, T, NK and CD11c+ cells. Using IL-12p40 cytokine reporter mice, the investigators showed that IL-12 is produced most prominently by CD11c+ cells, but also by CD11b+ cells and Gr1+ granulocytes. Joint tissue TGF-β transcript was higher and IFN-γ, IL-6 and IL-4 were lower in knockout mice. IL-17 and IL-23 were undetectable in wild-type and knockout mice, and joint inflammation and cytokine production were similar in B6 and IL-17-/- mice. Recombinant IL-12 restored cytokine levels to wild-type pattern. Both rmIFN-γ and anti-TGF-β restored arthritis severity in IL-12p35-/- mice. In joint tissue only NK1.1+TCR-β- NK and NK1.1+TCR-β+ NKT cells were found to express surface IL-12Rβ2. Adoptive transfer of splenocytes from B6 and Gr-1+ granulocyte-depleted B6 mice into IL-12Rβ2-/- mice restored arthritis severity and production of IFN-γ and IL-4, whereas transfer of splenocytes from iNKT-deficient Jα281-/- had no effect on arthritis severity and maintained higher levels of joint tissue TGF-β transcript. The investigators therefore suggested that IL-12p35 produced by CD11b+, CD11c+ and Gr-1+ cells promote antibody-induced inflammation by engaging IL-12 Rβ2 expressed on iNKT cells in joint tissues (Park et al., 2010).

3.4.2.2 Other models of autoimmune arthritis

Chiba et al. (2005) administered a mixture of four anti-CII mAb to C57BL/6 mice, followed 72h later by LPS. Jα281-/- and CD1d-/- knockout mice also showed reduced disease severity without any difference in susceptibility, in keeping with a role for iNKT cells during the effector as well as adaptive stages of CIA.
Antigen-induced arthritis (AIA) occurs when bovine serum albumin (BSA) is injected into the knee joint of B6 mice after priming with subcutaneous BSA injection, resulting in a week-long acute inflammatory arthritis (van den Berg et al., 2007). Teige et al. (2010) showed that CD1d-/- knockout mice experience a more severe AIA associated with a stronger splenocyte antigen-specific IFN-γ response without any difference in cell proliferation. Notably, NK1.1-depletion resulted in more severe arthritis.

3.4.3 Lessons learnt from animal models of autoimmune arthritis

CIA models using either C57BL/6 or the more susceptible DBA/1 mouse strains have consistently shown that iNKT cell deficient animals experience a reduced incidence and/or severity of arthritis. This therefore suggests that in contrast to other models of autoimmune disease and despite the apparent reduction in frequency of peripheral iNKT cells in RA, iNKT cells play a pathogenic role in animal models of autoimmune arthritis.
The increased incidence is a clue for an early role for iNKT cells in disease initiation, and this is supported by the observation of DLN cytokine deviation by day 11 in C57BL/6 mice (Yoshiga et al., 2008) and a reduction in incidence and disease amelioration when anti-CD1d is administered early, but not late in DBA1/J mice (Miellot-Gafsou et al., 2010). Ohnishi et al. (2005) found however no evidence of an effect on splenocyte cytokine deviation until day 26 in C57BL/6 mice, but given that they used the same mouse strains and CIA induction protocol as Yoshiga et al. (2008), the conflicting results are likely to be due to site and time-specific differences between DLN and splenocyte populations.
There is also reasonable evidence that iNKT cells play a role in later, effector stages of CIA too. IL-17 producing iNKT cells have been noted to steadily increase in numbers until the very late stages of disease in DBA/1 mice (Jung et al., 2009) and anti-CD1d administered to C57BL/6 mice on day 21 results in disease amelioration (Chiba et al., 2005). In addition, Jung et al. demonstrated that CD1d+/- but not CD1d-/- Tol-DC could suppress CIA in DBA/1 mice when administered as late as day 28 (Jung et al., 2010).
So how do iNKT cells influence the immune pathogenesis of CIA? Experimental data suggest that early on during induction and continuing into the effector stage of disease, iNKT cells skew the immune response to CII by promoting a Th1 and/or Th17 phenotype. It seems likely that by altering the cytokine environment, iNKT cells also influence the corresponding observed shift in autoantibody isotype from IgG1 to complement-fixing IgG2a. Furthermore, iNKT cells enhance both T and B cell responses as evidenced by the expression of activation markers and levels of circulating anti-CII autoantibodies, no doubt mediated in part by increased APC co-stimulatory molecule expression.
Whilst providing remarkable insight into the immunological role of iNKT cells in autoimmunity, murine models of CIA have also raised new issues and left us with many unanswered questions. It is unclear which particular iNKT cell subset is responsible for exacerbating disease, whether the same subsets are pathogenic at different stages or even whether some subsets play a protective role as suggested by Jung et al.'s Tol-DC experimental model (Jung et al., 2010). Neither do we know how iNKT cells become

activated or the mechanism(s) whereby they skew the phenotypic immune response to CII. Given that iNKT cells are found in diseased joints, do they play any direct role in terminal joint inflammation and tissue destruction?

Models of antigen and antibody-mediated arthritis are useful in clearly dissecting the role of iNKT cells during the induction and effector stages of autoimmune arthritis and confirm that iNKT cells play a pathogenic role during the terminal effector phase of disease. The work of Kim et al. (2006) and Park et al. (2010) was a particularly elegant demonstration of how iNKT cells appear to be stimulated through their IL-12Rβ2 and FcγRIII receptors, resulting in increased IL-4 and IFN-γ and suppressed TGF-β production, and subsequent modulation of arthritis severity. The only caveat to their work is the use of relatively non-specific markers which did not distinguish iNKT from other NKT cell subsets. It also still remains unclear which iNKT cell subsets are important and whether invariant TCR-self-lipid-CD1d interaction plays any role in iNKT cell activation during the effector stage. Further work is required to define the source of seemingly critical IL-4, IFN-γ and TGF-β, and ultimately, the extent to which these findings are applicable to rheumatoid arthritis in humans.

3.5 Clinical relevance of iNKT cells in RA

Despite the demonstrated pathogenicity of iNKT cells in animal models of autoimmune arthritis, their frequency and phenotype may yet serve as useful biomarkers, and their immune manipulation may serve a beneficial therapeutic purpose as shown in the context of infection, cancer immunity and other autoimmune diseases.

3.5.1 iNKT cells as diagnostic and prognostic tools

It seems that peripheral iNKT cell frequency is reduced in a range of autoimmune diseases including diabetes, multiple sclerosis and SLE. This may indicate a response to systemic inflammation or a generalised association with autoimmunity. As such, iNKT cells could in theory be used to distinguishing RA from other forms of arthritis. Furthermore, additional detailed analysis of iNKT subsets and function may provide prognostic information to guide individual treatment. Finally, it is tempting to speculate whether iNKT cells could serve as markers of self-tolerance to signal the safe withdrawal of long term immunosuppression in patients achieving clinical remission.

Our own work in this area showed that peripheral iNKT cell frequency was reduced among patients with RA, osteoarthritis (OA) and other inflammatory non-RA groups compared to patients with non-inflammatory, non-OA joint pain and healthy controls. This indicates that in practice iNKT cell frequency alone would prove of limited diagnostic or disease monitoring value. Whilst iNKT cell counts appear to improve with methotrexate therapy, we found no correlation with clinical response and therefore the significance of this observation remains unknown (Tudhope et al., 2010).

3.5.2 Manipulating iNKT cells for clinical benefit

OCH, a synthetic analogue of α-GalCer with a truncated sphingosine chain, has been shown to induce a Th2 bias in iNKT cytokine production and can efficiently inhibit EAE in C57BL/6 mice. Chiba et al. therefore studied the effects of intra-peritoneal α-GalCer and OCH administration, before and after induction of CIA in C57BL/6 mice. Unlike α-GalCer, OCH significantly reduced the clinical severity score of CIA from 13 to 4.6. When OCH was administered to Jα281-knockout mice, there was no difference in disease severity score as compared with vehicle alone, confirming the requirement for iNKT cells for OCH-mediated suppression of CIA. αGalCer injection induced a rapid rise in serum IL-4 and IFN-γ levels, while OCH increased IL-4 levels with much less IFN-γ production. Consistent with an iNKT cell derived source of cytokines, Jα281 knockout mice did not exhibit a rise in either IL-4 or IFN-γ (Chiba et al., 2004).

Miellot et al. (2005) explored the therapeutic potential of α-GalCer in the autoimmune prone DBA/1 model of CIA. Mice immunised with intra-peritoneal α-GalCer both before, at or after induction showed reduced disease severity but no difference in susceptibility or timing of disease onset. The optimal effect was noted with a single injection on day 0 and correlated with reduced histological inflammation and tissue destruction without any difference in levels of IgG1, IgG2a or IgG1/IgG2a ratio. Cytokine production by draining lymph node (DLN) $CD4^+$ T cells in response to CII stimulation showed no significant differences for IFN-γ or IL-4, but a significant increase in IL-10 production in α-GalCer/CII/CFA as compared to CII/CFA-immunised mice. Accordingly, the protective effect of α-GalCer on CIA was completely abrogated by blocking with anti-IL10R mAb.

Administration of a single dose of α-GalCer in a DBA/1 model of CIA on day 5 post-immunisation by Coppieters et al. (2007) resulted in an attenuated course of clinical disease and histological parameters. Splenic T-bet expression was reduced whilst GATA-3 was unchanged, suggesting an altered balance in favour of Th2 differentiation associated with a reduced antigen-specific CII proliferative response in DLN cells. Similar disease attenuation occurred following administration of the α-C-GalCer analog, a C-glycoside analogue of α-GalCer. Serum cytokine analysis after α-C-GalCer administration however showed marked differences as compared to α-GalCer administration, with negligible production of IL-2, TNF-α, IL-4 and IL-10, reduced IL-5 and IFN-γ, and increased IL-12p70 and IL-6. α-GalCer, but not α-C-GalCer, induced increased IgG1 levels with no difference in IgG2a between groups. T cell cytokine profiles induced with in vivo administration of anti-CD3 on day 14 after arthritis onset confirmed that mice treated with α-GalCer exhibited increased IL-10 production whilst mice treated with α-C-GalCer revealed lower levels of IL-4, IL-5 and IFN-γ. Furthermore, IL-10 production at 10 days post-immunisation was increased in α-GalCer-treated wild-type but not $J\alpha281^{-/-}$ mice, suggesting that the increased IL-10 in α-GalCer treated mice is iNKT cell-dependent. The authors therefore proposed that α-GalCer protection may be mediated by the development of an IL-10 producing population of regulatory cells whilst α-C-GalCer may operate by inducing a general hyporesponsive state as evidence by lower cytokine production.

α-carba-GalCer is another analogue of α-GalCer known to stimulate Th1 responses in iNKT cells. In DBA/1 mice, α-carba-GalCer can strongly induce IFN-γ, IL-2 and IL-12 but unlike α-GalCer, does not induce IL-4. When administered with CII/CFA on day 0, α-carba-GalCer reduced the incidence and severity of arthritis in an IFN-γ-dependent manner. This was associated with reduced CII-specific IgG2a antibody levels and inhibition of IL-17 production by CII-stimulated DLN cells. No change in apoptotic or regulatory FoxP3+ T cell frequency in DLN was noted. As early as day 3, DLN cells expressed reduced IL-6 and IL-23p19 with unchanged TGF-6 while CD1d-$tetramer^+$ iNKT cells produced higher IFN-γ in spleen, liver and DLN. On day 10, DLN T cells stimulated with PMA and ionomycin showed polarisation towards Th1 and suppression of Th17 cell differentiation, in keeping with protective Th1 deviation during the initiation phase of CIA (Yoshiga et al., 2011).

Screening a panel of analogs of α-GalCer for the ability to suppress the development of arthritis in a B6 model of K/BxN serum transfer-induced arthritis, Kaieda et al. (2007) found SGL-S23, an analog with a 5-carbon longer sphingosine base that could inhibit clinical and histological disease severity to a greater degree than α-GalCer by i.p. administration on days 0, 3 and 7. Furthermore, they showed a therapeutic effect when administered to mice with established arthritis. By injecting Jα281$^{-/-}$ knockout mice, they confirmed that SGL-S23-mediated disease suppression requires iNKT cells. Neutralisation of IL-4, IL-10 or TGF-β1 did not abolish the protective effect of SGL-S23. Instead, SGL-S23 was able to stimulate weaker in vitro cell proliferation and IFN-γ production than α-GalCer. Similarly, in vivo injection of SGL-S23 resulted in weaker IFN-γ serum responses. In keeping with the known essential role played by mast cells in the development of arthritis in the K/BxN serum transfer model, Kaieda et al. (2007) showed an elevation in serum histamine level five minutes after serum injection, abolished by pre-treatment with low-dose IFN-γ. SGL-S23 also suppressed histamine release, and more effectively so than α-GalCer or high dose IFN-γ.

Finally, CIA suppression through NKT cell manipulation can be accomplished with non-glycolipid stimulation as shown by Liu et al. (2011). Immunisation with murine CII induces a weaker responsethan heterologous collagen, characterised by multiple epitopes sharing a common motif, the strongest located at position 707-721. B10.Q or B6 mice immunised with $mCII_{707-721}$ mount a strong and specific immune response. In fact murine $mCII_{707-721}$ can bind to CD1d and partially competes with α-GalCer. B10.Q immunisation with $mCII_{707-721}$ resulted in significant expansion of $CD4^{+}NK1.1^{+}$ NKT cells. Reactive cells showed skewed TCR usage toward Vα14Jα18 with a diverse range of Vβ chains, with some skewing toward Vβ8.2. NKT cell proliferation was dependent on CD40-CD40L and B7-CD28 co-stimulation, while activated NKT cells produced IFN-γ, IL-4 and TGF-β but less TNF-α, peaking at 72h and thus resembling conventional T cell kinetics. Vaccination with $mCII_{707-721}$ ameliorated CIA, reducing clinical severity, joint inflammation, CD4 synovial infiltration and joint tissue IFN-γ, IL-4 and TNF-α production.

In summary, both α-GalCer and its analogues have been shown to modulate the severity of autoimmune arthritis in animal models during both the initiation and effector stages of disease. The mechanism of iNKT cell-mediated protection appears to be complex as evidenced by conflicting reports of Th1/Th2/Th17 polarisation, variable immunoglobulin isotype profiles and anergy induction by some agonists but not others. Immune alteration however is not restricted to the adaptive system, as shown by effects on mast cell activation in a serum transfer model of autoimmune arthritis. Before glycolipid ligands can be considered for use in rheumatoid arthritis, we will need to gain a better understanding of the factors important in predicting how these ligands will modulate the immune response, including ligand structure, dose, route of administration and timing of treatment.

4. Conclusion

Invariant NKT cells are powerful immune protagonists that can be engaged during innate immune system activation to amplify and direct subsequent adaptive immune responses by cytokine and cell contact-mediated cross-talk with a wide range of other immune players. In both rheumatoid arthritis and other autoimmune disorders, iNKT cells appear to be deficient in both number and function. Nevertheless, animal models of autoimmune arthritis consistently tell us that iNKT cells play a pathogenic rather than protective role.

Despite this, manipulating iNKT cell responses through the use of glycolipid or even peptide ligands has been shown to be effective both prophylactically and therapeutically. At the present time however our knowledge of iNKT cell mass, phenotype, function and significance in human disease remains limited. Furthermore, it is unclear whether animal models are truly representative and can be relied on to characterise iNKT cells in rheumatoid arthritis. Whilst pharmacological manipulation is evidently achievable, the general immunomodulatory governing principles are far from established. Future research will therefore need to address these issues in order to safely harness the full therapeutic potential of iNKT cells for effective clinical use.

5. References

Aggarwal, S., Ghilardi, N., Xie, M. H., de Sauvage, F. J., & Gurney, A. L. 2003, "Interleukin-23 promotes a distinct CD4 T cell activation state characterized by the production of interleukin-17", *J Biol.Chem.*, vol. 278, no. 3, pp. 1910-1914.

Ballas, Z. K. & Rasmussen, W. 1990, "NK1.1+ thymocytes. Adult murine CD4-, CD8- thymocytes contain an NK1.1+, CD3+, CD5hi, CD44hi, TCR-V beta 8+ subset", *J Immunol.*, vol. 145, no. 4, pp. 1039-1045.

Bettelli, E., Carrier, Y., Gao, W., Korn, T., Strom, T. B., Oukka, M., Weiner, H. L., & Kuchroo, V. K. 2006, "Reciprocal developmental pathways for the generation of pathogenic effector TH17 and regulatory T cells", *Nature*, vol. 441, no. 7090, pp. 235-238.

Brigl, M. & Brenner, M. B. 2004, "CD1: antigen presentation and T cell function", *Annu.Rev Immunol*, vol. 22, pp. 817-890.

Brigl, M. & Brenner, M. B. 2010, "How invariant natural killer T cells respond to infection by recognizing microbial or endogenous lipid antigens", *Semin.Immunol.*, vol. 22, no. 2, pp. 79-86.

Butler, D. M., Malfait, A. M., Maini, R. N., Brennan, F. M., & Feldmann, M. 1999, "Anti-IL-12 and anti-TNF antibodies synergistically suppress the progression of murine collagen-induced arthritis", *Eur.J Immunol.*, vol. 29, no. 7, pp. 2205-2212.

Chiba, A., Kaieda, S., Oki, S., Yamamura, T., & Miyake, S. 2005, "The involvement of V[alpha]14 natural killer T cells in the pathogenesis of arthritis in murine models", *Arthritis Rheum.*, vol. 52, pp. 1941-1948.

Chiba, A., Oki, S., Miyamoto, K., Hashimoto, H., Yamamura, T., & Miyake, S. 2004, "Suppression of collagen-induced arthritis by natural killer T cell activation with OCH, a sphingosine-truncated analog of alpha-galactosylceramide", *Arthritis Rheum*, vol. 50, no. 1, pp. 305-313.

Chu, C. Q., Swart, D., Alcorn, D., Tocker, J., & Elkon, K. B. 2007, "Interferon-gamma regulates susceptibility to collagen-induced arthritis through suppression of interleukin-17", *Arthritis Rheum.*, vol. 56, no. 4, pp. 1145-1151.

Coppieters, K. 2007, "A single early activation of invariant NK T cells confers long-term protection against collagen-induced arthritis in a ligand-specific manner", *J.Immunol.*, vol. 179, pp. 2300-2309.

Coquet, J. M. 2008, "Diverse cytokine production by NKT cell subsets and identification of an IL-17-producing CD4-NK1.1- NKT cell population", *Proc.Natl Acad.Sci.USA*, vol. 105, pp. 11287-11292.

D'Cruz, L. M., Yang, C. Y., & Goldrath, A. W. 2010, "Transcriptional regulation of NKT cell development and homeostasis", *Curr.Opin.Immunol.*, vol. 22, no. 2, pp. 199-205.

Ditzel, H. J. 2004, "The K/BxN mouse: a model of human inflammatory arthritis", *Trends Mol Med.*, vol. 10, no. 1, pp. 40-45.

Eberl, G., Lees, R., Smiley, S. T., Taniguchi, M., Grusby, M. J., & MacDonald, H. R. 1999, "Tissue-specific segregation of CD1d-dependent and CD1d-independent NK T cells", *J Immunol.*, vol. 162, no. 11, pp. 6410-6419.

Eberl, G. & MacDonald, H. R. 1998, "Rapid death and regeneration of NKT cells in anti-CD3epsilon- or IL-12-treated mice: a major role for bone marrow in NKT cell homeostasis", *Immunity.*, vol. 9, no. 3, pp. 345-353.

Fox, L., Hegde, S., & Gumperz, J. E. 2010, "Natural killer T cells: innate lymphocytes positioned as a bridge between acute and chronic inflammation?", *Microbes.Infect.*, vol. 12, no. 14-15, pp. 1125-1133.

Gapin, L. 2010, "iNKT cell autoreactivity: what is 'self' and how is it recognized?", *Nat Rev Immunol.*, vol. 10, no. 4, pp. 272-277.

Godfrey, D. I., MacDonald, H. R., Kronenberg, M., Smyth, M. J., & Van, K. L. 2004, "NKT cells: what's in a name?", *Nat Rev Immunol*, vol. 4, no. 3, pp. 231-237.

Godfrey, D. I., Stankovic, S., & Baxter, A. G. 2010, "Raising the NKT cell family", *Nat Immunol.*, vol. 11, no. 3, pp. 197-206.

Hegde, S., Fox, L., Wang, X., & Gumperz, J. E. 2010, "Autoreactive natural killer T cells: promoting immune protection and immune tolerance through varied interactions with myeloid antigen-presenting cells", *Immunology.*, vol. 130, no. 4, pp. 471-483.

Hegen, M., Keith, J. C., Jr., Collins, M., & Nickerson-Nutter, C. L. 2008, "Utility of animal models for identification of potential therapeutics for rheumatoid arthritis", *Ann Rheum Dis.*, vol. 67, no. 11, pp. 1505-1515.

Ho, L. P., Urban, B. C., Jones, L., Ogg, G. S., & McMichael, A. J. 2004, "CD4(-)CD8alphaalpha subset of CD1d-restricted NKT cells controls T cell expansion", *J Immunol.*, vol. 172, no. 12, pp. 7350-7358.

Ji, H., Gauguier, D., Ohmura, K., Gonzalez, A., Duchatelle, V., Danoy, P., Garchon, H. J., Degott, C., Lathrop, M., Benoist, C., & Mathis, D. 2001, "Genetic influences on the end-stage effector phase of arthritis", *J Exp.Med.*, vol. 194, no. 3, pp. 321-330.

Jung, S., Park, Y. K., Shin, J. H., Lee, H., Kim, S. Y., Lee, G. R., & Park, S. H. 2010, "The requirement of natural killer T-cells in tolerogenic APCs-mediated suppression of collagen-induced arthritis", *Exp.Mol Med.*, vol. 42, no. 8, pp. 547-554

Jung, S., Shin, H. S., Hong, C., Lee, H., Park, Y. K., Shin, J. H., Hong, S., Lee, G. R., & Park, S. H. 2009, "Natural killer T cells promote collagen-induced arthritis in DBA/1 mice", *Biochem.Biophys.Res Commun.*, vol. 390, no. 3, pp. 399-403.

Kaieda, S., Tomi, C., Oki, S., Yamamura, T., & Miyake, S. 2007, "Activation of invariant natural killer T cells by synthetic glycolipid ligands suppresses autoantibody-induced arthritis", *Arthritis Rheum*, vol. 56, no. 6, pp. 1836-1845.

Kim, H. Y. 2005, "NKT cells promote antibody-induced joint inflammation by suppressing transforming growth factor [beta]1 production", *J.Exp.Med.*, vol. 201, pp. 41-47.

Kim, H. Y., Kim, S., & Chung, D. H. 2006, "Fc[gamma]RIII engagement provides activating signals to NKT cells in antibody-induced joint inflammation", *J.Clin.Invest.*, vol. 116, pp. 2484-2492.

Koetz, K., Bryl, E., Spickschen, K., O'Fallon, W. M., Goronzy, J. J., & Weyand, C. M. 2000, "T cell homeostasis in patients with rheumatoid arthritis", *Proc.Natl.Acad.Sci.U.S.A*, vol. 97, no. 16, pp. 9203-9208.

Kojo, S., Adachi, Y., Keino, H., Taniguchi, M., & Sumida, T. 2001, "Dysfunction of T cell receptor AV24AJ18+, BV11+ double-negative regulatory natural killer T cells in autoimmune diseases", *Arthritis Rheum*, vol. 44, no. 5, pp. 1127-1138.

Kojo, S., Tsutsumi, A., Goto, D., & Sumida, T. 2003, "Low expression levels of soluble CD1d gene in patients with rheumatoid arthritis", *J Rheumatol.*, vol. 30, no. 12, pp. 2524-2528.

Kouskoff, V., Korganow, A. S., Duchatelle, V., Degott, C., Benoist, C., & Mathis, D. 1996, "Organ-specific disease provoked by systemic autoimmunity", *Cell*, vol. 87, pp. 811-822.

Langrish, C. L., Chen, Y., Blumenschein, W. M., Mattson, J., Basham, B., Sedgwick, J. D., McClanahan, T., Kastelein, R. A., & Cua, D. J. 2005, "IL-23 drives a pathogenic T cell population that induces autoimmune inflammation", *J Exp.Med*, vol. 201, no. 2, pp. 233-240.

Linsen, L., Thewissen, M., Baeten, K., Somers, V., Geusens, P., Raus, J., & Stinissen, P. 2005, "Peripheral blood but not synovial fluid natural killer T cells are biased towards a Th1-like phenotype in rheumatoid arthritis", *Arthritis Res Ther*, vol. 7, no. 3, p. R493-R502.

Liu, Y., Teige, A., Mondoc, E., Ibrahim, S., Holmdahl, R., & Issazadeh-Navikas, S. 2011, "Endogenous collagen peptide activation of CD1d-restricted NKT cells ameliorates tissue-specific inflammation in mice", *J Clin Invest.*, vol. 121, no. 1, pp. 249-264.

Lubberts, E., Joosten, L. A., Oppers, B., van den, B. L., Coenen-de Roo, C. J., Kolls, J. K., Schwarzenberger, P., van de Loo, F. A., & van den Berg, W. B. 2001, "IL-1-independent role of IL-17 in synovial inflammation and joint destruction during collagen-induced arthritis", *The Journal of Immunology*, vol. 167, no. 2, pp. 1004-1013.

Lubberts, E., Koenders, M. I., Oppers-Walgreen, B., van den, B. L., Coenen-de Roo, C. J., Joosten, L. A., & van den Berg, W. B. 2004, "Treatment with a neutralizing anti-murine interleukin-17 antibody after the onset of collagen-induced arthritis reduces joint inflammation, cartilage destruction, and bone erosion", *Arthritis Rheum.*, vol. 50, no. 2, pp. 650-659.

Luross, J. A. & Williams, N. A. 2001, "The genetic and immunopathological processes underlying collagen-induced arthritis", *Immunology.*, vol. 103, no. 4, pp. 407-416.

Malfait, A. M., Butler, D. M., Presky, D. H., Maini, R. N., Brennan, F. M., & Feldmann, M. 1998, "Blockade of IL-12 during the induction of collagen-induced arthritis (CIA) markedly attenuates the severity of the arthritis", *Clin Exp.Immunol.*, vol. 111, no. 2, pp. 377-383.

Mangan, P. R., Harrington, L. E., O'Quinn, D. B., Helms, W. S., Bullard, D. C., Elson, C. O., Hatton, R. D., Wahl, S. M., Schoeb, T. R., & Weaver, C. T. 2006, "Transforming growth factor-beta induces development of the T(H)17 lineage", *Nature.*, vol. 441, no. 7090, pp. 231-234.

Matsuda, J. L., Naidenko, O. V., Gapin, L., Nakayama, T., Taniguchi, M., Wang, C. R., Koezuka, Y., & Kronenberg, M. 2000, "Tracking the response of natural killer T cells to a glycolipid antigen using CD1d tetramers", *J Exp.Med.*, vol. 192, no. 5, pp. 741-754.

Matsumoto, I., Staub, A., Benoist, C., & Mathis, D. 1999, "Arthritis provoked by linked T and B cell recognition of a glycolytic enzyme", *Science*, vol. 286, no. 5445, pp. 1732-1735.

Matthys, P., Vermeire, K., Mitera, T., Heremans, H., Huang, S., & Billiau, A. 1998, "Anti-IL-12 antibody prevents the development and progression of collagen-induced arthritis in IFN-gamma receptor-deficient mice", *Eur.J Immunol.*, vol. 28, no. 7, pp. 2143-2151.

Miellot, A. 2005, "Activation of invariant NK T cells protects against experimental rheumatoid arthritis by an IL-10-dependent pathway", *Eur.J.Immunol.*, vol. 35, pp. 33704-33713.

Miellot-Gafsou, A., Biton, J., Bourgeois, E., Herbelin, A., Boissier, M. C., & Bessis, N. 2010, "Early activation of invariant natural killer T cells in a rheumatoid arthritis model and application to disease treatment", *Immunology*, vol. 130, no. 2, pp. 296-306.

Mitsuo, A., Morimoto, S., Nakiri, Y., Suzuki, J., Kaneko, H., Tokano, Y., Tsuda, H., Takasaki, Y., & Hashimoto, H. 2006, "Decreased CD161+CD8+ T cells in the peripheral blood of patients suffering from rheumatic diseases", *Rheumatology (Oxford).*, vol. 45, no. 12, pp. 1477-1484.

Murphy, C. A., Langrish, C. L., Chen, Y., Blumenschein, W., McClanahan, T., Kastelein, R. A., Sedgwick, J. D., & Cua, D. J. 2003, "Divergent pro- and antiinflammatory roles for IL-23 and IL-12 in joint autoimmune inflammation", *J Exp.Med*, vol. 198, no. 12, pp. 1951-1957.

Nakae, S., Nambu, A., Sudo, K., & Iwakura, Y. 2003, "Suppression of immune induction of collagen-induced arthritis in IL-17-deficient mice", *The Journal of Immunology*, vol. 171, no. 11, pp. 6173-6177.

Nandakumar, K. S. & Holmdahl, R. 2006, "Antibody-induced arthritis: disease mechanisms and genes involved at the effector phase of arthritis", *Arthritis Res Ther*, vol. 8, no. 6, p. 223.

Ohnishi, Y., Tsutsumi, A., Goto, D., Itoh, S., Matsumoto, I., Taniguchi, M., & Sumida, T. 2005, "TCR Valpha14 natural killer T cells function as effector T cells in mice with collagen-induced arthritis", *Clin Exp.Immunol.*, vol. 141, no. 1, pp. 47-53.

Parietti, V., Chifflot, H., Sibilia, J., Muller, S., & Monneaux, F. 2010, "Rituximab treatment overcomes reduction of regulatory iNKT cells in patients with rheumatoid arthritis", *Clin Immunol*, vol. 134, no. 3, pp. 331-339.

Park, Y., Kim, H. S., Ahn, J. Y., Yun, D., Cho, M. L., Hong, S., Kim, H. Y., & Chung, D. H. 2010, "IL-12p35 promotes antibody-induced joint inflammation by activating NKT cells and suppressing TGF-beta", *J Immunol.*, vol. 185, no. 3, pp. 1476-1484.

Ponchel, F., Morgan, A. W., Bingham, S. J., Quinn, M., Buch, M., Verburg, R. J., Henwood, J., Douglas, S. H., Masurel, A., Conaghan, P., Gesinde, M., Taylor, J., Markham, A. F., Emery, P., van Laar, J. M., & Isaacs, J. D. 2002, "Dysregulated lymphocyte proliferation and differentiation in patients with rheumatoid arthritis", *Blood*, vol. 100, no. 13, pp. 4550-4556.

Reilly, E. C., Wands, J. R., & Brossay, L. 2010, "Cytokine dependent and independent iNKT cell activation", *Cytokine.*, vol. 51, no. 3, pp. 227-231.

Salio, M., Silk, J. D., & Cerundolo, V. 2010, "Recent advances in processing and presentation of CD1 bound lipid antigens", *Curr.Opin.Immunol.*, vol. 22, no. 1, pp. 81-88.

Sarkar, S., Cooney, L. A., White, P., Dunlop, D. B., Endres, J., Jorns, J. M., Wasco, M. J., & Fox, D. A. 2009, "Regulation of pathogenic IL-17 responses in collagen-induced arthritis: roles of endogenous interferon-gamma and IL-4", *Arthritis Res Ther.*, vol. 11, no. 5, p. R158.

Scott, D. L., Wolfe, F., & Huizinga, T. W. 2010, "Rheumatoid arthritis", *Lancet*, vol. 376, no. 9746, pp. 1094-1108.

Segawa, S., Goto, D., Yoshiga, Y., Hayashi, T., Matsumoto, I., Ito, S., & Sumida, T. 2009, "Low levels of soluble CD1d protein alters NKT cell function in patients with rheumatoid arthritis", *Int.J Mol Med.*, vol. 24, no. 4, pp. 481-486.

Spadaro, A., Scrivo, R., Moretti, T., Bernardini, G., Riccieri, V., Taccari, E., Strom, R., & Valesini, G. 2004, "Natural killer cells and gamma/delta T cells in synovial fluid and in peripheral blood of patients with psoriatic arthritis", *Clin Exp.Rheumatol.*, vol. 22, no. 4, pp. 389-394.

Strominger, J. L. 2010, "An alternative path for antigen presentation: group 1 CD1 proteins", *J Immunol.*, vol. 184, no. 7, pp. 3303-3305.

Takahashi, T. 2002, "Cutting edge: analysis of human V[alpha]24+CD8+ NK T cells activated by [alpha]-galactosylceramide-pulsed monocyte-derived dendritic cells", *J.Immunol.*, vol. 168, pp. 3140-3144.

Teige, A., Bockermann, R., Hasan, M., Olofsson, K. E., Liu, Y., & Issazadeh-Navikas, S. 2010, "CD1d-dependent NKT cells play a protective role in acute and chronic arthritis models by ameliorating antigen-specific Th1 responses", *J Immunol.*, vol. 185, no. 1, pp. 345-356.

Tudhope, S. J., von, D. A., Falconer, J., Pratt, A., Woolridge, T., Wilson, G., Isaacs, J. D., & Ng, W. F. 2010, "Profound invariant natural killer T-cell deficiency in inflammatory arthritis", *Ann Rheum Dis*, vol. 69, no. 10, pp. 1873-1879.

van den Berg, W. B., Joosten, L. A., & van Lent, P. L. 2007, "Murine antigen-induced arthritis", *Methods Mol Med.*, vol. 136:243-53., pp. 243-253.

Van, K. L., Parekh, V. V., & Wu, L. 2011, "Invariant natural killer T cells: bridging innate and adaptive immunity", *Cell Tissue Res.*, vol. 343, no. 1, pp. 43-55.

Veldhoen, M., Hocking, R. J., Atkins, C. J., Locksley, R. M., & Stockinger, B. 2006, "TGFbeta in the context of an inflammatory cytokine milieu supports de novo differentiation of IL-17-producing T cells", *Immunity.*, vol. 24, no. 2, pp. 179-189.

Wang, C. R. 2003, "Involvement of natural killer T cells in C57BL/6 mouse model of collagen-induced arthritis", *J Microbiol.Immunol Infect.*, vol. 36, no. 1, pp. 15-20.

Wilson, M. T., Johansson, C., Olivares-Villagomez, D., Singh, A. K., Stanic, A. K., Wang, C. R., Joyce, S., Wick, M. J., & Van, K. L. 2003, "The response of natural killer T cells to glycolipid antigens is characterized by surface receptor down-modulation and expansion", *Proc.Natl Acad.Sci.U.S.A.*, vol. 100, no. 19, pp. 10913-10918.

Wooley, P. H., Luthra, H. S., Stuart, J. M., & David, C. S. 1981, "Type II collagen-induced arthritis in mice. I. Major histocompatibility complex (I region) linkage and antibody correlates", *J Exp.Med.*, vol. 154, no. 3, pp. 688-700.

Yanagihara, Y., Shiozawa, K., Takai, M., Kyogoku, M., & Shiozawa, S. 1999, "Natural killer (NK) T cells are significantly decreased in the peripheral blood of patients with rheumatoid arthritis (RA)", *Clin Exp.Immunol.*, vol. 118, no. 1, pp. 131-136.

Yoshiga, Y., Goto, D., Segawa, S., Horikoshi, M., Hayashi, T., Matsumoto, I., Ito, S., Taniguchi, M., & Sumida, T. 2011, "Activation of natural killer T cells by alpha-carba-GalCer (RCAI-56), a novel synthetic glycolipid ligand, suppresses murine collagen-induced arthritis", *Clin Exp.Immunol.*, vol. 164, no. 2, pp. 236-247.

Yoshiga, Y., Goto, D., Segawa, S., Ohnishi, Y., Matsumoto, I., Ito, S., Tsutsumi, A., Taniguchi, M., & Sumida, T. 2008, "Invariant NKT cells produce IL-17 through IL-23-dependent and -independent pathways with potential modulation of Th17 response in collagen-induced arthritis", *Int.J Mol Med.*, vol. 22, no. 3, pp. 369-374.

3

IL-12 Family Cytokines in Inflammation and Bone Erosion of Rheumatoid Arthritis

Ran Wei[1], Alastair J. Sloan[2] and Xiao-Qing Wei[2]
[1]*Chelsea and Westminster Hospital NHS Foundation Trust,*
[2]*Tissue Engineering and Reparative Dentistry, Dental School of Cardiff University, UK*

1. Introduction

Rheumatoid arthritis (RA) is an autoimmune disease characterised by chronic joint inflammation. The precise aetiology of this autoimmune process remains unclear. Soluble factors produced by infiltrating synovial cells play an important role in driving the inflammatory process that leads to inflammatory cell migration and proliferation in the synovial tissue. These soluble factors consist mainly of cytokines that either promote or suppress inflammation.

A number of cytokines have been identified in synovial fluid and the synovial membrane. Cytokines such as TNFα, IL-1 and IL-6 stimulate T-cells and induce subsequent cartilage and bone erosion (Kang et al., 2009). Along with IL-18, these cytokines are produced by synovial macrophages and synovial fibroblasts. IL-18 causes joint inflammation and subsequent bone destruction by facilitating T-cell activation and stimulating B-cell production of autoantibodies. Deletion of the IL-18 gene in mice has been shown to result in a significant reduction in the incidence of joint inflammation and bone destruction (Wei et al., 2001).

$CD4^+$ T-cells proliferate in inflamed synovial joints through stimulation of IL-15. Inhibition IL-15 results in a significantly lower production of TNFα and IL-1. As such, IL-15 blockade abolishes severe joint inflammation in collagen induced-arthritis mouse models (Ruchatz et al., 1998). In the $CD4^+$ T-cell population, Th17 has been demonstrated as a pathogenic T-cell that produces IL-17 to induce neutrophil migration (Shibata et al., 2009). IL-17 is known to stimulate receptor-activator of nuclear factor kappa-B ligand (RANKL) production by osteoblast cells to promote osteoclastogenesis in RA bone erosion (Joosten et al., 2003). Th17 development is governed by TGFβ, IL-1β and IL-23 (Paradowska-Gorycka et al., 2010; Santarlasci et al., 2009). Higher concentrations of IL-23 (a member of the IL-12 family cytokines) are detected in the serum and synovial fluid of patients with greater severity of RA (Melis et al., 2010). IL-23 can also be produced by osteoblast cells after stimulation with TNFα (unpublished data).

It is possible that remission of joint inflammation in RA patients can occur spontaneously. The fluctuation in inflammation within the joint results from auto-inhibition through the production of anti-inflammatory cytokines via regulatory T (Treg) cells (Raghavan et al.,

2009) and other regulatory mechanisms. Treg cells encompasse $CD4^+$ T-cells and produce anti-inflammatory cytokines - such as IL-10, TGFβ and IL-35 - to suppress Th17 and other T effector cells (Sabat et al., 2010). Recent studies have identified IL-35 (a member of the IL-12 family cytokines) as a potent suppressor of Th17 cells and promoter of Treg cell expansion (Collison et al., 2007; Niedbala et al., 2007). Injection of recombinant IL-35 into mice with collagen induced-arthritis has demonstrated effective suppression of the onset of joint inflammation (Niedbala et al., 2007). The mechanism of this model is thought to be through the promotion of Treg cell activity and suppression of Th17 function (Chaturvedi et al., 2011). Despite strong evidence from *in vivo* animal models demonstrating the therapeutic properties of IL-35 in the treatment of joint inflammation, there continues to be a lack of evidence from *in vitro* human bone inflammatory models. The efficaciousness of IL-35 as an immunomodulatory therapy against RA therefore remains to be proven.

In this chapter, we will concentrate on the role of the IL-12 family cytokines - namely IL-12, IL-23, IL-27 and IL-35 in the development of rheumatoid arthritis. We will present, analyse and summarise the most recent work in our field of research. We aim to provide an up-to-date and comprehensive overview of the compelling evidence and novel ideas paving way for a new generation of medical therapies against RA.

2. T cell activation and IL-12 family cytokines

2.1 T cell activation in rheumatoid arthritis

The main infiltrative inflammatory T cell in the synovial joint is the $CD4^+$ T cell. Dependent on cytokine production and cell linage control cell signalling, $CD4^+$ T cells can be divided into 4 sub-populations - Th1, Th2, Th17 and immune regulatory T (Treg) cells. These sub-types differ in function and activity. Th1, Th2 and Th17 cells act mainly as T effector cells whereas Treg cells display an immune suppressing role. T helper (Th) cell differentiation and expansion is controlled by maturated dendritic cells (DC) via three different means of signalling. The first is antigen presentation where MHC II (present on the surface of DCs) relay antigens to T cell receptors (TCR) found on T cells. In RA, pathological auto-antigen signalling mediated by DCs and other antigen presenting cells lead to auto-antigen induced T cell responses. The exact cause of this remains unclear, however, recent evidence has identified connective tissue protein and citrullinated vementin as likely mediators. Both have been shown to trigger an auto-immune T cell response following presentation by MHC II in RA patient (Snir et al., ; van Lierop et al., 2007). The second type of signalling is co-stimulation and is mediated via co-stimulation molecules found on DCs. An example of this is CD40 when it binds to T cell co-stimulation receptor (CD40L). The final means of signalling is mediated by cytokines or a group of cytokines and is the most important form of signalling generated by DCs. Cytokines produced by activated DCs bind to receptors on naïve T cells and drive T cell differentiation into Th1, Th2 or Th17. In some instances, it induces differentiation into Treg cells and suppresses over-reactive T cells. In patients with RA, this complex system can result in joint inflammation that is self-limiting and accounts for the fluctuating nature of the disease. Despite vast amounts of research dedicated to investigating the precise mechanism of T cell development, in health and in disease, it remains a mystery.

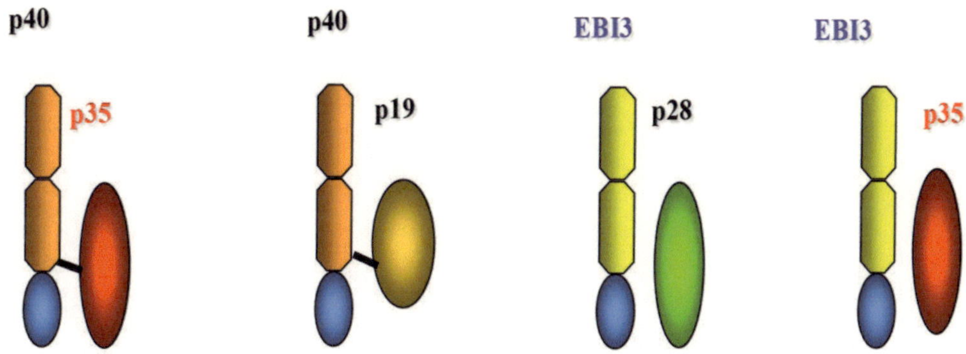

Fig. 1. Schematic representation of structure of members of the IL-12 family cytokines.

2.2 IL-12 family cytokines in inflammation

The cytokines involved in mediating T cell development belong to the IL-12 family cytokines. This family of cytokines are heterodimer secreted glycoproteins. One subunit is an IL-6 like protein and the other an IL-6 soluble receptor like protein. They are therefore also named IL-6/IL-12 family cytokines. IL-12, IL-23, IL-27 and IL-35 all belong to this IL-12 family cytokines and share certain protein subunits (Fig.1).

IL-12 consists of a p40 subunit and a p35 subunit. IL-23 consists of the same p40 subunit but couples with a p19 subunit. IL-12 was the first cytokine to be identified that had the capability of driving Th1 development (Hsieh et al., 1993; Murphy et al., 1994). IL-23 was discovered almost a decade later and was initially seen as a novel cytokine with the ability to aid Th1 development at the later stages of cell differentiation (Oppmann et al., 2000). Recent evidences suggest that IL-23 is in fact functionally very different from IL-12. Aside from its effects on Th1 cell development, IL-23 also stimulates production of IL-17 by Th17 cells (Horai et al., 2000; Zelante et al., 2007). Osteoclast formation has been shown to be up-regulated by IL-23 through its effects on macrophages (Chen et al., 2008). Unlike IL-12, IL-23 plays more of a pathological role in inflammatory and autoimmune diseases.

The cytokine IL-27 is composed of a p40-related protein called EBi3 (Epstein-Barr virus induced gene 3) and a p35-related protein known as p28. EBi3 was first identified in 1996 following its expression during infection of B-lymphocyte with the Epstein Barr Virus. The gene produced was a secreted glycoprotein related to p40 (Devergne et al., 1996). p28 was discovered some years later in a research investigation of IL-6 homologous proteins using bioinformatics. The p28 protein was found only to be efficiently secreted when coupled with EBi3. Following this discovery, the heterodimeric protein of EBi3 and p28 was named as IL-27 (Pflanz et al., 2002). The function of IL-27 was again, initially, thought to be similar to IL-12 in driving the early stages of Th1 cell development. Further study of IL-27 has shown it to be capable of inducing IL-10 production from Treg cells and subsequently inhibiting Th17 responses (Murugaiyan et al., 2009). In inflammatory mouse disease models, such as collagen induced arthritis (CIA) mouse model, IL-27 is able to suppress inflammation (Niedbala et al., 2008).

EBi3 can be coupled with the p35 subunit of IL-12 to form a heterodimeric protein (Devergne, Birkenbach and Kieff, 1997). The function of EBi3/p35 remained a mystery until relatively recently when studies used a recombinant EBi3/p35 protein in a rheumatoid arthritis mouse model. In these experiments, joint inflammation in CIA mice was effectively

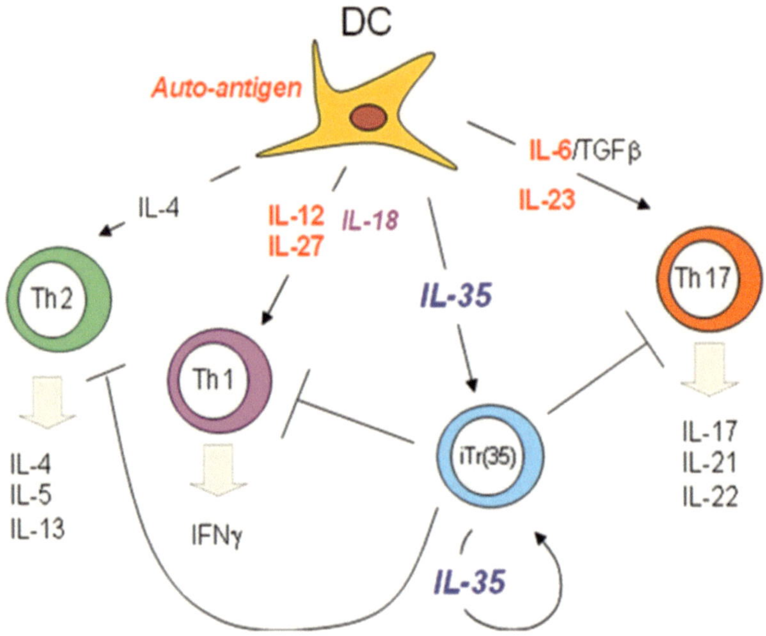

Fig. 2. Diagram showing CD4+ T cell differentiation resulting from production of IL-12 family cytokines produced by DCs. The presentation of auto-antigens by DCs and cytokine production result in T cell differentiation. The type of T cell response depends on the type of cytokine production in the inflammatory environment. Both DCs and iTr(35), a type of Treg cell, produce IL-35 to suppress Th1, Th17 and Th2 responses.

resolved by the EBi3/p35 recombinant protein. It was suggested that the therapeutic mechanism of this recombinant protein was through induction of Treg cell development and IL-10 expression leading to suppression of Th1 and Th17 responses (Niedbala et al., 2007).

EBi3 and p35 are also highly expressed in Treg cells thus seemingly a key component of the immune regulating function of mouse Treg cells. Deficiency in either EBi3 or p35 gene in Treg cells will result in a reduced ability to suppress effector T-cell proliferation. Without EBi3 or p35, Treg cells are unable to resolve gut inflammation in mouse inflammatory bowel disease (IBD). The EBi3/p35 heterodimeric protein has since been named IL-35 (Collison et al., 2007). The functional effects of IL-35 in mouse models have been clearly demonstrated by a number of research groups. The role of this particularly cytokine in immune regulation of humans has now been confirmed (Chaturvedi et al., 2011).

3. IL-12 family cytokines in joint inflammation of rheumatoid arthritis

3.1 IL-12 and IL-23 are the critical cytokines involved in joint inflammation

Involvement of IL-12 in joint inflammation has been demonstrated in Collagen-Induced Arthritis (CIA) mouse models in early studies. Injection of recombinant IL-12 into mouse induced severe joint inflammation in CIA mouse models. Severity was markedly increased with co-administration of IL-18 and IL-12 (Leung et al., 2000). In humans, IL-12p40 can be detected in serum of RA patients in more than 40% of cases. It is also present in osteoarthritic patients and even healthy individuals but in significantly lower instances (Kim et al., 2000). The number of collagen type II (CII) reactive T cell in the peripheral blood mononuclear cell (PBMC) and synovial fluid monocytes (SFMCs) from RA patients was significant higher than those from osteoarthritis and health control individuals. The higher IFNγ concentration in the culture supernatant was also associated with higher IL-12 production. This result indicated that CII reactive Th1 response is dominant in RA patients (Park et al., 2001).

Study of TNFα, TNFα-RI/II and IL-12 serum level in RA patients concluded that IL-12p40 levels have a stronger association with disease than TNFα levels (Ebrahimi et al., 2009). IL-12 binds to IL-12 receptor β1 and β2 to trigger STAT4 phosphorylation in T cells. RA patients not only produced more IL-12p40, but are also more sensitive to IL-12 stimulation, which based on the fact of T cells from RA patients showed earlier onset and higher levels of STAT4 phosphorylation in comparison with osteoarthritis and health controls (Sun et al., 2011). To date, anti-TNFα therapy has been proven as the most effective therapy in treatment of rheumatoid arthritis (Radovits et al., 2009;Salliot et al., 2011). $CD4^+$ T cells in peripheral blood mononuclear cells (PBMC) of RA patient have higher frequency of IL-12 receptor β and lower of IL-4 receptor. The frequency of IL-$12R^+$ T cell was remarkably reduced with both methothotrexate (MTX) therapy and anti-TNFα therapies (Herman et al., 2011). However another clinical study showed STAT4 phosphorylation was not induced in $CD4^+$ T cells from untreated RA patients by anti-CD3 and anti-CD28, but STAT4 activation was induced in healthy individuals and anti-TNFα treated patients (Aerts et al., 2010). This result disagreed with previous concepts of the role of IL-12 induced Th1 responses in RA. Since STAT4 phosphorylation was not induced by IL-12, but anti-CD3 and CD28 in this experimental setting, this result may indicate anti-TNFα altered T cell response in RA patients. Since IL-12 is the only cytokine that strongly drives Th1 cell development and subsequent production of IFNγ, the role of IL-12 in RA inflammation was challenged by the studies in Collagen induced arthritis (CIA) mouse model with IFNγ receptor gene knockout or IFNγ blockade (Boissier et al., 1995; Manoury-Schwartz et al., 1997). Mice with IFNγ gene deficiency and IFNγ blocker did not show reduced joint inflammation but rather enhanced inflammation. These may suggest that IL-12 stimulates other cytokines to induce autoimmune joint inflammation in disease. IFNγ production from Th1 responses is rather suppressing the joint inflammation which was seen in IL-27 suppressing joint inflammation (see section 3.2).

Comprehensive studies by using autoimmune disease mouse models with gene knockout mice have demonstrated the complexity of IL-12p40, p35 and its receptors β1 and β2 (Airoldi et al., 2005; Gran et al., 2002; Kikawada, Lenda and Kelley, 2003; Yoshida et al., 2009). IL-12p40 and IL-12 receptor β1 gene knockout mice showed resistance to joint inflammation in CIA mice while IL-12p35 and IL-12RII gene knockout mice are significantly more susceptible to joint inflammation induced by collagen type II (Hoeve et al., 2006; Murphy et al., 2003). Discovery of IL-23 provided a fully explanation for the confounding phenotype in these gene knockout mice (Ooi et al., 2009). Knockout of the IL-23p19 subunit in mice showed similar levels of resistance to joint inflammation as IL-12p40 knockout (Hoeve et al., 2006). Given that IL-23 shares the same protein subunit of IL-12p40, it can be concluded that IL-23 is the key pathological cytokine in joint inflammation. To support this theory is the discovery of significantly higher levels of IL-23 in both serum and synovial fluid of RA patients (Melis et al., 2010).

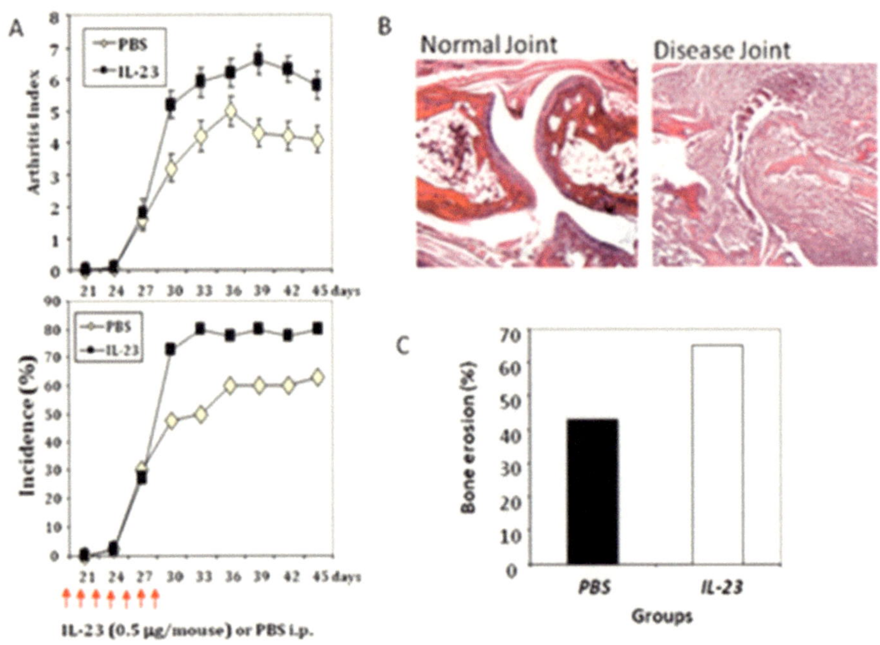

Fig. 3. IL-23 induced joint inflammation and pathology. A) Graph showing significantly higher incidence and index of severe joint inflammation in mice undergoing daily injections of 0.5μg/mouse of recombinant IL-23. B) Histology of normal and disease joints following injection of recombinant IL-23 injections. C) Incidence of bone erosion.

Results from our unpublished studies with recombinant IL-23 in CIA mice have yielded interesting findings. When recombinant IL-23 was injected into CIA mice severe joint inflammation ensued. The incidence of this was significantly higher when compared to mice injected with phosphate buffered saline (PBS). The degree of joint damage was also found to be greater in mice injected with recombinant IL-23 (Fig.3). Using *ex-vivo* bone slide culture models, IL-23 production has been found to increase in response to IL-1β, TNFα and LPS. Astonishingly, osteoblasts also seems to contribute to IL-23 production (*See section 4*). IL-23 is a crucial cytokine in the Th17 response of inflammatory disorders, including RA joint inflammation. Th17 differentiates from $CD4^+$ T cells in response to IL-1β, IL-6 and IL-23 combinational signaling. It is distinct from Th1 and Th2 cells. Investigations into the outcome of IL-23 and Th17 targeted therapies holds potential for novel therapies against RA.

3.2 IL-27 is dual-functional in joint inflammation

IL-27 (consisting of an EBi3 subunit and p28 subunit) was initially identified as a Th1 driving cytokine (Pflanzet al., 2002). IL-27 binds to gp130 which is a common cytokine receptor used by many cytokines as well as growth factors [e.g. IL-6, Granulocyte Macrophage Colony Stimulation Factor (GM-CSF) and leukemia inhibition factor (LIF) etc] (Pflanz et al., 2004; Sims and Walsh, 2010). The dominant feature of IL-27 is its use of its own receptor (WSX-1) for cell signal transduction (Pflanz et al., 2004; Takeda et al., 2003). This allows it to function both as a promoter and suppressor of joint inflammation (Crabe et al., 2009; Wong et al., 2010). IL-27 promotes development of pathology by stimulating fibroblast like synoviocytes (FLS) for IL-6, chemokines and MMPs expression (Wonget al., 2010). However it also suppresses joint inflammation by promoting Th1 cell responses and suppressing Th17 cell responses (Pickens et al., 2011). Because IL-17 production by Th17 cells induces inflammation through recruitment of neutrophils and macrophages (Ifergan et al., 2008; Xie, Jin and Yu, 2007), suppressing Th17 cell responses therefore results in protection against inflammation (Niedbala et al, 2008).

The effect of IL-27 on joint inflammation differs depending on the animal model. IL-27 expression was detected in the spleen and inflamed joints of proteoglycan-induced arthritis (PGIA) mice(Cao et al., 2008). IL-27R gene knockout mice showed more resistance to PGIA than wild-type control mice. This result indicates that IL-27 plays a role in promoting joint inflammation in mice (Caoet al., 2008). However, injection of IL-27 into onset collage-induced arthritis (CIA) mice suppressed joint inflammation. This reduction in inflammation was associated with a decrease in IL-6 and IL-17 production, and an increased in IL-10 production (Niedbala et al., 2008). IL-27 local expression by injection of adenovirus carrying IL-27 gene expression resulted in reduction of joint inflammation and bone erosion in CIA mice. This effect was associated with lower serum and joint levels of IL-17 (Pickens et al., 2011). The discrepancy in the effect of IL-27 on these two different mouse models likely indicates differing disease mechanisms in these models. It is possible that the PGIA model induces joint inflammation via stimulation of synoviocytes whilst the CIA model provokes joint inflammation through initiation of T cells.

A high concentration of IL-27 is found in the synovial fluid of RA patients and has a strong positive association with levels of IFNγ (a key cytokine produced by Th1) (Tanida et al., 2011). A negative association with IL-17 from Th17 cytokines can therefore be deduced. It would appear that IL-27 stimulates Th1 to suppress Th17 thereby prevents joint inflammation and bone/cartilage destruction (Tanida et al., 2011).

Fibroblast like synoviocyte (FLS) is a major player in generating joint inflammation in RA (Cooles and Isaacs, 2011). IL-27 receptors (gp130 and WSX-1) are expressed on FLS and render it capable of responding to IL-27 stimulation. Such stimulation leads to cell adhering molecule (ICAM-1 and VCAM-1) expression and chemokine (CXCL9 and CXCL10) production. The IL-27 response produced by FLS is synergistic with IL-1β and TNFα, both being key cytokines in RA pathology (Wong et al., 2010). Given the dual-action properties of IL-27, however, its potential in therapeutic use against RA is unappealing.

3.3 IL-35 has great potential in therapeutic treatment of RA

Unlike IL-27, IL-35 has great pharmaceutical potential in the treatment of RA. It is a novel cytokine consisting of an EBi3 subunit and IL-12p35 subunit. These two proteins are highly expressed in the placental trophoblast and exert an immune suppressing role during pregnancy to avoid foetal rejection (Devergne et al., 2001). Transfection of cells with EBi3 and p35 expressing vectors resulted in the secretion of a heterodimeric EBi3/p35 protein (Devergne, Birkenbach and Kieff, 1997). A recombinant EBi3-p35-Fc fusion protein has been constructed. When this purified protein was injected into onset CIA mice recently, joint inflammation was significantly suppressed. This response was strongly associated with an increase in IFNγ and IL-10 production, and a reduction in IL-17 production (Niedbala et al., 2007). Recombinant IL-35 also expands regulatory T cell (Treg) *in vitro*. The expanded Treg cells maintain the ability to suppress T effector cells for cell proliferation (Niedbala et al., 2007). IL-35 effectively inhibited IL-23 induced IL-17 production by Th17 cells *in vitro*. When compared to TNFα inhibitors, IL-35 showed greater efficacy in prevent the onset of joint inflammation in CIA model (Kochetkova et al., 2010; Niedbala et al., 2007). Both EBi3 and p35 are expressed in iTreg and contributes to its immune regulation functions (Collison et al., 2007). Treg cells from EBi3 and p35 gene knockout mice partially lost its immune suppression function in inflammatory bowel disease mice (Collison et al., 2007). Recent research found that IL-35 is able to induce a Foxp3⁻inducible regulatory T cell [iTr(35)] *in vitro*. This new type of iTr(35) plays a role immune tolerance (Collison et al., 2010). Unlike mice, human nature Treg (nTreg) cells do not constitutively express IL-35 (Bardel et al., 2008). However, IL-35 expressing Treg cells are induced by rhinovirus activated DCs independently of Foxp3 expression (Seyerl et al., 2010). EBi3 and p35 are both expressed in human Treg cells and are the molecules required for contact-independent T cell suppression (Chaturvedi et al., 2011). Research into IL-35 has demonstrated its role in immune suppression. Its potential in the therapeutic treatment of RA remains to be tested. Studies so far have mainly focused on IL-35 producing T cells (Ning-Wei, 2010; Wei et al., 2011). IL-35 can be produced by a variety of cell types, such as stromal cells, macrophages and DCs. Further research using these cells may yield great insight into the actions of IL-35.

All members of the IL-12 family of cytokines can be expressed by DCs, with the type of cytokine produced dependent on the stimulus (Maroof and Kaye, 2008; van Seventer, Nagai and van Seventer, 2002). DCs are professional antigen presenting cells that drive $CD4^+$ T cell differentiation into Th1, Th2, Th17 and Treg cells with the aid of the IL-12 family of cytokines (Collison et al., 2010; Xu et al., 2010). The interplay between expression levels and competition coupling of the IL-12 family of cytokines is complex. Alteration of this intricate system to promote or resolve joint inflammation in RA may prove to be tedious and tricky. Nonetheless, therapies that either up-regulate IL-35 production or down-regulate IL-23 should remain at the forefront of research into the treatment of RA.

4. Inflammation induced bone and cartilage destruction in RA

4.1 Breaking the balance of osteoblast/osteoclast in joint inflammation

4.1.1 Osteoclastogenesis in rheumatoid arthritis

In health, the homeostasis between osteoclasts and osteoblasts results in constant renewal of bone. Osteoclasts remove old bone matter whilst osteoblasts produce new bone. This homeostasis is maintained and controlled by a number of factors. Osteoblasts respond to changes in hormone levels, calcium concentration and interact with bone matrix protein degradation and growth factors as well as cytokines (Clarke and Khosla, 2010; Gurlek and Kumar, 2001; Izu et al., 2011). Osteoblasts produce cell membrane and soluble factors in order to direct osteoclast differentiation and maturation. The essential factors produced by osteoblasts are macrophage colony stimulatory factor (M-CSF) and receptor-activator of nuclear factor kappa-B ligand (RANKL) (Gori et al., 2000). M-CSF drives a myeloid cell linage precursor into macrophages and stimulates expression of RANK, a receptor for RANKL (Granchi et al., 2005). Further activation of macrophages by RANK mediated cell signal, on the bone surface, result in the formation of multinuclear giant cell as a result of macrophage fusion (Hofbauer et al., 2000). Fully matured osteoclasts are multinuclear tartrate resistant acitic phosphotase (TRAP) positive and express cathepsin K (Ishikawa et al., 2001). *In vitro* culturing of bone marrow macrophage or peripheral blood monocytes with M-CSF and soluble RANKL results in full maturation of osteoclasts with bone erosion properties (Chen et al., 2008; Granchi et al., 2005). In addition to the production of M-CSF and RANKL, osteoblasts also produce osteoprotegerin (OPG) that acts as a decoy receptor for RANKL. This protein suppresses osteoclast formation by blocking RANKL activity (Granchi et al., 2005). Reduction of OPG expression by osteoblasts allows up-regulation of osteoclast formation. It is the balance between RANKL and OPG expression that regulates osteoclastogenesis (Fig. 3).

In RA joints, RANKL is also produced by infiltrative T cells and FLS (Fig.4) (Dai, Nishioka and Yudoh, 2004; Okamoto and Takayanagi, 2011a; Takayanagi, 2009). RANKL production is stimulated by cytokines present in synovial fluid (Dai, Nishioka and Yudoh, 2004). RANKL is an essential factor in inflammation-induced bone erosion. Mice deficient in the RANKL gene are resistant to bone erosion in all antibody induced arthritis models (Pettit et al., 2001). Higher quantities of osteoclasts exist in the joint of RA and arthritis mouse models (Gravallese et al., 1998; Suzuki et al., 1998). Using histological staining of joint tissue, fully matured osteoclasts with multinuclear expression of TRAP and cathepsin K can be found at the pannus-bone interface and subchondral site (Gravalleseet al., 1998). Elevated soluble RANKL (sRANKL) are present in the synovial fluid of RA patients (Hein et al., 2008). FLS produces sRANKL in response to number of cytokine stimulation (Kim et al., 2007). Synovial T cells also produce sRANKL, however the specific subset of T cell responsible for this has not yet been identified. Cytokines produced by FLS and macrophages further stimulate sRANKL production by synovial T cells (Gracie et al., 1999). *In vitro* IL-18 is able to stimulate sRANKL production in isolated synovial T cells from a RA joint (Dai, Nishioka and Yudoh, 2004).

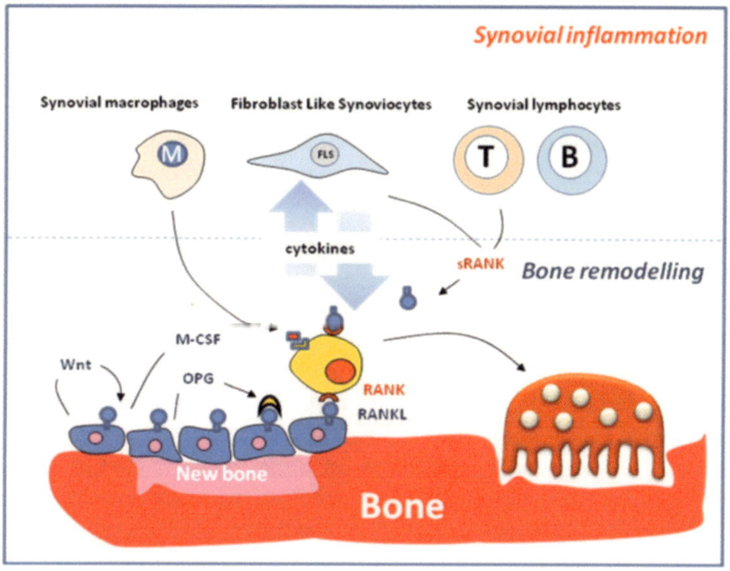

Fig. 4. Schematic diagram showing the influence of cytokines on bone remodeling in synovial joint inflammation. Synovial macrophages, fibroblast like synoviocytes, T and B cells are the main cytokine producing cells involved in RA joint inflammation. The cytokines produced by these inflammatory cells influence osteoblast and osteoclast differentiation and function. Osteoblasts produce M-CSF, RANKL and OPG in order to control TRAP$^+$ multinuclear osteoclast formation. Osteoblast maturation and function is control by autocrine / paracrine Wnt signaling.

4.1.2 Osteoblast maturation in RA

Synergistic to enhanced osteoclastogenesis in RA joints, a reduction in osteoblast activity was observed in animal models and RA patients (Cejka et al., ;Walsh et al., 2009b). Roughly 10% of RA patients on DARMs, an anti-inflammatory therapy, showed evidenced of bone regeneration (Ideguchi et al., 2006). Bone re-absorption provides strong stimulation for bone production by osteoblasts in inflamed joints (Davis et al., 2010). In RA, this response is significantly dampened in areas of inflammation when compared with healthy areas bone (Walsh and Gravallese, 2010). This indicates that cell signaling for osteoblast maturation is suppressed in inflammatory sites (Walsh et al., 2009). In healthy bone, osteoblast precursor expresses Runx2 and leads to full maturation of non-proliferative osteoblasts with expression of alkaline phosphatase, collagens and mineralization cell matrix proteins - such as osteocalcin, osteopontin and bone salioprotein (Komori, 2010).

The canonical Wingless (Wnt) signal is vital in the control of osteoblast maturation (Tamura et al., 2010). Wnt proteins are a group of secreted glycoproteins. Bone Morphogenic Proteins (BMPs) stimulate immature osteoblasts to produce Wnt proteins (Sethi and Kang, 2011). Wnt protein receptors have been identified as Frizzlrd (FZD) and low density lipoprotein receptor-related protein 5 and 6 (LRP5/6) (Takahashi et al., 2011). Osteoblasts produce endogenous inhibitors, such Dickkopf1 (DKK1), to competitively bind to LRP5 and LRP6 (Walsh et al., 2009). TNFα stimulates DKK1 production and therefore suppresses osteoblast development (Diarra et al., 2007). Levels of DKK1 are raised in both arthritis mouse models and human RA synovial fluid (Diarraet al., 2007). In arthritis animal models, blockade of DKK1 *in vivo* results in enhanced bone formation (Diarraet al., 2007). Recent clinical research into the effects of B cell depletion using Rituximab (anti-B cell antibody) on suppression of inflammation in RA patients yielded interesting results. It showed that treatment with Rituximab resulted in a reduction of bone re-absorption as well as a marked increase in bone formation (Wheater et al., 2011). These findings contribute greatly to the new and fast developing field of osteoimmunology (study of bone remodeling in inflammation). The role of the IL-12 family cytokines in regulating bone turnover is currently unclear. So far, the majority of research in this field has focused on osteoclastogenesis. In order to understand osteoblast maturation in the inflammatory environment, a greater understanding of the mechanisms behind inflammation induced joint destruction must be achieved.

4.2 Role of IL-12 family cytokine in regulation of inflammatory bone erosion

In RA, two key biological processes contribute to joint destruction - synovial inflammation and altered bone remodelling. Synovial inflammation results from infiltration by large numbers inflammatory cells, such as neutrophils, macrophages and T cells. These cells produce proteinases to degrade cell matrix proteins in both cartilage and bone. More importantly, they produce large numbers of cytokines that influence bone remodelling via effects on osteoclast and osteoblast activities. Osteoblasts and its precursors also produce cytokines in response to this stimulation (Cornish et al., 2003). The IL-12 family cytokines stimulate T cell responses that subsequently act on osteoclast/osteoblast precursors to promote or suppress cell differentiation (Kamiya et al., 2011). Certain members of the IL-12 family cytokines can also act on osteoclast precursors directly (Chen et al., 2008).

4.2.1 IL-12 inhibits osteoclastogenesis *in vitro* and *in vivo*.

The majority of research into the effect of IL-12 on osteoclastogenesis has been studied in *in vitro* cell culture models. Bone marrow macrophages or splenic cells have the ability to differentiate into fully matured $TRAP^+$ multinuclear functional osteoclasts in a culture with M-CSF and sRANKL (Chen et al., 2008). In earlier studies, IL-12 synergised with IL-18 to inhibit osteoclast formation (Yamada et al., 2002). Given that GM-CSF stimulation of bone marrow cells and splenic cells results in its differentiation into DCs, inhibition of osteoclastogenesis can be explained by GM-CSF production stimulated by IL-12 and IL-18 (Horwood et al., 2001). Bone marrow cells differentiate into macrophage 1 (M1) in response to GM-CSF and macrophage 2 (M2) in response to M-CSF (Krausgruber et al., 2011). M2 expresses higher RANK and is capable of osteoclast formation in response to RANKL. M1 and M2 are phenotypically plastic. Functional M2 cells can convert into M1 cells in a culture medium containing GM-CSF (Krausgruber et al., 2011). The reverse is also true. It can therefore be theorised that, in inflammatory joints, osteoclasts responsible for bone erosion cannot form if levels of GM-CSF and M1 cells exist. Osteoclastogenesis could occur as a result of M2 migration into inflamed joints during the inflammation resolution stage of joint disease. TNFα can also induce osteoclastogenesis *in vivo* (Kitaura et al., 2006). Injection of IL-12 and TNFα results in reduced osteoclast formation and lower serum TRAP levels. This demonstrates that IL-12 inhibits TNFα stimulation of osteoclasts (Yoshimatsu et al., 2009).

4.2.2 IL-23 promotes bone erosion via direct and indirect mechanisms

IL-23 promotes osteoclast formation indirectly via IL-17/Th17. IL-23 is an essential cytokine in the production and maintenance of Th17 cells. IL-17 induces RANKL production in both osteoblasts and FLS (Okamoto and Takayanagi, 2011b;Yago et al., 2007). IL-17 also stimulates osteoclast precursor cells to up-regulate RANK expression and subsequently promote osteoclast formation in the presence of RANKL. Recent experiments have suggested a more direct effect of IL-23 on osteoclastogenesis. In our laboratory, we have shown IL-23 to drive osteoclast formation independent of IL-17 production in culture. IL-23 induces RANK expression in osteoclast precursor cells thereby sensitising the cells to RANKL stimulation and resulting in osteoclast development (Chen et al., 2008). Further support arose from experiments investigating osteoclastogenesis using bone marrow cells from IL-23p19 knockout mice. The direct osteoclastogenic effect of IL-23 was evidenced by greatly reduced osteoclast formation in IL-23p19 gene deficient mice (Li et al., 2010). Experiments using FLS from RA patients found that IL-23 stimulated RANKL expression with subsequent up-regulation of osteoclastogenesis and bone erosion (Li et al., 2010). IL-23 has also been suggested to stimulate GM-CSF production by T cells thereby inhibiting osteoclastogenesis (Quinn et al., 2008). The contradictory roles of IL-23 in bone loss secondary to inflammation are perplexing and in desperate need of further research. Interestingly, IL-23p19 knockout mice have lower bone mass (Quinn et al., 2008). This suggested that, in health, IL-23 aids the function of osteoblasts in bone formation . In our laboratory, osteoblasts have been found to induce IL-23p19 expression (unpublished data). In terms of bone remodelling in RA, these results suggest that IL-23 play multiple roles. Not only does it contribute to the functioning of osteoblasts but it also acts as a signal for communication between osteoblasts and osteoclasts.

4.2.3 IL-27 protects joint from inflammatory bone erosion

IL-27 has a dual-effect in the regulation of joint inflammation. In RA, IL-27 proteins can be detected in both serum and synovial fluid (Tanida et al., 2011). In synovial fluid, $CD14^+$ mono-nuclear cells (MNC), not FLS, contribute to IL-27 production (Tanida et al., 2011). The effects of IL-27 on osteoclast formation are either direct (on osteoclast precursors) or indirect (via T cells). IL-27 acts on osteoclast precursor cells to down regulate RANK expression and suppress RANKL induced cell signalling (Kalliolias et al., 2010). IL-27 inhibits oseteoclastogensesis through blockade of M-CSF cell signalling via STAT1 dependent mechanisms (Furukawa et al., 2009). $CD4^+$ T cells produce cell surface and soluble RANKL to promote osteoclast formation in joint inflammation (Kamiya et al., 2011). IL-27 suppresses both cell surface and soluble RANKL expressions in $CD4^+$ T cells through suppression of the STAT3 dependent mechanism, rather than STAT1 (Kamiyaet al., 2011). These results suggest that IL-27 suppress osteoclastogenesis indirectly, via T cells.

IL-27 also acts on osteoblast cells. Osteoblasts express both receptor chains (gp130 and WSX-1) for IL-27 signalling (Sims and Walsh, 2010). Cultures of human osteoblast cells in a medium containing IL-27 for 14 days showed increased production of osteoblast terminal markers, alkaline phosphatase and bone nodules (Cocco et al., 2010). Results published by a number of independent studies have shown IL-27 to protect the joint from damage in inflammatory joint disease of CIA mice (Niedbala et al., 2008).

The role of IL-35 in inflammatory bone loss is poorly understood and is yet to be studied. IL-35 is capable of suppressing IL-17 production by Th17 cells (Niedbala et al., 2007; Wei et al., 2011). Both IL-27 and IL-35 appear to play salient roles in the protection against joint damage in RA. IL-35 has strong therapeutic potential in the treatment of arthritis in CIA mouse models. In order to further this potential, urgent attention on studies investigating the biological functions of IL-35 in the control of RA bone loss must be paid.

Cytokines	$CD4^+$ T cell	Effects on Joint inflammation	Osteoclast formation	Osteoblast maturation
IL-12	Th1	Promote	Suppress	?
IL-23	Th17	Promote	Promote	?
IL-27	Th1	Promote or Suppress	Suppress	?
IL-35	Treg	Suppress	?	?

Table 1. Summary the effects of IL-12 family cytokines in joint inflammation and bone remodelling of rheumatoid arthritis.

5. Conclusion

The changes in synovial joints with RA begin with inflammatory cell migration. T cell activation results in chronic inflammation and extra cellular matrix protein production by fibroblast-like synoviocytes. Macrophages transform into bone resorptive osteoclast cells and erode both joint cartilage and bone. In response to this, osteoblast cells mature and produce bone matrix. This leads to healing of joint destruction. IL-12 family cytokines can influence the responses produced by T cells and fibroblast like synoviocytes, and thus influence bone remodelling within inflamed joints. IL-12 family cytokines also bind to osteoblast and osteoclast precursors to either promote or suppress bone formation and erosion. Although IL-12 family cytokines have protein homology, with certain members sharing the same protein subunits, its functions in T cell induced inflammation and bone loss remain distinctly different (Table 1). Unlike IL-35, which suppresses the inflammatory joint response in RA, IL-12, IL-23 and IL-27 promote it. The mechanisms of action behind some of these cytokines are known whilst others are waiting to be uncovered. IL-12 drives a Th1 response whereas IL-23 promotes a Th17 response. These T cell responses lead to chronic joint inflammation. IL-12 is also a potent inducer of IFNγ production. The immune suppression role of IFNγ in osteoclastogenesis deems IL-12 to have a protective role against joint destruction caused by RA. On the other hand, IL-23 promotes joint inflammation and osteoclastogensis thereby causing bone erosion. IL-27 stimulates fibroblast like synoviocytes to produce a number of inflammatory factors that trigger joint inflammation. IL-27 also suppresses Th17 and therefore prevents bone loss in RA. The discovery of IL-35 in recent years has spawned a new area of research. This novel cytokine suppresses T cell activation and has impressive therapeutic potential against joint inflammation in RA. Its role against bone loss is unknown and requires further investigation. The role of IL-12 family cytokines in the regulation of osteoblast functions is another area in need of research. Bone erosion and joint destruction are debilitating and irreversible consequences of RA. Further exploration of IL-12 family cytokines (in particular IL-35) and their role in osteoclastogenesis needs to be undertaken without delay. Only then will the therapeutic potential of IL-35 be ready and safe to test in humans. With new therapies against RA, and potentially other autoimmune disorders, the future looks bright in this field of research.

6. References

Aerts, N. E., Ebo, D. G., Bridts, C. H., Stevens, W. J., and De Clerck, L. S. (2010). *Clinical and experimental rheumatology* 28, 208.

Airoldi, I., Di Carlo, E., Cocco, C., Sorrentino, C., Fais, F., Cilli, M., D'Antuono, T., Colombo, M. P., and Pistoia, V. (2005). *Blood* 106, 3846.

Bardel, E., Larousserie, F., Charlot-Rabiega, P., Coulomb-L'Hermine, A., and Devergne, O. (2008). *Journal of immunology* 181, 6898.

Boissier, M. C., Chiocchia, G., Bessis, N., Hajnal, J., Garotta, G., Nicoletti, F., and Fournier, C. (1995). *European journal of immunology* 25, 1184.

Cao, Y., Doodes, P. D., Glant, T. T., and Finnegan, A. (2008). *Journal of immunology* 180, 922.

Cejka, D., Hayer, S., Niederreiter, B., Sieghart, W., Fuereder, T., Zwerina, J., and Schett, G. *Arthritis Rheum* 62, 2294.

Chaturvedi, V., Collison, L. W., Guy, C. S., Workman, C. J., and Vignali, D. A. (2011). *Journal of immunology* 186, 6661.

Chen, L., Wei, X. Q., Evans, B., Jiang, W., and Aeschlimann, D. (2008). *European journal of immunology* 38, 2845.

Clarke, B. L., and Khosla, S. (2010). *Arch Biochem Biophys* 503, 118.

Cocco, C., Giuliani, N., Di Carlo, E., Ognio, E., Storti, P., Abeltino, M., Sorrentino, C., Ponzoni, M., Ribatti, D., and Airoldi, I. (2010). *Clinical cancer research : an official journal of the American Association for Cancer Research* 16, 4188.

Collison, L. W., Chaturvedi, V., Henderson, A. L., Giacomin, P. R., Guy, C., Bankoti, J., Finkelstein, D., Forbes, K., Workman, C. J., Brown, S. A., Rehg, J. E., Jones, M. L., Ni, H. T., Artis, D., Turk, M. J., and Vignali, D. A. (2010). *Nature immunology* 11, 1093.

Collison, L. W., Workman, C. J., Kuo, T. T., Boyd, K., Wang, Y., Vignali, K. M., Cross, R., Sehy, D., Blumberg, R. S., and Vignali, D. A. (2007). *Nature* 450, 566.

Cooles, F. A., and Isaacs, J. D. (2011). *Current opinion in rheumatology* 23, 233.

Cornish, J., Gillespie, M. T., Callon, K. E., Horwood, N. J., Moseley, J. M., and Reid, I. R. (2003). *Endocrinology* 144, 1194.

Crabe, S., Guay-Giroux, A., Tormo, A. J., Duluc, D., Lissilaa, R., Guilhot, F., Mavoungou-Bigouagou, U., Lefouili, F., Cognet, I., Ferlin, W., Elson, G., Jeannin, P., and Gauchat, J. F. (2009). *Journal of immunology* 183, 7692.

Dai, S. M., Nishioka, K., and Yudoh, K. (2004). *Ann Rheum Dis* 63, 1379.

Davis, J., Tucci, M., Russell, G., and Benghuzzi, H. (2010). *Biomed Sci Instrum* 46, 63.

Devergne, O., Birkenbach, M., and Kieff, E. (1997). *Proceedings of the National Academy of Sciences of the United States of America* 94, 12041.

Devergne, O., Coulomb-L'Hermine, A., Capel, F., Moussa, M., and Capron, F. (2001). *The American journal of pathology* 159, 1763.

Devergne, O., Hummel, M., Koeppen, H., Le Beau, M. M., Nathanson, E. C., Kieff, E., and Birkenbach, M. (1996). *Journal of virology* 70, 1143.

Diarra, D., Stolina, M., Polzer, K., Zwerina, J., Ominsky, M. S., Dwyer, D., Korb, A., Smolen, J., Hoffmann, M., Scheinecker, C., van der Heide, D., Landewe, R., Lacey, D., Richards, W. G., and Schett, G. (2007). *Nature medicine* 13, 156.

Ebrahimi, A. A., Noshad, H., Sadreddini, S., Hejazi, M. S., Mohammadzadeh Sadigh, Y., Eshraghi, Y., and Ghojazadeh, M. (2009). *Iranian journal of immunology : IJI* 6, 147.

Furukawa, M., Takaishi, H., Takito, J., Yoda, M., Sakai, S., Hikata, T., Hakozaki, A., Uchikawa, S., Matsumoto, M., Chiba, K., Kimura, T., Okada, Y., Matsuo, K., Yoshida, H., and Toyama, Y. (2009). *Journal of immunology* 183, 2397.

Gori, F., Hofbauer, L. C., Dunstan, C. R., Spelsberg, T. C., Khosla, S., and Riggs, B. L. (2000). *Endocrinology* 141, 4768.

Gracie, J. A., Forsey, R. J., Chan, W. L., Gilmour, A., Leung, B. P., Greer, M. R., Kennedy, K., Carter, R., Wei, X. Q., Xu, D., Field, M., Foulis, A., Liew, F. Y., and McInnes, I. B. (1999). *J Clin Invest* 104, 1393.

Gran, B., Zhang, G. X., Yu, S., Li, J., Chen, X. H., Ventura, E. S., Kamoun, M., and Rostami, A. (2002). *Journal of immunology* 169, 7104.

Granchi, D., Amato, I., Battistelli, L., Ciapetti, G., Pagani, S., Avnet, S., Baldini, N., and Giunti, A. (2005). *Biomaterials* 26, 2371.

Gravallese, E. M., Harada, Y., Wang, J. T., Gorn, A. H., Thornhill, T. S., and Goldring, S. R. (1998). *The American journal of pathology* 152, 943.

Gurlek, A., and Kumar, R. (2001). *Crit Rev Eukaryot Gene Expr* 11, 299.

Hein, G. E., Meister, M., Oelzner, P., and Franke, S. (2008). *Rheumatology international* 28, 765.

Herman, S., Zurgil, N., Machlav, S., Shinberg, A., Langevitz, P., Ehrenfeld, M., and Deutsch, M. (2011). *Clinical and vaccine immunology : CVI.*

Hoeve, M. A., Savage, N. D., de Boer, T., Langenberg, D. M., de Waal Malefyt, R., Ottenhoff, T. H., and Verreck, F. A. (2006). *European journal of immunology* 36, 661.

Hofbauer, L. C., Khosla, S., Dunstan, C. R., Lacey, D. L., Boyle, W. J., and Riggs, B. L. (2000). *J Bone Miner Res* 15, 2.

Horai, R., Saijo, S., Tanioka, H., Nakae, S., Sudo, K., Okahara, A., Ikuse, T., Asano, M., and Iwakura, Y. (2000). *The Journal of experimental medicine* 191, 313.

Horwood, N. J., Elliott, J., Martin, T. J., and Gillespie, M. T. (2001). *Journal of immunology* 166, 4915.

Hsieh, C. S., Macatonia, S. E., Tripp, C. S., Wolf, S. F., O'Garra, A., and Murphy, K. M. (1993). *Science* 260, 547.

Ideguchi, H., Ohno, S., Hattori, H., Senuma, A., and Ishigatsubo, Y. (2006). *Arthritis research & therapy* 8, R76.

Ifergan, I., Kebir, H., Bernard, M., Wosik, K., Dodelet-Devillers, A., Cayrol, R., Arbour, N., and Prat, A. (2008). *Brain : a journal of neurology* 131, 785.

Ishikawa, T., Kamiyama, M., Tani-Ishii, N., Suzuki, H., Ichikawa, Y., Hamaguchi, Y., Momiyama, N., and Shimada, H. (2001). *Mol Carcinog* 32, 84.

Izu, Y., Sun, M., Zwolanek, D., Veit, G., Williams, V., Cha, B., Jepsen, K. J., Koch, M., and Birk, D. E. (2011). *J Cell Biol* 193, 1115.

Joosten, L. A., Radstake, T. R., Lubberts, E., van den Bersselaar, L. A., van Riel, P. L., van Lent, P. L., Barrera, P., and van den Berg, W. B. (2003). *Arthritis and rheumatism* 48, 339.

Kalliolias, G. D., Zhao, B., Triantafyllopoulou, A., Park-Min, K. H., and Ivashkiv, L. B. (2010). *Arthritis and rheumatism* 62, 402.

Kamiya, S., Okumura, M., Chiba, Y., Fukawa, T., Nakamura, C., Nimura, N., Mizuguchi, J., Wada, S., and Yoshimoto, T. (2011). *Immunology letters.*

Kang, J. W., Choi, S. C., Cho, M. C., Kim, H. J., Kim, J. H., Lim, J. S., Kim, S. H., Han, J. Y., and Yoon, D. Y. (2009). *Immunology* 128, e532.

Kikawada, E., Lenda, D. M., and Kelley, V. R. (2003). *Journal of immunology* 170, 3915.

Kim, K. W., Cho, M. L., Lee, S. H., Oh, H. J., Kang, C. M., Ju, J. H., Min, S. Y., Cho, Y. G., Park, S. H., and Kim, H. Y. (2007). *Immunol Lett* 110, 54.

Kim, W., Min, S., Cho, M., Youn, J., Min, J., Lee, S., Park, S., Cho, C., and Kim, H. (2000). *Clin Exp Immunol* 119, 175.

Kitaura, H., Tatamiya, M., Nagata, N., Fujimura, Y., Eguchi, T., Yoshida, N., and Nakayama, K. (2006). *Immunol Lett* 107, 22.

Kochetkova, I., Golden, S., Holderness, K., Callis, G., and Pascual, D. W. (2010). *Journal of immunology* 184, 7144.

Komori, T. (2010). *Cell Tissue Res* 339, 189.

Krausgruber, T., Blazek, K., Smallie, T., Alzabin, S., Lockstone, H., Sahgal, N., Hussell, T., Feldmann, M., and Udalova, I. A. (2011). *Nat Immunol* 12, 231.

Leung, B. P., McInnes, I. B., Esfandiari, E., Wei, X. Q., and Liew, F. Y. (2000). *Journal of immunology* 164, 6495.

Li, X., Kim, K. W., Cho, M. L., Ju, J. H., Kang, C. M., Oh, H. J., Min, J. K., Lee, S. H., Park, S. H., and Kim, H. Y. (2010). *Immunol Lett* 127, 100.

Manoury-Schwartz, B., Chiocchia, G., Bessis, N., Abehsira-Amar, O., Batteux, F., Muller, S., Huang, S., Boissier, M. C., and Fournier, C. (1997). *Journal of immunology* 158, 5501.

Maroof, A., and Kaye, P. M. (2008). *Infection and immunity* 76, 239.

Melis, L., Vandooren, B., Kruithof, E., Jacques, P., De Vos, M., Mielants, H., Verbruggen, G., De Keyser, F., and Elewaut, D. (2010). *Annals of the rheumatic diseases* 69, 618.

Murphy, C. A., Langrish, C. L., Chen, Y., Blumenschein, W., McClanahan, T., Kastelein, R. A., Sedgwick, J. D., and Cua, D. J. (2003). *The Journal of experimental medicine* 198, 1951.

Murphy, E. E., Terres, G., Macatonia, S. E., Hsieh, C. S., Mattson, J., Lanier, L., Wysocka, M., Trinchieri, G., Murphy, K., and O'Garra, A. (1994). *J Exp Med* 180, 223.

Murugaiyan, G., Mittal, A., Lopez-Diego, R., Maier, L. M., Anderson, D. E., and Weiner, H. L. (2009). *J Immunol* 183, 2435.

Niedbala, W., Cai, B., Wei, X., Patakas, A., Leung, B. P., McInnes, I. B., and Liew, F. Y. (2008). *Annals of the rheumatic diseases* 67, 1474.

Niedbala, W., Wei, X. Q., Cai, B., Hueber, A. J., Leung, B. P., McInnes, I. B., and Liew, F. Y. (2007). *European journal of immunology* 37, 3021.

Ning-Wei, Z. (2010). *Revista medica de Chile* 138, 758.

Okamoto, K., and Takayanagi, H. (2011a). *International immunopharmacology* 11, 543.

Okamoto, K., and Takayanagi, H. (2011b). *Arthritis research & therapy* 13, 219.

Ooi, J. D., Phoon, R. K., Holdsworth, S. R., and Kitching, A. R. (2009). *Journal of the American Society of Nephrology : JASN* 20, 980.

Oppmann, B., Lesley, R., Blom, B., Timans, J. C., Xu, Y., Hunte, B., Vega, F., Yu, N., Wang, J., Singh, K., Zonin, F., Vaisberg, E., Churakova, T., Liu, M., Gorman, D., Wagner, J., Zurawski, S., Liu, Y., Abrams, J. S., Moore, K. W., Rennick, D., de Waal-Malefyt, R., Hannum, C., Bazan, J. F., and Kastelein, R. A. (2000). *Immunity* 13, 715.

Paradowska-Gorycka, A., Grzybowska-Kowalczyk, A., Wojtecka-Lukasik, E., and Maslinski, S. (2010). *Scandinavian journal of immunology* 71, 134.

Park, S. H., Min, D. J., Cho, M. L., Kim, W. U., Youn, J., Park, W., Cho, C. S., and Kim, H. Y. (2001). *Arthritis and rheumatism* 44, 561.

Pettit, A. R., Ji, H., von Stechow, D., Muller, R., Goldring, S. R., Choi, Y., Benoist, C., and Gravallese, E. M. (2001). *Am J Pathol* 159, 1689.

Pflanz, S., Hibbert, L., Mattson, J., Rosales, R., Vaisberg, E., Bazan, J. F., Phillips, J. H., McClanahan, T. K., de Waal Malefyt, R., and Kastelein, R. A. (2004). *Journal of immunology* 172, 2225.

Pflanz, S., Timans, J. C., Cheung, J., Rosales, R., Kanzler, H., Gilbert, J., Hibbert, L., Churakova, T., Travis, M., Vaisberg, E., Blumenschein, W. M., Mattson, J. D., Wagner, J. L., To, W., Zurawski, S., McClanahan, T. K., Gorman, D. M., Bazan, J. F., de Waal Malefyt, R., Rennick, D., and Kastelein, R. A. (2002). *Immunity* 16, 779.

Pickens, S. R., Chamberlain, N. D., Volin, M. V., Mandelin, A. M., 2nd, Agrawal, H., Matsui, M., Yoshimoto, T., and Shahrara, S. (2011). *Arthritis and rheumatism*.

Quinn, J. M., Sims, N. A., Saleh, H., Mirosa, D., Thompson, K., Bouralexis, S., Walker, E. C., Martin, T. J., and Gillespie, M. T. (2008). *Journal of immunology* 181, 5720.

Radovits, B. J., Fransen, J., Eijsbouts, A., van Riel, P. L., and Laan, R. F. (2009). *Rheumatology* 48, 906.

Raghavan, S., Cao, D., Widhe, M., Roth, K., Herrath, J., Engstrom, M., Roncador, G., Banham, A. H., Trollmo, C., Catrina, A. I., and Malmstrom, V. (2009). *Annals of the rheumatic diseases* 68, 1908.

Ruchatz, H., Leung, B. P., Wei, X. Q., McInnes, I. B., and Liew, F. Y. (1998). *Journal of immunology* 160, 5654.

Sabat, R., Grutz, G., Warszawska, K., Kirsch, S., Witte, E., Wolk, K., and Geginat, J. (2010). *Cytokine & growth factor reviews* 21, 331.

Salliot, C., Finckh, A., Katchamart, W., Lu, Y., Sun, Y., Bombardier, C., and Keystone, E. (2011). *Annals of the rheumatic diseases* 70, 266.

Santarlasci, V., Maggi, L., Capone, M., Frosali, F., Querci, V., De Palma, R., Liotta, F., Cosmi, L., Maggi, E., Romagnani, S., and Annunziato, F. (2009). *European journal of immunology* 39, 207.

Sethi, N., and Kang, Y. (2011). *Bone* 48, 16.

Seyerl, M., Kirchberger, S., Majdic, O., Seipelt, J., Jindra, C., Schrauf, C., and Stockl, J. (2010). *European journal of immunology* 40, 321.

Shibata, S., Tada, Y., Komine, M., Hattori, N., Osame, S., Kanda, N., Watanabe, S., Saeki, H., and Tamaki, K. (2009). *Journal of dermatological science* 53, 34.

Sims, N. A., and Walsh, N. C. (2010). *BMB reports* 43, 513.

Snir, O., Rieck, M., Gebe, J. A., Yue, B. B., Rawlings, C. A., Nepom, G., Malmstrom, V., and Buckner, J. H. *Arthritis Rheum.*

Sun, Z. J., Zhang, Y. J., Sun, T. Z., Xiong, A., Liu, R. B., and Lu, H. S. (2011). *Zhongguo gu shang = China journal of orthopaedics and traumatology* 24, 295.

Suzuki, Y., Nishikaku, F., Nakatuka, M., and Koga, Y. (1998). *The Journal of rheumatology* 25, 1154.

Takahashi, N., Maeda, K., Ishihara, A., Uehara, S., and Kobayashi, Y. (2011). *Front Biosci* 16, 21.

Takayanagi, H. (2009). *Nat Rev Rheumatol* 5, 667.

Takeda, A., Hamano, S., Yamanaka, A., Hanada, T., Ishibashi, T., Mak, T. W., Yoshimura, A., and Yoshida, H. (2003). *Journal of immunology* 170, 4886.

Tamura, M., Nemoto, E., Sato, M. M., Nakashima, A., and Shimauchi, H. (2010). *Front Biosci (Elite Ed)* 2, 1405.

Tanida, S., Yoshitomi, H., Ishikawa, M., Kasahara, T., Murata, K., Shibuya, H., Ito, H., and Nakamura, T. (2011). *Cytokine.*

van Lierop, M. J., den Hoed, L., Houbiers, J., Vencovsky, J., Ruzickova, S., Krystufkova, O., van Schaardenburg, M., van den Hoogen, F., Vandooren, B., Baeten, D., De Keyser, F., Sonderstrup, G., Bos, E., and Boots, A. M. (2007). *Arthritis and rheumatism* 56, 2150.

van Seventer, J. M., Nagai, T., and van Seventer, G. A. (2002). *Journal of neuroimmunology* 133, 60.

Walsh, N. C., and Gravallese, E. M. (2010). *Immunol Rev* 233, 301.

Walsh, N. C., Reinwald, S., Manning, C. A., Condon, K. W., Iwata, K., Burr, D. B., and Gravallese, E. M. (2009). *J Bone Miner Res* 24, 1572.

Wei, X. Q., Leung, B. P., Arthur, H. M., McInnes, I. B., and Liew, F. Y. (2001). *Journal of immunology* 166, 517.

Wei, X. Q., Rogers, H., Lewis, M. A. O., and Williams, D. W. (2011). *Clinical & developmental immunology.*

Wheater, G., Hogan, V. E., Teng, Y. K., Tekstra, J., Lafeber, F. P., Huizinga, T. W., Bijlsma, J. W., Francis, R. M., Tuck, S. P., Datta, H. K., and van Laar, J. M. (2011). *Osteoporosis international : a journal established as result of cooperation between the European Foundation for Osteoporosis and the National Osteoporosis Foundation of the USA.*

Wong, C. K., Chen da, P., Tam, L. S., Li, E. K., Yin, Y. B., and Lam, C. W. (2010). *Arthritis research & therapy* 12, R129.

Xie, Y. D., Jin, L., and Yu, Q. W. (2007). *Xi bao yu fen zi mian yi xue za zhi = Chinese journal of cellular and molecular immunology* 23, 536.

Xu, M., Mizoguchi, I., Morishima, N., Chiba, Y., Mizuguchi, J., and Yoshimoto, T. (2010). *Clin Dev Immunol* 2010.

Yago, T., Nanke, Y., Kawamoto, M., Furuya, T., Kobashigawa, T., Kamatani, N., and Kotake, S. (2007). *Arthritis Res Ther* 9, R96.

Yamada, N., Niwa, S., Tsujimura, T., Iwasaki, T., Sugihara, A., Futani, H., Hayashi, S., Okamura, H., Akedo, H., and Terada, N. (2002). *Bone* 30, 901.

Yoshida, K., Yang, G. X., Zhang, W., Tsuda, M., Tsuneyama, K., Moritoki, Y., Ansari, A. A., Okazaki, K., Lian, Z. X., Coppel, R. L., Mackay, I. R., and Gershwin, M. E. (2009). *Hepatology* 50, 1494.

Yoshimatsu, M., Kitaura, H., Fujimura, Y., Eguchi, T., Kohara, H., Morita, Y., and Yoshida, N. (2009). *Bone* 45, 1010.

Zelante, T., De Luca, A., Bonifazi, P., Montagnoli, C., Bozza, S., Moretti, S., Belladonna, M. L., Vacca, C., Conte, C., Mosci, P., Bistoni, F., Puccetti, P., Kastelein, R. A., Kopf, M., and Romani, L. (2007). *Eur J Immunol* 37, 2695.

4

The Role of Neutrophils in Rheumatoid Arthritis – Experiments *In Vitro*: A Change of Conception?

Michal Gajewski[1], Przemyslaw Rzodkiewicz[1,2] and Slawomir Maslinski[1,2]
[1]*Department of Biochemistry, Institute of Rheumatology, Warsaw,*
[2]*Department of General and Experimental Pathology, Warsaw Medical University, Warsaw, Poland*

1. Introduction

Essential cells of innate immunity, neutrophils are often considered to be a homogenous population of terminally differentiated cells (Chakravarti et al., 2009). These cells represent the body's primary line of defence against invading pathogens such as bacteria, and constitute 40-60% of the white blood cell population. Neutrophils are short-lived polymorphonuclear phagocytes. They are known as first-responding inflammatory cells migrating towards the site of inflammation (Chakravarti et al., 2009; Edwards et al., 1997).
In the circulation of healthy adults, neutrophils exist in a resting state, which ensures that their toxic intracellular contents are not accidentally released to damage host tissues. Neutrophils become activated by agents that include bacterial products and cytokines or chemokines, such as TNF-α, IL-8 or IFN-γ. The primed neutrophils are then mobilized to the site of infection or inflammation and encounter activating signals to trigger bacterial killing. (Wright et al., 2010; Cascao et al., 2009)
It must be noted, that the functions of resting blood neutrophils and primed neutrophils may be very different. Thus, many of the regulatory functions of macrophages are shared by primed (but not resting) neutrophils (Wright et al., 2010). For this reason, *in vitro* experiments using freshly isolated blood neutrophils often fail to recognize the full functional repertoire and capacity of neutrophils.

2. Oxidative metabolism of neutrophils

In a chronic inflammatory process, such as rheumatoid arthritis (RA), large numbers of neutrophils are attracted across the synovial membrane, and become activated. The number of neutrophils in synovial fluid (SF) of patients with RA can reach $5x10^{-9}$ (Edwards et al., 1997). Neutrophils possess a range of potent proteinases and hydrolases, and have the ability to generate a series of reactive oxygen intermediates (ROI) via the combined activities of NADPH (reduced form) oxidase and myeloperoxidase (MPO) (Robinson et al., 1992; Duluray et al., 1990; Nurcombe et al., 1991a). If the neutrophils are not efficiently depleted, their production of inflammatory mediators, such as ROI, could prolong the inflammatory reaction. In fact, inappropriate release of ROI from activated neutrophils is responsible for joint damage observed in RA (Edwards et al., 1997). Beside ROI and inflammatory mediators, neutrophils are also an important source of proteolytic enzymes which play a role in degradation of articular structures. Wojtecka-Lukasik et al. were the first to isolate collagenase from peripheral blood neutrophils to a degree which allowed determination of its physicochemical properties and assessment of its effects on the biological activity of some drugs used in treatment of rheumatic diseases (Wojtecka-Lukasik et al., 1974). In addition to the active enzyme, its latent form and activator were discovered and described in the rheumatoid joint fluids (Dancewicz et al., 1978).

Neutrophils are able to form extracellular structures, named neutrophils extracellular traps (NETs). NETs are composed by nuclear components, such as chromatin DNA (i.e. histones anchored to this molecular backbone), and cytoplasmic components, such as granular peptides and enzymes. Upon activation, the induction of activation of NADPH oxidase was reported, suggesting that formation of NETs is ROI-dependent (Cascao et al., 2009). Neutrophils die upon release of these structures. However, this is a form of cell death different from apoptosis and necrosis, named "NETosis" (Steinberg et al., 2007). NETs represent an unconventional form of immune response, because these structures remain active even after the neutrophil's death. The presence of nucleic acid can contribute to the development of autoimmune diseases, such as systemic lupus erythematosus (SLE) in which there is an exacerbated reaction against the host DNA (Wartha et al., 2007).

As was shown by Wenthworth (Wenthworth et al., 2002), antibodies catalyze the generation of hydrogen peroxide from singlet molecular oxygen and water. This process can lead to efficient killing of bacteria, regardless of the antigen specificity of the antibody. Hydrogen peroxide production by antibodies alone was found to be not sufficient for bacterial killing. Wenthworth et al. suggested that the antibody-catalyzed water-oxidation pathway produced an additional molecular species with a chemical signature similar to that of ozone. This species is also generated during the oxidative burst of activated human neutrophils and during inflammation. These observations suggest that alternative pathways may exist for biological killing of bacteria that are mediated by potent oxidants previously unknown to biology (Wentworth et al., 2002).

More recently (Yamashita et al., 2008), it was discovered that four amino acids themselves (tryptophan, methionine, cysteine and histidine) are able to catalyze the production of an oxidant with the chemical signature of ozone from singlet oxygen in the water-oxidation pathway. The resultant oxidant with the chemical signature of ozone exhibited significant bactericidal activity in human neutrophils. These results also suggest that an oxidant with the chemical signature of ozone produced by neutrophils might potentiate a host defence system, when the host is challenged by high doses of infectious agents. These findings provide biological insights into the killing of bacteria by neutrophils (Yamashita et al., 2008).

From a different point of view, it is believed that ROI function as second messengers (Hitchon & El-Gabalawy, 2004). Typically, second messengers are short-lived molecules that at the time of activation of a receptor, act specifically on effectors to alter their activity transiently. Indeed, ROI can be generated at the time of receptor activation and they are short-lived, as the other second-messengers (Fillipin et al., 2008). ROI produced by phagocytes are critical for protection against invading microorganisms but also seem to have important physiological roles in priming the immune system. It has been demonstrated that exposure to ROI down-regulate the activity of T lymphocytes: ROI produced by phagocytes also seem to have essential physiological roles in priming the immune system as second messengers (Jones, 2006). Hitchon and El-Gabalawy propose that the physiological production of ROI by phagocytes in response to an antigen affects T-cell antigen interactions and possibly induces apoptosis in autoreactive arthritogenic T cells, thereby preventing autoimmune responses (Hitchon & El-Gabalawy, 2004).

3. Oxidative metabolism and apoptosis of neutrophils cultured in physiological concentrations of SF, oxygen and cyclic loaded pressure

Although the presence of activated neutrophils in SF is well documented, it is still unknown how the neutrophils are activated, how they interact with other cells, and how long they persist at the site of inflammatory joint.

It was identified that addition of SF to neutrophils results in activation of neutrophils measured by a rapid chemiluminescence (CL) response (luminol- and lucigenin-dependent). Luminol-dependent CL is capable of monitoring both intracellular and extracellular ROI generation (NADPH oxidase and MPO), as luminol freely penetrates the neutrophil's cell membrane. Lucigenin-dependent CL, on the other hand, measures only the rate of extracellular ROI secretion (NADPH oxidase dependent) because lucigenin does not penetrate neutrophils, and light emission detected is independent of the activity of MPO. Pre-incubation of normal blood neutrophils in 10% SF enhanced the luminol- and lucigenin-CL, suggesting that both MPO and NADPH oxidase activity were activated in parallel during exposure to 10% SF from RA patients (Bender et al., 1986). Synovial fluid (20% concentration) isolated from RA patients activated blood neutrophils, leading to increase of luminol dependent CL over a 50 range (Nurcombe et al., 1991b). In contrast, the same fluid activated to a much lower range (two or three fold) of maximal rates of lucigenin dependent CL. All the mentioned reports were performed with SF in concentrations that did not exceed 20%. Other studies, confirmed that SF (used in concentration of 25%) produced rapid and parallel responses (luminol- and lucigenin-CL) in neutrophils.

Our recent results (Gajewski et al., 2009), in contrast to earlier studies, indicate that higher concentrations of SF (up to 80%) have a quite different effect on lucigenin-dependent and luminol-dependent CL response. Increased concentrations of SF resulted in a reduction of luminol-dependent CL response and a very significant increase of lucigenin-dependent CL, reflecting extracellular ROI generation. This effect was observed irrespective of the stimulator used and whether neutrophils were isolated from SF or blood from either RA patients or healthy subjects. This indicates that increasing SF concentration results in higher extracellular ROI secretion and lower MPO-dependent ROI production. The promotion of extracellular release of ROI observed in this experiment is likely to be associated with the high concentrations of SF used, and raises the possibility that extracellular activity of neutrophils may be a general characteristic which prolongs the inflammatory process (Gajewski et al., 2009).

Similar studies were performed by Bell et al. (1995). In these studies they examined the hypothesis that persistent inflammatory responses in RA may result from inhibition of neutrophils apoptosis by factors in SF. The effects of aging in culture and addition of SF on apoptosis was investigated using SF in a concentration range 0-75%. A significant effect of SF on promotion of apoptosis of synovial fluid neutrophils was observed at concentrations of 50% and above (Bell et al., 1995).

It has been proposed that the process of hypoxic reperfusion injury contributes to the persistence of synovitis in the inflamed joint. The generation of pathological, exercise induced intra-articular pressure leading to occlusion of the microcirculation is central to this mechanism (Hitchon & El-Gabalawy, 2004). Several observations show that neutrophils-mediated lysis of surrounding cells during ischemia-reperfusion is largely mediated by ROI (Smith et al., 1989). Superoxide dismutase (SOD) can significantly reduce cellular lysis and damage. Treatment with SOD prior the reperfusion reduces the concentration of the potentially injurious ROI. Similarly, administration of catalase decreases hydrogen peroxide concentration and reduces tissue damage during reperfusion (Smith et al., 1989). In the investigation of Nguyen (Nguyen et al., 2005) it was concluded that neutrophils play a significant role in injuring cell membranes reloading following periods of unloading, and that this membrane damage was mediated by MPO. A substantial, synergistic effect on the level of muscle lysis when both mechanical loading and neutrophils were applied to muscle cells *in vitro* was found. Loading alone caused only a 1.7% lysis of muscle cells, while co-culturing with neutrophils in the absence of loading resulted in only 3.5% lysis. However, loading in the presence of neutrophils resulted in 12.6% lysis of muscle cells under otherwise identical culture conditions in the presence of SOD (Nguyen et al., 2005). These observations provide a direct link between changes in mechanical loads applied to tissue, and an increase in damage that is induced by inflammatory cells. According to these results, pressure could be also considered as an important factor in *in vitro* experiments.

Another factor that is not often considered and influences neutrophils metabolism and survival is the concentration of molecular oxygen used to incubate the cell suspensions. Most *in vitro* experiments are performed in air or air mixtures of 21% O_2. Rarely, if ever, will such high concentration of oxygenation occur *in vivo*. For example, the O_2 tension within SF has been reported to be low as 1-2%. It was recently showed that local O_2 concentration affects neutrophils apoptosis. Only under hypoxic conditions, such as those typically found in RA joints, anti-apoptotic pathways are trigged. Neutrophils normally have a short life in the circulation (8-12h), whereas within SF with physiological oxygen concentration, neutrophils lifetime can be extended, increasing their potential to cause damage and promote inflammation (Cross et al., 2006).

The arguments that the prolonged lifespan of activated neutrophils in patients with RA may contribute to the progression of the inflammatory process to chronicity were supported by experiments in which neutrophils were exposured to SF (50%). In these conditions, in whole blood, neutrophils were stimulated with equal volume of SF and trans-differentiation of neutrophils into dendritic like cells was observed (Iking-Konert et al., 2005). It may be suggested that neutrophils from SF undergo major alterations, including trans-differentiation to cells with dendritic-like characteristics, probably induced by T cell derived cytokines. Exposure of SF, which contained considerable amounts of cytokines, induced a similar receptor pattern on blood derived neutrophils of healthy donors. This effect was also achieved by T cell supernatant alone (Iking-Konert et al., 2005).

Antigen-presenting dendritic cells provide the reducing extracellular microenvironment required for T lymphocyte activation. The mutual activation of neutrophils and T cells might contribute to perpetuation of the local inflammatory process, and eventually to the destructive process in RA (Angellini et al., 2002).

Actual findings confirm that extreme conditions within the joint have influence on neutrophils metabolism. Neutrophils in synovial tissues have different features than blood neutrophils. The proposal to use conditions, as close as possible to physiological conditions, is strongly recommended for *in vitro* experiments on neutrophils role in RA.

4. Immune cells – a new, diffusely expressed adrenergic and cholinergic organ? The neuromodulatory aspects of inflamed joint cavity: the importance of cholinergic system

One of the truly remarkable discoveries in modern biology is the finding that the nervous system and the immune system use a common language for intra- and inter-system communication (Blalock, 2005). This biochemical information circuit between neurons and immune cells allows the immune system to function as a sensory organ, and completes our ability to be cognizant not only of the world we can seen hear, taste, touch and smell, but also of bacteria, viruses, antigens or tumor cells. Recognition of such "non-cognitive stimuli" by the immune system results in transmission of information to the central nervous system to cause a physiological response that is ultimately beneficial to the host and detrimental to the infectious agent (Blalock, 2002, 2005).

The idea that immune cells were a source of neuropeptides was viewed by many as heretical; as is often the case when fundamental and unexpected discoveries are made (Blalock, 2005). Concurrent with early observation on production of neuropeptides by immune cells emerging studies reported that neuropeptide/neurotransmitter receptor were present on the same cells (Wybran et al., 1979).

It has been proposed that activity of neutrophils in RA may be influenced by neurotransmitters, including agonists of adrenergic and cholinergic receptors. This conclusion was based on the results of pharmacological studies that suggested the existence of several subtypes of functional adrenergic and cholinergic receptors of human neutrophils. An important modulatory mechanism in neutrophils is the interplay between stimulatory and inhibitory receptors. For example, activation of neutrophils is antagonized by agents that stimulate adenylate cyclase (AC). These agents include Β-adrenergic agonists, prostaglandins of the E series, adenosine and histamine. These effects appear to be mediated through adrenergic receptors, activating AC, which leads to an increase in cyclic AMP. Based on the hypothesis of the opposing actions of cAMP and cGMP, it was suggested that the agonists of cholinergic receptors might stimulate leukocyte activation (Gajewski et al., 1995).

The effect of the adrenergic receptors isoproterenol (ISO) and the cholinergic receptor carbachol on ROI production was measured by CL. Activation of neutrophils by OZ (stimulating phagocytosis), PMA (activation of NADPH oxidase) and fMLP (stimulation of chemotactic receptors) leads to elevation of the CL reponse (Gajewski et al., 1997).

The adrenergic receptor antagonist ISO has inhibitory effects on the CL of both peripheral blood neutrophils and SF neutrophils, preactivated by all three stimulators. The inhibitory effect was unchanged after addition of carbachol. Carbachol itself does not influence the CL of neutrophils isolated from either blood or SF, and preactivated by OZ, but PMA modulates the response of fMLP stimulated cells. It causes a significant increase of both luminol-and lucigenin CL expressed by peripheral blood neutrophils, whereas it reduces the response of SF neutrophils. For the first time, to our knowledge, we showed that the cholinergic agonist, carbachol, has been able to increase CL of peripheral human blood neutrophils. In contrast, the same treatment resulted in a decreased CL of neutrophils isolated from SF of patients with RA. These results support the hypothesis that neutrophils, upon cholinergic stimulation may affect the parasympathetic system - both its pro-inflammatory, and its anti-inflammatory activities. With the milieu of the cells determining the nature of the stimulation (Gajewski et al., 1997).

The observed opposite effects may suggest that different subtypes of muscarinic receptors are expressed on neutrophils presented in blood and synovial fluid, respectively. Because there are five distinct genes encoding muscarinic cholinergic receptors subtypes, we investigated the expression of mRNA encoding these receptors subtypes (i.e. m1-m5) in neutrophils isolated from healthy blood donors and patients with RA. Our results demonstrated for the first time the presence of m3, m4 and m5 muscarinic receptor subtypes in human blood neutrophils (Bany et al., 1999). The lack of mRNA for m4 muscarinic receptor subtype in neutrophils isolated from SF, may contribute to the opposite responses to cholinergic stimuli observed in neutrophils from blood and SF (Gajewski et al., 1997, Bany et al., 1999).

These findings were partially confirmed by Tracey (Tracey, 2002). The molecular dovetail between the cholinergic nervous system and the innate immune system is a nicotinic α-bungarotoxin-sensitive macrophage acetylcholine receptor. Exposure of human macrophages, but not peripheral blood monocytes, to nicotine or acetylcholine inhibits the release of TNF-α, IL-1 and IL-8 in response to endotoxin. Tissue macrophages, but not circulating monocytes, produce most of the TNF-α which appears systemically during an excessive inflammatory response. Interaction between the macrophage cholinergic receptor and its ligand inhibits the synthesis of pro-inflammatory cytokines (TNF-α, IL-1 and IL-18) but not anti-inflammatory cytokines (such as IL-10). Acetylcholine inhibits the expression of TNF-α protein in macrophages, but not the induction of TNF-α mRNA levels, indicating that activation of the cholinergic receptor transduces intracellular signals that inhibit cytokine synthesis at a post-transcriptional stage. As compared with macrophages, monocytes are refractory to the cytokine-inhibiting effects of acetylcholine: only supra-physiological concentrations of cholinergic agonist inhibit cytokine synthesis in monocytes (Tracey, 2002).

Further studies on the "reprogramming" of blood neutrophils (contradictory effects of adrenergic and cholinergic systems) into other cell types, SF neutrophils, (both systems inhibiting CL response) are expected to yield new insight into event related to RA therapy.

5. Long-lived dedifferentiated neutrophils

In the clinical setting it was observed, that neutrophils are present in high number in the synovial tissues during the initial stages of RA, and are described to persist in the SF during the course of this disease (Cascao et al., 2009). Patients in an active disease state may have in the SF cellular infiltrate up to 90% of neutrophils (Edwards et al., 1997).

Neutrophils that enter a joint are exposed to multiple factors such as cytokines and extreme physical conditions (low oxygen concentration, high pressure conditions). Recent achievements in neutrophil research indicate that certain inflammatory conditions induce a phenotyphic switch in circulating neutrophils toward a resident neutrophil with different functions (Chakravarti et al., 2009).

Neutrophils isolated from RA patients contain high levels of class II MHC RNA (Cross et al., 2003). It was identified that neutrophils isolated from SF express different types and numbers of surface receptors like CD49, CD80, CD83, CD86, HLA-DR, have increased cell surface ICAM-1 (Iking-Konert et al., 2005).

There are many differences in protein expression between SF and blood-derived neutrophils in RA patients. Neutrophils from RA SF have mobilized pre-formed molecules from intracellular stores to the cell surface and activated genes expression resulting from enhanced transcription and translation (Quayle et al., 1997). Consequently, several gene products, such as IL-8 and MMP-9, are up-regulated, allowing not only the up-regulation of cell function but also development of new cellular responses, such as antigen-presentation to T cell via activated MHCII expression (Cascao et al., 2009). Neutrophils isolated from the SF of RA patients expressing MHCII, CD80 and CD86 are able to stimulate T-cell proliferation (Wright et al., 2010). Indeed, the levels of expression of MHCII and co-stimulatory molecules on neutrophils from SF have been reported to be equivalent to or greater than the levels of expression on monocytes and B cells (Sandilands et al., 2005). Apart from their ability to stimulate T-cells in this way, it is also possible that neutrophils can expose cryptic epitopes, as they possess different proteases than other antigen-presenting cells. Thus, their function within SF could be different from that of other antigen-presenting cells (Wright et al., 2010).

Inflammatory reprogramming may increase neutrophil viability. As was shown, 8-17% neutrophils of the global neutrophil population have the potential to persist for more than 72 h under inflammatory conditions (Chakravarti et al., 2008). This is in contrast to the circulating neutrophils whose survival is measured in hours. The mechanism of this persistence remains unknown, but it seems that the protein kinases are largely implicated in survival of these long-lived neutrophils (Cronstein et al., 1992). The phospholipids metabolic pathway leading to leukotriene B4 (LTB4) synthesis also illustrates differences between these long-lived neutrophils and circulating neutrophils. As was shown, a significant amount of the 5-lipoxygenase (5-LO) is localized to the nuclear membrane in long-lived neutrophils, in basal conditions, a phenomenon absent in circulating neutrophils (Chakravarti et al., 2008).

As was mentioned, neutrophils exposure to SF (50%) induces transdifferentiation of neutrophils into dendritic like cells (Iking-Konert et al., 2005). When the neutrophils were cultured with TNF-α, IFN-γ and IL-4, the resultant cells had morphologic, cytochemical, and phenotypic features of macrophages. In contrast to the starting population, they were negative for myeloperoxidase, specific esterase and lactoferrin. It appears that, in response to the cytokines present in SF, postmitotic neutrophils can become macrophages (Araki et al., 2004).

Neutrophils are known to phagocytose invading pathogens and harmful particles. However, in the study of Rydel-Tormanen et al. (Rydel-Tormanen et al., 2006) it was demonstrated that neutrophils are also able to engulf apoptotic neutrophils or cell debris resulting from secondary necrosis of neutrophils. Previously, neutrophils phagocytosing apoptotic cells and nuclei have been described in blood smears from patients with systemic lupus erythematosus (SLE), a feature called LE cells (Bohm, 2004). Moreover, in inflammatory foci, apparently viable neutrophils with phagosomes enclosing were found with what appeared to be whole apoptotic neutrophils and apoptotic nuclei. Neutrophils may thereby contribute to clearance and resolution of inflammation, thus acting as a back up system in situations when the macrophages clearance system is insufficient and/or overwhelmed. It is apparent that neutrophils have the abilities needed to mimic macrophage behavior and express most, if not all, surface receptors used by macrophages in the process of phagocytosis, suggesting the mechanisms to be similar in the two types of cells (Rydell-Tormanen et al., 2006).

6. Long-density granulocytes (LDG) and endothelial progenitor cells (EPC)

Two studies (Denny et al., 2010, Hacbarth & Kajdacsy-Bella, 1986) have reported the presence of an abnormal subset of neutrophils in the peripheral circulation of SLE patients.

Low density granulocytes (LDG) are present in PBMC preparations derived from lupus patients. LDGs display an activated phenotype, induce significant endothelial cytotoxicity and synthesize sufficient levels of type I IFNs to disrupt the capacity of endothelial progenitor cells (EPC) to differentiate into mature endothelial cells.

EPCs have been shown to play a role in the neovascularization that occurs in diseased tissues. Given the extensive neovascularization that occurs in RA, it was suggested by Denny (Denny et al., 2010) that EPCs are recruited to the arthritic synovium, where they might contribute to expansion of the synovial microcirculation. The VCAM-1/very late activation antigen 4 adhesive system critically mediated EPC adhesion to cultured RA fibroblasts. As was shown, in 3 diverse animal models used to investigate cell homing in arthritis, EPCs preferentially localized to inflamed synovium compared to normal synovium (Silverman et al., 2007). This correlates well with earlier observations that the number of EPCs per mm^2 identified immunihistochemically in postsurgical human RA synovial tissue (ST) was elevated ~25-fold over the number of EPCs localized in normal ST (Ruger et al., 2004).

The findings provide evidence of a possible role of EPC in the synovial neovascularization that is critical to RA pathogenesis; and it may be suggested that neutrophils play a crucial role in this phenomenon. As was showed by Schruefer (Schruefer et al., 2004), neutrophils are critically involved in angiogenesis. Growing evidences indicates that angiogenesis can be initiated by inflammatory cytokines, including IL-8. Human neutrophils release a variety of proinflamatory cytokines, including IL-8, which was originally identified as a potent activator of human neutrophils (Baggiolini et al., 1989). Subsequently, IL-8 was shown to stimulate angiogenesis by promoting proliferation of endothelial cells, moreover IL-8 inhibits endothelial cell apoptosis and induces the upregulation of endothelial matrix metalloproteinase-2 and -9, which also play an important role in angiogenesis.

Neovascularization is a hallmark of diverse pathological conditions, including RA. Microcirculatory expansion occurs either through angiogenesis (the proliferation and branching off of pre-existing microvessels, by IL-8 from neutrophils), or by vasculogenesis (the de novo formation of blood vessels from circulating EPCs). This phenomenon may be restored by LDG depletion (Denny et al., 2010).

Inhibition of neovascularization and thus inhibition of the expansion of invasive tissue in RA is the desired effect. A clearer understanding of the role of neutrophils in biologic processes that guide EPCs to the angiogenic tissue and exert contradictory effects on mirocirculatory expansion may lead to the development of the novel tools to modulate these activities (Silverman et a., 2007).

7. Neutrophil-mediated monocyte recruitment. View on neutrophil-monocyte axis

The sequence of phagocyte recruitment to the site of inflammation comprises initial extravasation of neutrophils followed by a subsequent emigration of monocytes. The experiments of Gallin (Gallin et al., 1982) pointed to the importance of ready made neutrophil granule proteins in the recruitment of monocytes. Granule proteins are stored in 4 distinct sets of granules. Primary and secondary granules discharged from emigrated neutrophils contain mainly antimicrobial polypeptides. Rapidly mobilized secretory vesicles contain mainly receptors important for adhesion and recognition of foreign particles. Tertiary granules released during transendothelial migration contain mainly proteases (Soehlein et al., 2009).

It has been shown that neutrophils that have migrated to the site of inflammation can up-regulate their production of chemokines, supporting the notion that, in this way, neutrophils participate in the regulation of leukocyte accumulation (Soehlein et al., 2009). In terms of production, the principal chemokine produced by neutrophils is IL-8, which activates neutrophils in an autocrine loop. IL-8 binds to CXCR2 expressed not just on neutrophils, but also monocytes. IL-8 also mediates adhesion both human neutrophils and monocytes to the endothelium (Soehlein et al., 2009).
Adhesion of neutrophils to the endothelial cells results in rapid release of secretory vesicles: proteinase-3 and azurocidin (also known as cationic antimicrobial protein). Both azurocidin and proteinase-3 are strongly positively charged and may therefore act with negatively charged endothelial proteoglycans. Azuricidin was recently shown (Soehnlein et al., 2009) to induce monocyte extravasation, it has been demonstrated that depletion of neutrophils reduces the recruitment of inflammatory monocytes. Interestingly, this deficiency in recruitment can be almost completely rescued by the local application of the supernatant from activated human neutrophils (Soehlein et al., 2009).
Activated neutrophils are short-lived cells. Their apoptosis is a tightly regulated process involving ROI and pathogens. Once neutrophils migrate toward the site of inflammation, their life span increases because of the presence of survival signals in the inflammatory milieu. In response to pro-inflammatory signals, neutrophils not only extend their life span, but also release a web of DNA in which granule proteins are enweaved (Brinkmann et al., 2004). Exposure of granule proteins and entrapment within a net of DNA may contribute to creating a gradient of chemotactic stimuli relevant to monocyte recruitment. Apart from release of granule proteins, apoptotic neutrophils may release attraction signals leading to influx monocytes. In recent years, several apoptotic cell-derived "find-me" signals were identified. Among them is lysophosphatidylcholine (LPC), of which the latter has received much attention. LPC was identified (Kim et al., 2002) as an "eat-me" signal on the apoptotic cell surface. More recently, it has been shown that changes in membrane composition of apoptotic cells (negative surface charges) in initiate attractive signals for phagocytes including monocyte. It is feasible that apoptotic neutrophils generate such electric signals resulting in electrotaxis of monocytes (Zhao et al., 2006).
In addition, neutrophil granule proteins enhance the production of ROI by monocytes (Soehnlein et a., 2008). Thus, various experimental setups provide evidence that the axis of neutrophils and inflammatory monocytes promotes and sustained inflammation. Taken together, the multifaceted action of neutrophils in recruiting and activating monocytes may offer a powerful target for interfering with the sustained inflammatory reponse in RA (Soehnlein et al., 2009).

8. Summary

The research conditions of most neutrophil experiments differ considerably from the physiological environment of the joint, i.e. the presence and concentration of cytokines such as TNF-α, IL-1β, IL-6, IL-8, IL-12, IL-17, IL-18, IL-23 and IFN-γ (McInnes et al., 2007), and physical factors such as viscosity, oxygen concentration, and pressure. Each of these differences can influence neutrophil metabolism and activation (Gajewski et al., 2006, 2010a; Cross et al., 2006). Reasoning that conditions imitating physiological environment are required for proper conclusions, we developed and used culture systems which more accurately simulated conditions in the joint (Gajewski, et al., 2010b). The proposal to conduct studies in more physiological conditions, is strongly recommended for *in vitro* experiments on neutrophil's role in RA.

Findings confirm that neutrophils in synovial tissues have different features than blood neutrophils. The old view of neutrophils as a terminally differentiated cell completely focused on destroying pathogens and tissues is no longer held (Cascao et al., 2009). Our understanding of the role of neutrophils in inflammation has changed fundamentally over recent years. The initial perception of the neutrophil playing a passive role and merely responding to external signals has now been replaced by an appreciation that activated neutrophils can perform most, if not all, the functions of macrophages (Cascao et al., 2009).

Neutrophils are key cells in the immune response due to their dual anti-infection and pro-inflammatory roles, being critical effectors in both innate and humoral immunity. Neutrophils generate chemotactic signals and cytokines that recruit, differentiate and activate B and T lymphocytes and antigen presentating cells (APCs), thus establishing a "bridge" between the innate and adaptive immune system. Neutrophils seem to be important "decision-shapers" (Cascao et al., 2009) in this complex system and further understanding of the specific roles of these cells may help to answer one of the main questions in the immune system domain; "What triggers an immune response?" (Cascao et al., 2009).

The knowledge about neutrophil complex biology and their role in immune-mediated inflammatory diseases is expected to reveal promising new therapeutic targets.

9. References

Angellini G, Gardella S, Ardy M, Ciriolo MR, Filomeni G, Di Trapani G, Clarke F, Sitia R, Rubartelli A. (2002). Antigen-presenting dendritic cells provide the reducing extracellular microenvironment required for T lymphocyte activation. *Proceedings of the National Acadademy of Sciences* Vol. 99, No. 3, (February 2002), pp. (1491-1496),

Araki H, Katayama N, Yamashita Y, Mano H, Fujieda A, Usui E, Mitani H, Ohishi K, Nishii, K,Masuya M, Minami N, Nobori T, Shiku H. (2004) Reprogramming of human postmitotic neutrophils into macrophages by growth factors. *Blood* Vol. 103, No. 8, (April 2004), pp. (2973-2980),

Baggiolini M, Walz A, Kunkel SL. (1989). Neutrophil-activating peptide-1/interleukin 8, a novel cytokine that activates neutrophils. *The Journal of Clinical Investigation* Vol. 84, No. 4, (October 1989), pp. (1045 1049),

Bany U; Gajewski M; Ksiezopolska-Pietrzak K; Jozwicka M; Klimczak E; Ryzewski J; Chwalinska-Sadowska H; Maslinski W. (1999). Expression of mRNA Encoding Muscarinic Receptor Subtypes in Neutrophils of Patients with Rheumatoid Arthritis. *Annals of The New York Academy of Sciences.* Vol 876, (Jun 1999), pp. (301-304),

Bell AL, Magill MK, McKane R, Irvine AE. (1986) Human blood and synovial fluid neutrophils cultured in vitro undergo programmed cell death which is promoted by the addition of synovial fluid. *Annals of Rheumatoid Diseases* Vol. 54, No. 11 , (November 1986), pp. (910-915),

Bender JG, Van Epps DE, Searles R, Williams RC. (1986). Altered functions of synovial fluid granulocytes in patients with acute inflammatory arthritis: evidence for activation of neutrophils and its mediation by a factor present in synovial fluid. *Inflammation.* Vol 10, No. 4, (December 1986), pp. (443-453),

Blalock JE. (1984). The immune system as a sensory organ. *The Journal of Immunology.* Vol 132, No. 3, (March 1984), pp. (1067-1076),

Blalock JE. (2005). The immune system as the sithx sense. *Journal of Internal Medicine.* Vol 257, No. 1, (January 2005), pp. (126-138),

Bohm I. (2004). LE cell phenomenon: nuclear IgG deposits inhibits enzymatic cleavage of the nucleus of damaged cells and support its phagocytic clearance by PMN. *Biomedicine and Pharmacotherpy.* Vol 58, No. 3, (April 2004), pp. (196-201),

Brinkmann V, Reichard U, Grosmann C, Fauler B, Uhlemann Y, Weiss DS, Weinrauch Y, Zychlinsky A. (2004) Neutrophil extracellular traps kill bacteria. *Science.* Vol 303, No. 5663, (March 2004), pp. (1532-1535),

Cascao R, Rosario HS,Fonseca JE. (2009) Neutrophils: warriors and commanders in immune mediate inflammatory diseases. *Acta Reumatologica Portuguesa* Vol. 34, No. 2B, (April-Jun 2009), pp. (313-26),

Chakravarti A, Rusu D, Flamand N, Borgeat P, Poubelle PE. (2009). Reprogramming of a subpopulation of human blood neutrophils by prolonged exposure to cytokines. *Labolatory Investigation.* Vol. 89, No. 10, (October 2009), pp. (1084-1099),

Cronstein BN, Kimmel SC, Levin RI, Martiniuk F, Wiessmann G. (1992) A mechanisms for the anti-inflammatory effects of corticosteroids: the glucocorticoid receptor regulates leukocyte adhesion to endothelial cells and expression of endothelial-leukocyte adhesion molecule 1 and intracellular adhesion molecule 1. *Proceedings of the National Acadademy of Sciences* Vol. 89, No. 21, (November 1992), pp. (9991-9995),

Cross A, Bucknall RC, Cassatella MA, Edwards SW, Moots RJ. (2003). Synovial fluid neutrophils transcribe and express class II major histocompatibility complex molecules in rheumatoid arthritis. *Arthritis & Rheumatism.* Vol. 48, No. 10, (October 2003), pp. (2796-2806),

Cross A, Barnes T, Bucknall RC, Edwards SW, Moots RJ. (2006). Neutrophil apoptosis in rheumatoid arthritis is regulated by local oxygen tensions within joints. *Journal of Leukocyte Biology.* Vol. 80, No. 3, (September 2006), pp. (521-528),

Dancewicz AM, Wize J, Sopata I, Wojtecka-Lukasik E, Ksiezny S. (1978). Specific and nonspecific activation of latent collagenolytic proteases of human polymorphonuclear leukocytes. In: *Neutral Proteases of Human Polymorphonuclear Leukocytes* (Havemann, K. & Janoff, A., eds.) pp. (373 -383), Urban & Schwarzenberg, Inc. Baltimore—Munich,

Denny MF, Yalavarthi S, Zhao W, Thacker SG, Anderson M, Sandz AR, McCune WJ, Kaplan MJ. (2010). A distinct subset of proinflammatory neutrophils isolated from patients with systemic lupus erythematosus induces vascular damage and synthetize type I interferons. *The Journal of Immunology.* Vol 184, No. 6, (March 2010), pp. (3284-3297),

Duluray B, Badesha JS, Dieppe PA, Elson CJ. (1990). Oxidative response of polymorphonuclear leucocytes to synovial fluid from patients with rheumatoid arthritis. *Annals of Rheumatoid Diseases.* Vol. 49, No. 9, (September 1990), pp. (661-664),

Edwards SW, Hallett MB. (1997) Seeing the wood for the trees: the forgoten role of neutrophils in rheumatoid arthritis. *Immunology Today* Vol. 18, No. 7, (July 1997), pp. (320-324),

Fierl MA, Rittirsch D, Huber-Lang M, Sarma JV, ward PA. (2008). Catecholamines-crafty weapons in the inflammatory arsenal of immune/inflammatory cells or opening Pandora's box? *Molecular Medicine,* Vol.14, No. 3-4, (March-april 2008), pp. (195-204),

Fillipin LI, Vercelino R, Marroni NP, Xavier RM. (2008) Redox signaling and the inflammatory response in rheumatoid arthritis. *Clinical and Experimental Immunology* Vol. 152, No. 3, (Jun 2008), pp. (415-22),

Gajewski M, Moutiris JA, Maśliński S, Ryżewski J. (1995) The neuromodulation aspects of ichemic myocardium: the importance of cholinergic system. *Journal of Physiology and Pharmacology* Vol. 46, No. 2, (Jun 1995), pp. (107-125),

Gajewski M, Gujski M, Ksiezopolska-Pietrzak K; Jozwicka M, Maslinski S. (1997). The influence of adrenergic and cholinergic agents on respiratory burst of human neutrophils from peripheral blood and synovial fluid. *Journal of Physiology and Pharmacology.* Vol. 48, Suppl 2, (April 1997), pp. (72-79),

Gajewski M, Warnawin E, Gajewska J, Sygitowicz G, Rell-Bakalarska M, Burakowski T, Dziewczopolski W, Szczepanik S, Wysocki L, Pachecka J, Maslinski W, Maslinski S. (2006) Experimental study of the to cytotoxic effects of neutrophils on chondrocytes cultivated in different oxygen concentrations. *Reumatologia.* Vol.44, No.2, (March 2006), pp.(76-86),

Gajewski M, Szczepanik S,Wysocki L, Dziewczopolski W, Gajewska J, Maslinski S. (2009). The effect of increasing amounts of synovial fluid isolated from patients with rheumatoid arthritis on the respiratory burst of human neutrophils. *Reumatologia.* Vol.47, No.5, (September 2009), pp.(273-281),

Gajewski M, Rzodkiewicz P, Szczepanik S, Wysocki L, Dziewczopolski W, Gajewska J, Szacillo-Kosowski J, Wichniak J, Maslinski S. (2010). Interactions between neutrophils and chondrocytes seeded on scaffolds in an environment supplemented with synovial fluid exposed to the influence of variable atmospheric pressure. *Reumatologia.* Vol. 48, No. 5, (September 2010), pp. (307–316),

Gajewski M, Szacillo-Kosowski J, Wichniak J, Rzodkiewicz P, Szczepanik S, Wysocki L, Gajewska J, Maslinski S. (2010). The disposable incubator for tissue engineering. *Reumatologia.* Vol. 48, No. 5, (September 2010), pp. (317–319),

Gallin JL, Flechter MP, Seligmann BE, Hoffstein S, Cehrs K, Mounessa N. (1982). Human neutrophil-specific granule deficiency: a model to assess the role of neutrophil-specific granules in the evolution of the inflammatory response. *Blood.* Vol 59, No. 6, (Jun 1983), pp. (1317-1329),

Hacbarth E, Kajdacsy-Bella A. (1986). Low density neutrophils in patients with systemic lupus erythematosus, rheumatoid arthritis, and acute rheumatic fever. *Arthritis & Rheumatism.* Vol 29, No. 11, (November 1986), pp. (1334-1342),

Hitchon CA, El-Gabalawy HS. (2004) Oxidation in rheumatoid arthritis. *Arthritis Research and Therapy* Vol. 6, No. 6, (October 2004), pp. (265-278),

Iking-Konert C, Ostendorf B, Sander O, Jost M, Wagner C, Joosten L, Schneider M, Hansch GM. (2005) Trans-differentiation of polymorphonuclear neutrophils to dendritic-like cells at the site of inflammation in rheumatoid arthritis: evidence for activation by the T cells. *Annals of Rheumatid Diseases* Vol. 64, No. 10, (October 2005), pp. (1436-42),

Jones DP. (2006), Disruption of mitochondrial redox circuitry in oxidative stress. *Chemico Biological Interactions* Vol. 163, No. 1-2, (October 2006) pp. (38-53),

Kim SJ, Gershov D, Ma X, Brot N, Elkon KB. (2002). I-PLA(2) activation during apoptosis promotes the exposure of membrane lysophosphatidylcholine leading to binding by natural immunoglobulin M antibodies and complement activation. *The Journal of Experimental Medicine.* Vol 196, No. 5 (September 2002), pp. (655-665),

McInnes IB, Schett G. (2007) Cytokines in the pathogenesis of rheumatoid arthritis. *Nature Reviews Immunology.* Vol. 7, No. 6, (June 2007) pp. (429-442),

Nguyen HX, Lusis AJ, Tidball JG. (2005). Null mutation of myeloperoxidase in mice prevents mechanical activation of neutrophils lysis of muscle cell membranes in vitro and in vivo. *The Journal of Physiology.* Vol. 565, No. 2, (Jun 2005), pp. 403-413,

Nurcombe HL, Bucknall RC, Edwards SW. (1991) Neutrophils isolated from the synovial fluid of patients with rheumatoid arthritis: priming and activation in vitro. *Annals of Rheumatoid Diseases* Vol. 50, No. 3, (March 1991), pp. (147-153).

Nurcombe HL, Bucknall RC, Edwards SW. (1991) Activation of the neutrophil myeloperoxidase H_2O_2 system by synovial fluid isolated from patients with rheumatoid arthritis. *Annals of Rheumatoid Diseases.* Vol. 50, No. 3, (March 1991), pp. (237-242),

Quayle JA, Watson F, Bucknall RC, Edwards SW. (1997) Neutrophils from the synovial fluid of patients with rheumatoid arthritis express the high affinity immunoglobulin G receptor, Fc gamma RI (CD64): role of immune complexes and cytokines in induction of receptor expression. *Immunology* Vol. 91, No. 2, (Jun 1997), pp. (266-273),

Ruger B, Giurea A, Wanivenhaus AH, Zehetgruber H.,Hollemann D, Yanagida G. (2004). Endothelial precursor cells in the synovial tissue of patients with rheumatoid arthritis and osteoarthritis. *Arthritis & Rheumatism.* Vol 50, No. 7, (July 2004), pp. (2157-2166),

Rydell-Tormanen K, Uller L, Erjefalt JS. (2006) Neutrophil cannibalism –a back up when macrophage clearance system is insufficient. *Repiratory Research* Vol. 7:143, (December 2006), Retrieved from <http://www.ncbi.nlm.nih.gov/pmc/articles/PMC1716176/>

Sandilands GP, Ahmed Z, Perry N, Davison M, Lupton A, Young B. 2005) Cross-linking of neutrophil CD11b results in rapid cell surface expression of molecules required for antigen presentating and T-cell activation. *Immunology* Vo. 114, No.3 , (March 2005), pp. (354-68),

Silverman MD, Haas CS, Rad AM, Arbab AS, Koch AE. (2007). The role of vascular cell adhesion molecule 1/very late activation antigen 4 I endothelial progenitor cell recruitment to rheumatoid arthritis synovium. *Arthritis & Rheumatism.* Vol.56, No.6, (June 2007), pp. (1817-1826),

Schruefer R, Lutze N, Schymeinsky J, Walzog B. (2005). Human neutrophils promote angiogenesis by a paracrine feedforward mechanisms involving endothelial interleukin-8. *American Journal of Physiology - Heart and Circulatory Physiology.* Vol 288, No. 3, (March 2005), pp. (H1186-H1192)

Smith J,Grisham M, Granger N, Korthuis R. (1989). Free radical defence and neutrophil infiltration in postischemic skeletal muscle. *American Journal of Physiology - Heart and Circulatory Physiology.* Vol 256, No. 3, (March 1989), pp. (H789-H793),

Soehnlein O, Kenne E, Rotzius P, Eriksson EE, Lindboom L. (2008). Neutrophil secretion products regulate anti-bacterial activity in monocytes and macrophages. *Clinical & Experimental Immunology*. Vol 151, No. 1, (January 2008), pp. (139-145),

Soehnlein O, Lindborn L, Weber C. (2009). Mechanisms underlying neutrophil-mediated monocyte recruitment. *Blood*. Vol 114, No. 21, (November 2009), pp. (4613-4623),

Steinberg BE, Grinstein S. (2007) Unconventional roles of the NADPH oxidase: signaling, ion homeostasis, and cell death. *Science`s STKE* Vol. 2007, Issue 379, (March 2007): pp11.

Tracey KJ. (2002) The inflammatory reflex. *Nature* Vol. 420, No. 6917, (December 2002), pp. (853-859)

Wartha F, Beiter K, Normark S, Hnriques-Normark B. (2007) Neutrophil extracellular traps: casting the NET over pathogenesis. *Current Opinon in Microbiology* Vol. 10, No. 1, (February 2007), pp. (52-56),

Wenthworth PJr, McDunn JE,Wenthworth AD, Takeuchi C, Nieva J, Jones T, Bautista C, Ruedi JM, Gutierrez A, Janda KD, Babior BM, Eschenmoser A, Lerner RA. (2002). Evidence for antibody-catalyzed ozone formation in bacterial killing and inflammation. *Science*. Vol 298, No. 5601, (December 2002), pp. (2195-2199),

Wojtecka-Lukasik E, Dancewicz AM. (1974) Inhibition of human leukocyte collagenase by some drugs used for therapy of rheumatic diseases. *Biochem Pharmacol* Vol. 23, No. 15, (August 1974), pp. (2077-2081),

Wright HL, Moots RJ, Bucknall RC, Edwards RC. (2010) Neutrophil function in inflammation and inflammatory diseases. *Rheumatology (Oxford)* Vol. 49, No. 9, (September 2010), pp. (1618-1631).

Wybran J, Appleboom T, Famaey JP, Govaerts A. (1979). Suggestive evidence for receptors for morphine and methionine-enkephalin on normal human blood T lymphocytes. *The Journal of Immunology*. Vol 123, No. 3, (September 1979), pp. (1068-1070),

Yamashita K, Miyoshi T, Arai T, Endo N, Itoh H, Makino K, Mizugishi K, Uchiyama T, Sasada M. (2008). Ozone production by amino acids contributes to killing of bacteria. *Proceedings of the National Academy of Sciences of the United States of America*. Vol 105, No. 44, (November 2008), pp.(16912-16917),

Zhao M, Song B, Pu J, Wada T, Reid B, Tai G, Wang F, Guo A, Walczysko P, Gu Y, Sasaki T, Suzuki A, Forrester JV, Bourne HR, Devreotes PN, McCaig CD, Penninger JM. (2006). Electrical signals control wound healing through phosphatidylinositol-3-OH kinase-gamma and PTEN. *Nature*. Vol 442, No. 7101, (July 2006), pp. (457-460).

5

Molecular Mechanisms of Rheumatoid Arthritis Revealed by Categorizing Subtypes of Fibroblast-Like Synoviocytes

Katsuhiko Ishihara and Hideya Igarashi
Kawasaki Medical School
Japan

1. Introduction

The immune system is a highly organized defense system, which recognizes invading microorganisms and aims to exclude them. In order to do this effectively and safely, the immune system must distinguish between self- and non-self-antigens, and be tolerant of self-antigens. Autoimmune diseases develop through the breakdown of self-tolerance, as a result of immune deregulation. This is caused by the combined influence of genetic and environmental factors, including infectious microorganisms. Rheumatoid arthritis (RA) is a systemic autoimmune disease, characterized by synovial hyperplasia leading to the destruction of bones and joints. This severely impairs the life of patients. RA is a relatively common autoimmune disease, occurring in approximately 1% of the population. However, its etiology and pathophysiology are not completely understood. The incidence of RA is correlated with certain human leukocyte antigen (HLA)-DR haplotypes, and the production of autoantibodies such as rheumatoid factor and anticitrullinated protein autoantibody. Thus, the involvement of the deregulated immune system is strongly implicated. Various molecules, including type II collagen, gp39, citrullinated peptides, and glucose-6-phosphoisomerase, have been reported as potential pathogenic autoantigens. However, their involvement explains only a proportion of RA cases. Autoantigens are abundant in the body and, theoretically, the immune response to them continues indefinitely. Thus, systemic autoimmune diseases exhibit the characteristics of chronic inflammation.

In the pathological condition of RA, the joints are infiltrated with T cells, B cells, macrophages, and plasma cells, all of which are characteristic chronic inflammation cells driven by the immune system. Recently, Th17, a novel helper T-cell subset producing interleukin (IL)-17, has been recognized as a pivotal player in the local inflammation driven by acquired immunity. In addition to immune-competent cells, there is accumulating evidence for abnormalities in non-hematopoietic cells, especially fibroblast-like synoviocytes (FLSs) (Bartok & Firestein, 2010; Firestein, 2009; Mor *et al.*, 2005; Pap & Gay, 2009). The cartilage and bone are destroyed by the invasion of pannus, which is formed from proliferating FLSs and multi-nucleated osteoclasts. Osteoclasts are specialized to resolve bone, and play a major role in bone destruction in RA. However, there is strong evidence that FLSs themselves are aggressive enough to destroy bone. When cultured FLSs derived from RA or osteoarthritis (OA) were co-implanted with human cartilage under the renal capsule of a severe combined immunodeficiency (SCID) mouse, the FLSs derived from RA, but not from OA, destroyed the cartilage (Muller-Ladner *et al.*, 1996; Pierer *et al.*, 2003). In RA, cytokines produced by surrounding cells in the inflamed joints, such as basic fibroblast growth factor (FGF), platelet-derived growth factor (PDGF), transforming growth factor (TGF)-β, tumor necrotizing factor (TNF)-α, and IL-1β, are thought to be responsible for the hyperplasia of FLSs. On the other hand, activated FLSs produce TNF-α, IL-1β, IL-6, chemokines, and matrix metalloproteinases (MMPs), thereby establishing the chronic and destructive inflammatory circuit driven by cellular interaction. Thus, it appears that some passively activated FLSs may be changed to be in a distinctly activated state, autonomously destroying bone and joints.

The critical roles of inflammatory cytokines are evidenced by the effectiveness of cytokine-blockade therapies for RA, using anti-TNF-α or anti-IL-6 receptor antibodies (Brennan & McInnes, 2008; Nishimoto & Kishimoto, 2006). In spite of the promising effects shown by these anti-cytokine therapies, several problems remain, such as suppression of the normal immunity and substantial numbers of resistant cases (Firestein, 2007). To overcome these difficulties, increased knowledge of the molecular mechanisms involved in the complex and multi-factorial pathophysiology of RA is required. In this context, our research on the disease-associated genes of RA is based on the theory that FLSs are heterogeneous in physiological, and also in pathological situations. In this chapter, we briefly overview the current understanding of FLSs in RA, and introduce the pathophysiological natures of FLSs as revealed by our subtyping studies.

2. Fibroblast-like synoviocytes

2.1 Fibroblast-like synoviocytes in the normal synovium

The syovium is a membranous structure that extends from the margins of articular cartilage and lines the capsule of diarthrodial joints. The synovium supports the joint structure, provides nutrition to the cartilage and lubricates the surface. The synovial membrane has 2 compartments: the initimal lining layer and the sublining layer. The initimal lining layer is the superficial layer that faces the intra-articular cavity, and produces synovial fluid as lubricant. This lining layer is normally 2 to 3 cells thick and consists of 2 types of synovial cells: macrophage-like synoviocytes (Type A synoviocytes), and fibroblast-like synoviocytes (Type B synoviocytes). Type A synoviocytes are hematopoietic in origin, bone marrow-derived, and terminally differentiated, as are other tissue-resident macrophages. Type B synoviocytes are mesenchymal cells with vimentin in the cytoskeleton, and Thy-1 (CD90) on their surface. Type B synoviocytes display many characteristics of fibroblasts, such as the production of extracellular matrix, and collagen type IV and V. Specific characteristics for FLSs in the intimal lining layer include expression of cadherin-11 for homotypic aggregation (Lee *et al.*, 2007) and uridine diphosphoglucose dehydrogenase for synthesis of hyaluronic acid, an essential joint lubricant. Expression of decay accelerating factor, CD55, and adhesion molecules (VCAM-1 and ICAM-1) is also characteristic.

2.2 Fibroblast-like synoviocytes in the synovium of RA

In the synovium of RA, the histopathological characteristics are hyperplasia of FLSs, and infiltration with inflammatory cells. The pathophysiological reactions are joint destruction and perpetuation of inflammation.

2.2.1 Hyperplasia

Hyperplasia of FLSs exhibits features of stable activation—the so-called tumor-like transformation. Features of tumor-like transformation include anchorage-independent growth, adhesion to the extracellular matrix of cartilage, resistance to apoptotic signaling, and invasiveness to cartilage and bone. Tumor-like transformation may be cell-autonomous or non-cell-autonomous. The non-cell-autonomous pathway is indirectly driven by factors produced by autoimmune-competent cells in the microenvironment. These include cytokines, growth factors, lipid mediators, and reactive oxygen species. By contrast, the cell-autonomous pathway results from the cell-intrinsic changes of FLSs themselves.

Reflecting cell-intrinsic changes, FLSs in RA have a characteristic morphology, i.e., an abundant cytoplasm; a dense, rough endoplasmic reticulum; and large, pale nuclei with several prominent nucleoli (Pap & Gay, 2009). One of the important molecular characteristics of FLSs in RA is the expression of proto-oncogenes (Bartok & Firestein, 2009), including c-fos, (Aikawa et al., 2008), *ras, raf, sis, myb*, and *myc* (Roivainen *et al.*, 1999). Interestingly, proto-oncogenes are predominantly expressed by FLSs attached to cartilage and bone (Muller-Ladner *et al.*, 2000). Furthermore, some of these proto-oncogenes regulate gene expression of MMPs or cathepsin L. Thus, in the SCID mouse, inhibition of c-Raf-1 or c-Myc significantly reduced the expression of *MMP-1* and *MMP-3*, resulting in decreased invasiveness of FLSs to the cartilage (Pap *et al.*, 2004).

Among the various cells in the inflamed synovium, macrophages and T cells are thought to be most responsible for producing various stimuli for stable activation of FLSs. Various combinations of PDGF, TGF-β, TNF-α, IL-1, and the arachidonic acid metabolites induce the proliferation of FLSs (Konttinen *et al.*, 1999). On the other hand, FLSs in RA have been shown to exhibit defective apoptosis, rather than enhanced proliferation (Jacob *et al.*, 1995; Korb *et al.*, 2009). Apoptosis was rapidly induced in RA-derived FLSs by retroviral transduction of a combination of dominant-negative c-Raf-1 and dominant-negative c-Myc (Pap *et al.*, 2004), indicating that some proto-oncogenes are involved. Death receptor Fas is expressed and is functional in FLSs *in vitro*. However, apoptosis induced by anti-Fas antibody was prevented by TNF-α, IL-1β, and IL-6, suggesting that FLSs in the inflamed joints are resistant to apoptosis (Ohshima *et al.*, 2000; Wakisaka *et al.*, 1998). The anti-apoptotic function of nuclear factor (NF)-κB activated by TNF-α signaling, and the induction of the anti-apoptotic molecule Bcl-xL by IL-1β are involved (Jeong *et al.*, 2004). In addition to the effects of cytokines, the adhesion molecule VLA-5 (integrin α5β1), upon ligation with fibronectin, is involved in this resistance to Fas-mediated apoptosis (Kitagawa *et al.*, 2006). Under conditions of genotoxic stress, the tumor-suppressor p53 induces cell-cycle arrest, followed by either DNA repair or apoptosis, depending on the degree of DNA damage (Gudkov & Komarova, 2010). A main effector of p53-dependent apoptosis, PUMA (p53 up-regulated modulator of apoptosis) is present in very low concentrations in the synovium. Adenovirus-mediated transfer of the *p53* gene into FLSs induced production of the p53 protein, leading to p21 expression; however, PUMA expression was not enhanced and apoptosis was not induced (Cha *et al.*, 2006). This suggests that, under conditions of genotoxic stress, the FLSs in RA tend to undergo cell-cycle arrest rather than apoptosis.

2.2.2 Infiltration with inflammatory cells

Infiltration with inflammatory cells mainly involves chemokines, cytokines, lipids of chemical mediators, and adhesion molecules. It comprises the mutual activation of interacting cells of distinct lineages, leading to the perpetuation of inflammation.

Inflammatory mediators produced by FLSs include IL-15 (Miranda-Carus *et al.*, 2004), IL-16 (Pritchard *et al.*, 2004), IL-18 (Gracie *et al.*, 1999), TNF-α, TGF-β (Pohlers *et al.*, 2007), NO, and prostagrandin E2 (Kojima *et al.*, 2003). Various chemokines are reported to be produced by FLSs in RA (Iwamoto *et al.*, 2008). The production of IL-8/CXCL8 and GROα/CXCL1, which recruit neutrophils, is induced by stimulation of FLSs with IL-1α, IL-1β, TNF-α, or IL-17 (Hosaka *et al.*, 1994; Kehlen *et al.*, 2002; Koch *et al.*, 1991, 1995). Neutrophils are abundant in the synovial fluid of RA, but rare in the synovial tissue. The levels of lymphotactin/XCL1 are elevated in the synovial fluid and tissues of RA. Moreover, infiltrating mononuclear cells and FLSs in the tissues of RA express XCR1, a receptor for lymphotactin/XCL1 (Wang *et al.*, 2004). The levels of macrophage inflammatory protein (MIP)-1α/CCL3 (a ligand of CCR1 and CCR5) are higher in the synovial fluid of RA. Furthermore, upon stimulation with lipopolysaccharide and TNF-α, isolated FLSs produce MIP-1α/CCL3 (Koch *et al.*, 1994). The migration of $CD4^+$ memory T cells to the synovium of RA, and the inhibition of activation-induced apoptosis of T cells, are induced by stromal cell-derived factor (SDF)-1/CXCL12. Thus, the accumulation of $CD4^+$ memory T cells in the synovium plays an important role in RA (Nanki *et al.*, 2000). The production of RANTES (Regulated upon Activation, Normal T cell Expressed and Secreted)/CCL5 is histologically detected in the synovial lining and sublining layers of affected rheumatoid joints (Robinson *et al.*, 1995). All these suggest that, in microenvironments rich with TNF-α and IL-1β, FLSs themselves recruit monocytes, neutrophils, Th1 cells, eosinophils, and basophils (Rathanaswami *et al.*, 1993).

In addition to the regulation of migration, stimulation with MCP-1/CCL2, SDF-1/CXCL12, IP-10/CXCL10, Mig/CXCL9, and MCP-4/CCL13 enhances the proliferation of FLSs, leading to synovial hyperplasia (Garcia-Vicuna *et al.*, 2004; Iwamoto *et al.*, 2007). Furthermore, continuous infusion of human IL-8/CXCL8 into the knee joints of rabbits for 14 days led to severe arthritis, characterized by erythema, joint pain, infiltration of leucocytes and mononuclear cells in the synovial tissue, and hypervascularization in the synovial lining layer (Endo *et al.*, 1994). Thus, the angiogenic properties of chemokines, such as IL-8/CXCL8, GROα/CXCL1, MCP-1/CCL2, SDF-1/CXCL12, and fractalkine/CX3CL1 (Koch *et al.*, 1992; Salcedo *et al.*, 1999, 2000; Volin *et al.*, 2001) may play an important role in the development of RA. Angiogenic factors, including FGF (Thomas *et al.*, 2000), vascular endothelial growth factor (VEGF) (Cho *et al.*, 2002), IL-18, and angiopoietin (Scott *et al.*, 2002), are also produced by FLSs. This suggests that FLSs are involved in neovascularization, and may cause critical pathological changes to sustain pannus formation in RA (Szekanecz & Koch, 2007).

2.2.3 Joint destruction

Proteinases, such as MMPs and cathepsins, are produced by FLSs attached to cartilage and bone, and play an important role in joint destruction. The expression of *MMP-1/interstitial collagenase* and *MMP-3/stromelysin* correlates with the invasive growth of FLSs in RA (Tolboom *et al.*, 2002). MMP-1 is found in the synovial membranes of all RA patients. Moreover, the levels of MMP-1 in the synovial fluid, but not in the sera, correlate with the degree of synovial inflammation (Konttinen *et al.*, 1999; Maeda *et al.*, 1995; Sorsa *et al.*, 1992). MMP-3 plays a key role in joint destruction, not only by degrading matrix molecules, but also by activating other pro-MMPs into their active forms (Okada, 2009). The major source of MMP-3 is FLSs in the lining layer (Tetlow *et al.*, 1993). High concentrations of MMP-3 have been detected in the synovial fluid and sera of RA patients (Beekman *et al.*, 1997; Taylor *et al.*, 1994). Moreover, elevated serum levels of MMP-3 are correlated with systemic inflammation at the clinical and also the serologic level (Manicourt *et al.*, 1995; Yoshihara *et al.*, 1995). Although expression of MMP-13/collagenase-3 correlates with elevated levels of systemic inflammatory markers, this is not specific to RA (Lindy *et al.*, 1997; Westhoff *et al.*, 1999). MT1-MMT/MMP-14 degrades the extracellular matrix, and activates MMP-2/gelatinase A and MMP-13 (Pap *et al.*, 2000a).

The expression of MMPs in synovial cells is regulated by several extracellular signals, including inflammatory cytokines, growth factors, and molecules of the extracellular matrix, such as collagen and fibronectin (Pap & Gay, 2009). Among these, IL-1 is the most potent inducer of MMPs, including MMP-1, MMP-3, MMP-8, MMP-13, and MMP-14. FGF and PDGF also act as potent inducers for MMPs, by enhancing the effects of IL-1. TNF-α and TGF-β induce MMP-1 and MMP-13, respectively, while IL-17 induces MMP-1 and MMP-9.

Another group of proteinases involved in joint destruction is the cathepsins, which cleave cartilage types II, IX, and XI, and proteoglycan. The expression of the cysteine proteases, cathepsins B and L, was increased in the synovium of RA, especially at the sites of cartilage invasion (Keyszer *et al.*, 1995, 1998). Similarly to MMPs, the production of cathepsins is induced by proto-oncogene, IL-1, and TNF-α (Joseph *et al.*, 1987; Huet *et al.*, 1993; Lemaire *et al.*, 1997). Cathepsin K, which plays an important role in bone resorption by osteoclasts, is also expressed by FLSs and macrophages at the site of synovial invasion into the articular bone (Min *et al.*, 2004).

2.2.4 Perpetuation of inflammation

When cells producing soluble factors or expressing ligands on their surfaces are located close to cells that receive signals through the specific receptor, a circuit of chronic inflammation may be generated through an exchange of cell roles. For example, activated Th1 cells produce IFNγ, which activates macrophages. The activated macrophages produce IL-1 and TNF-α, which in turn activate T cells. In cases of RA, IL-1 and TNF-α from macrophages can activate FLSs, creating another circuit with a distinct cellular combination. Although one can easily imagine the operation of such a circuit at a certain time point of autoimmune diseases, it is difficult to demonstrate the mechanism by a suitable model system. Recently, Ogura *et al.* (2008) proposed that IL-17 secreted from Th17 cells induces fibroblasts to produce more IL-6, in a manner dependent on the transcription factor NF-κB, and the signal transducer and activator of transcription (STAT) 3. The mechanism, designated as "IL-17A-triggered positive-feedback loop of IL-6 signaling", is thought to amplify the inflammatory responses mediated by interactive cytokines. Enhancement of this loop was shown to be involved in the development of RA-like arthritis or experimental autoimmune encephalomyelitis in knock-in mice gp130F759, which are defective in the negative regulation of signaling through a common receptor subunit of IL-6 family cytokines, gp130. The identification of such a powerful circuit, specific to each autoimmune disease, will facilitate the development of a critical target point for effective therapy.

3. Progress in the study of RA by the molecular genetic approach

3.1 Genome-wide screening for disease-related genes

The risk of developing RA and the severity of the disease are significantly affected by genetics. It has long been recognized that certain HLA alleles, especially HLA-DR4, are associated with increased risk of onset and severity of RA (Weyand *et al.*, 1992). A shared epitope on certain HLA haplotypes is thought to affect the binding of peptides derived from self-antigens, leading to autoimmune responses by T cells (Wordsworth *et al.*, 1989). To identify non-HLA genes that regulate the development and severity of RA, human genome-wide studies have been performed. Some of these studies have used a combined approach, with factors such as microsatellites (Tamiya *et al.*, 2005), or disease subsets; serum autoantibody alone (Stahl *et al.*, 2010) or combined with a shared epitope (Sugino *et al.*, 2010); race, or nation (Freudenberg *et al.*, 2011; Martin *et al.*, 2010); correlation with other autoimmune diseases (Cui *et al.*, 2009; Zhernakova *et al.*, 2011); or responsiveness to therapies targeting specific cytokines (Liu *et al.*, 2008; Plant *et al.*, 2011). Single nucleotide polymorphisms that may be involved in the development of RA include protein tyrosine phosphatase, nonreceptor-type 22 (*PTPN22*), cytotoxic T-lymphocyte antigen 4 (*CTLA4*), *STAT4*, and peptidylarginine deiminase type 4 (*PADI4*). Among these, *PADI4* has been identified by genome-wide screening (Suzuki *et al.*, 2003) as being able to modify self-antigens by citrullination. Moreover, the presence of anti-cyclic citrullinated antibody in the serum is highly specific to RA and has a high diagnostic value. The role of PADI4 in the pathogenesis of RA, especially with respect to "autoimmunity" to modified self-antigens, will be intriguing to clarify.

Large-scale, genome-wide association studies, based firmly on statistics, have provided valuable information on the candidate genes for RA. Nevertheless, to understand the complex pathophysiology of RA, data from studies on additional aspects must be integrated. Such studies should include molecular and cell-biological analyses of clinical materials from individual RA cases, and functional analyses of candidate genes *in vitro* and *in vivo*, including experimental system using engineered mutant mice.

3.2 Transcription profiling reveals disease-specific genes and heterogeneity in RA tissues

Gene expression profiling of FLSs, comparing RA and OA, has revealed disease-specific genes. The genes highly and exclusively expressed in RA were *HOXD10, HOXD11, HOXD13, CCL8*, and *LIM homeobox* 2. Further analysis of the relationships between gene expression on RA-FLSs and clinical disease parameters revealed specific and unique correlations as follows; *HLA-DQA2* with Health Assessment Questionnaire (HAQ) score; *Clec12A* with rheumatoid factor; *MAB21L2, SIAT7E, HAPLN1*, and *BAIAP2L1* with C-reactive protein level; and *RGMB* and *OSAP* with erythrocyte sedimentation rate (Galligan *et al.*, 2007). The data indicated the heterogeneity of gene expression in patients with the same disease. These RA-specific or clinical state-related genes differ from those identified by genome-wide screening, indicating that the complete pathophysiology of RA, as a multi-factorial disease, involves genomic and also epi-genomic regulation of genes. The functional roles of these genes remain to be determined.

Evidence for the heterogeneity of gene expression in synovial tissues from erosive RA cases has been demonstrated by large-scale profiling studies. Systemic characterization of the differentially expressed genes highlighted the existence of at least 2 molecularly distinct forms of RA tissues (van der Pouw Kraan *et al.*, 2003). The first is RA tissue with high-grade inflammation (RA^{high}), which exhibits abundant expression of gene clusters indicative of adaptive immune responses, such as genes expressed by T cells, B cell, and antigen-presenting cell (APC). The second form of RA tissue is a low-grade inflammatory gene

expression signature (RA^{low}), common to the tissues from patients with OA, and characterized by increased expression of genes involved with tissue remodeling activity. Importantly, the cluster of RA^{high} showed an increased expression of STAT1-pathway related genes;STAT1-inducing receptors (*IL-2Rγ, CCR5*), and STAT1 target genes (*MMP-1, MMP-3, caspase-1, TAP-1, and IRF-1*), suggesting a prominent role for this pathway. Furthermore, patients with the high-grade inflammation tissue type had higher Disease Activity Scores in 28 joints, higher C-reactive protein levels, higher erythrocyte sedimentation rates, increased numbers of platelets, and shorter disease durations (van Baarsen *et al.*, 2010).
Several trials have profiled gene expression in the synovial tissues of RA patients undergoing molecular-targeting therapy (Lindberg *et al.*, 2006; Wijbrandts *et al.*, 2008). Further analysis is expected to yield valuable data on cytokine activity in the human body, facilitating the development of effective therapy with a clear target point.

4. Mouse models for RA

The generation of RA-like joint diseases in engineered mutant mice appears to reflect the heterogeneous and complicated mechanisms of human arthritis, diagnosed simply as rheumatoid arthritis. In contrast to previous years, when animal models for human diseases rarely emerged by point mutations in nature, current research on autoimmune diseases such as RA benefits from the existence of various engineered mutant mice models. For example, mechanisms for RA-like disease revealed by murine models include, the abnormal T-cell receptor (TCR) signaling by a natural mutant ZAP70 in SKG mouse (Sakaguchi *et al.*, 2003), an autoantibody to glucose-6-phosphoisomerase in K/BxN TCR transgenic mouse (Korganow *et al.*, 1999), defective autoantigen clearance in *DNaseII-/-* moue (Kawane *et al.*, 2006), overexpression of the viral gene in HTLV-1 *pX* transgenic mouse (Iwakura *et al.*, 1991), and excessive amounts or activity of cytokines. RA-like disease developed in TNF-α transgenic mice (Keffer *et al.*, 1991) and IL-1α transgenic mice (Niki *et al.*, 2001) with overproduction of inflammatory cytokines and in TNF AU-rich elements-deficient (ΔARE) mice (Kontoyiannis *et al.*, 1999) with increased stability of cytokine messenger RNA. Excessive activities of arthritogenic cytokines were evoked in IL-1 receptor antagonist knock-out mouse (Horai *et al.*, 2000) lacking a physiological negative feedback molecule, and in gp130F759 with a defective, intracellular negative-regulatory signaling pathway (Atsumi *et al.*, 2002; Ohtani *et al.*, 2000).
These wide variety of murine arthritis models with a defined genetic defect will be useful for analyzing the mechanisms for the synergistic action of genetic and environmental factors in RA development (Ishihara *et al.*, 2004), and also the mechanisms for initiation or perpetuation of joint inflammation (Murakami *et al.*, 2011; Ogura *et al.*, 2008). Furthermore, bone marrow transplantation experiment revealed a unique feature of gp130F759 that non-hematopoietic cells with a point mutation Y759F in gp130 are sufficient to induce passive but arthritogenic activation of wild type $CD4^{+}$T cells (Sawa *et al.*, 2006). In human TNF-α transgenic mouse, arthritogenic FLSs showed increased expression of *MMP-1* and *MMP-9*, and also diminished adhesion to extracellular matrix components. These changes could induce increased proliferation and migration, which are critical for the spread of hyperplasia in the joints (Aidinis *et al.*, 2003). Dispensable roles for *RAG* in arthritis have been observed in $TNF^{\Delta ARE}$ mouse (Kontoyiannis *et al.*, 1999) and *DNaseII-/-* mouse (Kawane *et al.*, 2010), indicating that synovial hyperplasia may develop independently of acquired immunity.

5. Fibroblast-like synoviocytes and mesenchymal stem cells

FLSs are characterized mainly by *in vitro* analyses. The synovial membranes are easily obtained by joint surgery. The cells liberated from the synovial tissues by treatment with collagenase can be cultured under the appropriate conditions. Although primary FLSs are useful, experiments must be carefully designed, because the composition of the cells in the culture changes after 4 passages, when contaminated hematopoietic cells disappear (Zimmermann *et al.*, 2001).

The source of pathogenic FLSs proliferating in the synovium of RA is an intriguing issue, and several possibilities can be considered. Growth of FLSs can be stimulated by adjacent hematopoietic cells in the microenvironment, or initiated by the acquisition of cell-intrinsic properties for unregulated growth. Alternatively, growing FLSs can be derived from resident FLSs in the normal synovial membrane, or migrated from other organs. The latter possibility was demonstrated by experiments to inject FLSs from human TNF-α transgenic mice into the knee joint, and to transplant human synovial fibroblasts into SCID mice (Aidinis *et al.*, 2003; Lefevre *et al.*, 2009).

Fibroblast-like cells that initiate growth during the very early stages of RA can originate from mature FLSs or from other mesenchymal cells at the primitive stage, such as mesenchymal stem cells (MSCs). The presence of MSCs in the synovium has been reported by several researchers. MSCs with the potential to differentiate into 3 lineages, osteogenic, adipogenic, and chondrogenic cells, were obtained from the synovial membrane following digestion with collagenase and more than 3 passages (De Bari *et al.*, 2001). Fibroblast-like MSCs expressing fibroblast marker D7-FIB, but not CD45, were detected in the synovial fluid (Jones *et al.*, 2004). The number of these MSCs was lower in the synovial fluid of RA than in that of OA. In addition to the synovium, MSCs have been derived from blood (Zvaifler *et al.*, 2000), adipose tissue (Zuk *et al.*, 2002), and the periosteal region (De Bari *et al.*, 2006). Although not genuine MSCs, circulating $CD14^+$ monocytes may contain progenitors with the potential to differentiate into mesenchymal cells (Kuwana *et al.*, 2003).

In terms of the underlying mechanism for the transformation-like phenotype of FLSs, and the involvement of MSCs, Li & Makarov (2006) reported intriguing data from animal models of RA. Arthritic FLSs contained a substantial fraction of bone marrow-derived precursors, with the ability to differentiate *in vitro* into various mesenchymal cell types. However, inflammation prevented multilineage differentiation. The transcription factor NF-κB played a key role in repressing osteogenic and adipogenic differentiation of arthritic FLSs. On the other hand, specific activation of NF-κB profoundly enhanced proliferation, motility, and matrix-degrading activity of FLSs by the induction of MMPs. These data suggest an intriguing mechanism, namely, that arthritic FLSs are bone marrow-derived MSCs, which are arrested during the early stages of differentiation, by the activation of NF-κB induced by inflammatory cytokines (Li & Makarov, 2006).

6. Search for RA-related genes through the classification of fibroblast-like synoviocytes

6.1 Subtypes of fibroblast-like synoviocytes in RA

Kasperkovitz *et al.* (2005) reported that subtypes of FLSs in RA differ in their gene expression. Complementary DNA microarrays of the synovial tissues and cultured FLSs obtained from RA patients revealed that the gene expression profiles of high- and low-grade inflammation synovial tissues were characterized by high and low expression of genes of immune-competent cells (T cells, B cells, and APCs), respectively. Furthermore, hierarchical clustering identified 2 groups of FLSs, characterized by distinctive gene expression profiles and correlation with the inflammatory profiles of the synovial tissues. The first group correlated with the high-grade inflammation tissue, and exhibited increased expression of a TGF-β/activin A-inducible gene profile, which is characteristic of myofibroblasts, a cell type involved in wound healing. The second group correlated with the low-grade inflammation tissue, and showed increased expression of the genes involved in autocrine growth regulation, cell transformation, complement activation, and oxidative stress. Reflecting the gene expression profile, an increased proportion of myofibroblast-like cells in the heterogeneous population of FLSs were immunohistochemically detected in the high-grade inflammation tissue. These data suggest that the inflammatory state of the synovium is determined by the composition of heterogeneous FLSs.

6.2 Transformed fibroblast-like synoviocyte lines reveal heterogeneity irrespective of arthritis types

The data of Kasperkovitz *et al.* (2005), Galligan *et al.* (2007) and others indicate that combining gene expression profiling with other parameters, such as clinical data or characteristics of FLS lines, constitutes a powerful tool for identifying novel disease-related genes. To identify the cell-intrinsic abnormalities of RA-FLSs, we established transformed cell lines from the synovium of RA or OA cases, by immortalization with SV40 large T Ag (unpublished data of Ishihara *et al.*). Characterization of FLSs from 2 types of arthritis revealed no significant differences in surface molecules, growth rates, patterns of tyrosine-phosphorylated proteins, or expression of the genes related to inflammation (*IL-1β, IL-6, MMP-1, MMP-3,* etc.). Since the expression levels of these genes vary (ranges exceeding 1,000-fold) among FLS lines from each type of arthritis, we tentatively categorized them into 2 subtypes reflecting resting (r) and active (a) stages, based on the expression levels of *IL-1β* and *MMP-1*. Next, we performed a micro DNA array to obtain the gene expression profiles for 4 representative cell lines, r-OA-FLS, a-OA-FLS, r-RA-FLS, and a-RA-FLS, and obtained 10 gene clusters. Although no disease-specific clusters were obtained, 2 reciprocal, stage-specific clusters were detected, suggesting the validity of our hypothesis for the presence of subtypes in FLSs. Using these data we are presently searching for 2 types of candidate genes; master genes that determine the states of FLSs, and genes that could play a role in the pathophysiology of RA by inference based on our current understanding of FLSs. In the following sections, we will review the potential roles of activation-induced cytidine deaminase (*AID*) (Igarashi *et al.*, 2010) and the *A20/ABIN* family.

6.3 Ectopic expression of *AID* and acquisition of a tumor-like phenotype by fibroblast-like synoviocytes

6.3.1 *P53* mutation in fibroblast-like synoviocytes of RA and *AID* expression in inflammation

In addition to the properties described above, the expression of the tumor-suppressor gene *p53* with somatic mutations (Firestein *et al.*, 1997; Inazuka *et al.*, 2000; Kullmann *et al.*, 1999; Reme *et al.*, 1998; Yamanishi *et al.*, 2002), and the down-regulation of the tumor suppressor *PTEN*, a protein phosphatase gene, have been demonstrated in RA-FLSs (Pap *et al.*, 2000b).

In particular, the somatic mutation of the *p53* gene appears consistent, not only in terms of increased resistance to apoptosis, but also with respect to pro-inflammatory responses such as production of IL-6 and MMP-1 (Han *et al.*, 1999; Sun *et al.*, 2004; Yamanishi *et al.*, 2005). However, little is known about the mechanism by which the somatic mutations are introduced into the *p53* gene in RA-FLSs.

AID is a member of the APOBEC family, which is a cellular cytidine deaminase involved in protection from retroviral infection or regulation of cholesterol metabolism (Goila-Gaur & Strebel, 2008). AID was originally identified as an indispensable molecule for somatic hypermutation at the immunoglobulin variable region, and also for class-switch recombination in germinal center B lymphocytes (Di Noia & Neuberger, 2007; Honjo *et al.*, 2004). Recently, several investigators have demonstrated up-regulation of *AID* in non-lymphoid tumor cells such as breast cancer, cholangiocarcinoma, hepatoma, and colorectal cancer cells (Babbage *et al.*, 2006; Chan-On *et al.*, 2009; Endo *et al.*, 2007, 2008; Komori *et al.*, 2008; Kou *et al.*, 2007; Morisawa *et al.*, 2008). During the process of oncogenesis, NF-κB activation in inflammation is thought to be important for aberrant expression of *AID*. For example, the infection of gastric mucosal cells with *Helicobacter pylori*, or of hepatocytes with hepatitis C virus, activates NF-κB and successfully induces local production of pro-inflammatory cytokines such as TNF-α and IL-1β. Together, these secreted cytokines also activate NF-κB, and lead to the induction of AID. In fact, stimulation with TNF-α or IL-1β induces *AID* expression even in non-tumor hepatocyte or colon epithelial cells. Moreover, the somatic mutations of *p53* found in these cancer cells appeared to be a direct target of AID (Endo *et al.*, 2008; Kou *et al.*, 2007; Takai *et al.*, 2009).

RA is characterized by an environment rich in pro-inflammatory cytokines and the existence of mutations in the *p53* gene. Thus, under chronic inflammatory circumstances, it is possible that aberrant expression of *AID* could introduce mutations into the *p53* gene of FLSs.

6.3.2 Aberrant expression of *AID* in RA-FLSs

First, we assessed the expression of the *AID* gene in the transformed FLS cell lines described in 6.2, by real-time reverse transcription polymerase chain reaction (RT-PCR). *AID* was transcribed in more than half of the RA-FLS cell lines (5 out of 9) and in none of the OA-FLS cell lines. Quantitative assay by RT-PCR showed 7- to 18-fold higher *AID* transcription in the RA-FLS lines compared to the OA-FLS lines that expressed a low but detectable level of *AID* transcription. The possibility of contaminated signals from *AID*-expressing B cells was excluded by the absence of pan B cell marker transcription. The translation of AID was further confirmed by the detection of protein in the cell lysate from RA-FLSs, with western blot analysis.

Patients who provided *AID*-expressing FLSs showed a tendency toward higher levels (approximately 2.7 times) of CRP in the serum. Regarding gender, the number of female patients with *AID*$^+$ FLSs was approximately 1.9 times higher than the number of male patients. Although our data are not statistically significant because of the small sample numbers used, it appears that *AID* expression in FLSs is facilitated under conditions of inflammation in female patients. Indeed, we observed that estrogen, a representative female hormone, or TNF-α, a representative pro-inflammatory cytokine, augmented the transcription of *AID* in *AID*$^+$ RA-FLSs to more than 20-fold higher levels compared with the basal levels in OA-FLSs. These results are similar to those previously reported for other cells

(Endo *et al.*, 2007, 2008; Pauklin *et al.*, 2009). The transcription levels of *TNF-α*, or the pro-inflammatory cytokines *IL-6* and *IL-1β*, did not correlate with that of *AID*, suggesting that *AID* transcription is not induced by autocrine cytokines. No clear relationship was observed between aberrant expression of *AID* and other clinical parameters, such as age, serum MMP-3 levels, or medication.

6.3.3 Accumulation of *p53* gene mutations in *AID*-expressing RA-FLSs

The mutations of the *p53* tumor-suppressor gene frequently found in RA-FLSs could contribute to the tumor-like, and also the pro-inflammatory properties of RA-FLSs, such as aggressive growth, invasion, and destruction of cartilage and bone (Firestein *et al.*, 1997; Inazuka *et al.*, 2000; Kullmann *et al.*, 1999; Reme *et al.*, 1998; Sun *et al.*, 2004; Yamanishi *et al.*, 2002). Although genotoxic and oxidative stresses have been speculated to be causative candidates for the somatic mutation in the *p53* gene in RA-FLSs, the molecular mechanism has not yet been elucidated. As mentioned in 6.3.1, a clear relationship between *AID* expression and the frequency of *p53* somatic mutations has been demonstrated in some non-B lymphocytes, such as hepatocytes and colon epithelial cells (Chan-On *et al.*, 2009; Endo *et al.*, 2008; Komori *et al.*, 2008; Kou *et al.*, 2007; Morisawa *et al.*, 2008). Thus, we speculated that aberrant expression of *AID* might be involved in the introduction of the *p53* gene mutation. We amplified the coding region of *p53* from 3 *AID*+ RA-FLS cell lines with high-fidelity polymerase. We then determined the nucleotide sequence corresponding to that region and compared it with the intact *p53* gene sequence.

AID+ RA-FLSs harbored approximately 2- to 3.5-fold more mutations than the control RA-FLS subsets, which expressed *AID* at a lower level. In addition, the frequency of non-silent mutations was 3 times more than that of silent mutations. Notably, the base substitution pattern in *p53* was biased toward the transition type, which is typical for AID-mediated mutations at the variable region of the immunoglobulin gene (Di Noia & Neuberger, 2007). The mutations were distributed intensively at the DNA-binding domain of the *p53* gene, where the hotspot of somatic mutations is found in some malignant tumors. The Arg^{248} mutation, one of the cancer hotspot mutations (Ko & Prives, 1996), was found in *p53* from our *AID*+ RA-FLSs. In addition, among the amino acid mutations that we identified, 17% were identical to those previously reported. A further 33% were distinct amino acid mutations; however, the positions of base change were located in the same codons as previously reported. The apparent correlation between ectopic expression of *AID* and increased frequency of somatic mutations of *p53* strongly suggests that AID may be involved in the introduction of mutations to *p53*. Such mutations could lead to reductions or increases in the function of p53, which in turn may result in the tumor-like or anti-apoptotic phenotypes of FLSs in RA.

6.3.4 AID is produced by non-transformed RA-FLSs and in the RA synovium outside the B-cell follicles

The aberrant expression of *AID* in some RA-FLS transformed cell lines is not caused by the effects of transformation with SV40 large T Ag. Indeed, 3 to 8 times higher transcription levels of *AID* were observed, even in non-transformed primary FLS cell lines (4 out of 11 RA-FLSs, but none of the 6 OA-FLSs). In addition, cyto-staining with anti-AID antibody revealed a positive signal in *AID*-expressing primary RA-FLSs. Furthermore, dual-color immunohistostaining of the synovial sections from *AID*+ RA patients clearly demonstrated the production of AID by FLSs in the RA synovial tissues (Figure 1), providing definitive evidence for the occurrence of ectopic and aberrant expression of *AID* in RA.

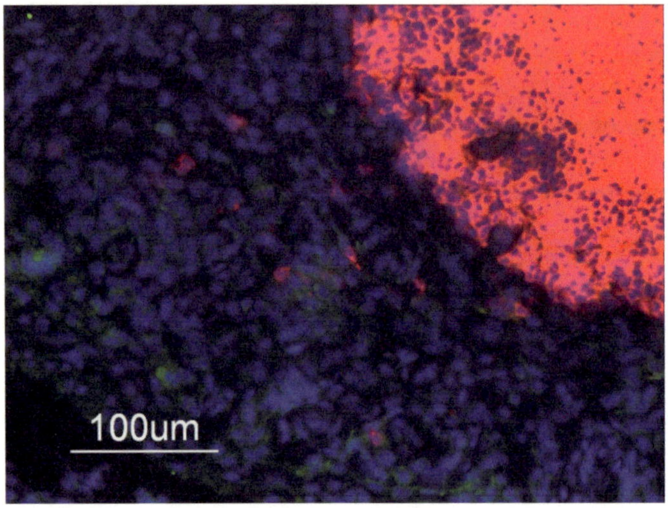

Fig. 1. Immunofluorescence staining of AID on synovial tissue sections from a representative RA patient. Sections were stained simultaneously with rat mAb for AID and anti-CD20 (B-cell marker) mAb. AID was visualized with alexa 488 fluoro-dye conjugated anti-rat secondary Ab (green); CD20 was visualized with alexa 594 fluoro-dye conjugated anti-mouse secondary Ab (red). The nucleus was stained with 4',6-diamino-2-phenylindole (blue). Scale bar is 100 μm.

We concluded that AID is selectively expressed by a proportion of RA-FLSs and that its expression is associated with an increased frequency of somatic mutations in *p53* (Igarashi *et al.*, 2010). Thus, it is possible that the aberrant expression of AID within certain RA-FLSs induces somatic mutations in *p53*, leading to the acquisition of pro-inflammatory or tumor-like phenotypes.

6.4 Heterogeneous responsiveness of fibroblast-like synoviocytes to TNF-α

6.4.1 RA-FLS cell lines differentially respond to TNF-α

The chronic inflammation circuit in the joints of RA is initiated by the production of inflammatory cytokines by FLSs, following stimulation with TNF-α secreted from the surrounding inflammatory cells. In this context, the TNF-α/NF-κB pathway plays an essential role in the transcription of pro-inflammatory cytokines. However, the regulation of NF-κB activity downstream of TNF-α in FLSs is not fully understood. To investigate the heterogeneous responsiveness of RA-FLS cell lines to TNF-α stimulation, we examined the panels of primary RA-FLS cell lines for their induction levels of pro-inflammatory cytokines following TNF-α stimulation. Interestingly, RA-FLS cell lines can be clearly categorized into 2 types based on the responsiveness to TNF-α, namely, whether the transcription levels of pro-inflammatory cytokine gene are high (designated as the high-responder group) or not (designated as the low-responder group). This facilitated production of pro-inflammatory cytokines can be explained by the significant elevation of NF-κB activity in the high-responder FLS lines compared with that in the low-responder lines.

6.4.2 Possible positive effect of A20/ABINs on pro-inflammatory cytokine induction

A20, also termed TNFAIP3 (TNFα-induced protein 3), was originally identified as an inducible zinc finger protein in human umbilical vein endothelial cell lines following stimulation with TNF-α. A20 has dual enzymatic activities, namely, ubiquitination and deubiquitination (Dixit *et al.*, 1990). The induction of A20 upon stimulation with TNF-α is NF-κB dependent; moreover, induced A20 reversely suppresses the activation of NF-κB through the regulation of ubiquitin-mediated degradation of NF-κB activator (Vereecke *et al.*, 2009). This negative feedback loop is thought to be necessary to terminate inflammation and protect tissues from unnecessary damage. Recently, it was reported that the expression level of A20 in RA-FLSs was lower than that in OA-FLSs (Elsby *et al.*, 2010). Although the difference was not significant, this finding could provide *in vitro* evidence of altered *A20* transcription by 6q23 intergenic SNPs associated with RA (Dieguez-Gonzalez *et al.*, 2009; Orozco *et al.*, 2009). Thus, we speculated that the down-regulation of NF-κB inhibitors might be a possible mechanism for enhanced activation of NF-κB in high-responder FLSs. Contrary to our speculation, the high-responder group with abundant mRNA levels of pro-inflammatory cytokines also exhibited marked induction of *A20* following stimulation with TNF-α. Furthermore, the transcription of the NF-κB inhibitory molecules *ABIN* (A20-binding inhibitor of NF-κB activation, also called TNIP, TNFAIP3 interacting protein)-*1* and *ABIN-3*, but not of *ABIN-2*, was increased (Igarashi et al., in press).
These observations indicate that there is heterogeneity of RA-FLSs in the responsiveness to TNF-α stimulation and suggest that these "inhibitors" might not play negative regulatory roles in RA-FLS. The precise mechanism, cell-lineage specificity, disease specificity, and significance in cell biology of this unexpected possible positive role for A20/ABINs are currently under investigation.

7. Conclusion

Anti-cytokine therapy for RA is a prominent achievement in the field of autoimmune diseases. Accumulated evidence from clinical and basic medical research indicates pivotal roles for FLS in the pathogenesis and pathophysiology of RA. Data from genome-wide screening, transcriptional profiling, and animal models indicate that RA consists with heterogeneous disease subsets. Together with several other researchers, we have presented evidence for heterogeneity in FLS. Based on this finding, we have successfully searched for disease-related genes by subtyping FLS. We have identified 2 groups of genes, *AID* and *A20/ABINs*. *AID* is involved in the irreversible transformation of FLS, whereas *A20/ABINs* participate in the reversible, but potentially harmful, responsiveness of them. Both groups of genes are constituent elements for distinct levels of heterogeneity in FLS, which may be involved in resistance to anti-cytokine therapies. Subtyping of FLS based on expression of AID did not coincide with that based on responsiveness to signal-utilizing NF-κB, which is reasonable because RA is a multi-factorial disease. We believe that our approach to categorizing subsets of FLS based on differential gene expression, or on responsiveness to inflammatory stimuli, will facilitate a comprehensive understanding of the pathogenesis and pathophysiology of RA.

8. Acknowledgment

We are grateful to Dr. Jun Hashimoto, Dr. Tetsuya Tomita, and Professor Hideki Yoshikawa in Department of orthopaedics (Osaka University) for collaboration on our study of FLS in

RA. We thank Dr. Masaaki Murakami and colleagues in the Laboratory for Developmental Immunology (Osaka University) for co-operation in the study of gp130F759. We are indebted to Professor Toshio Hirano (Osaka University) for instruction, encouragement, and long-term collaboration on our research into RA. We also thank Ms. Reina Tanaka and Ms. Yuka Kenmotsu for technical assistance. This work was partly supported by Research Project Grants from Kawasaki Medical School, and Grants-in-Aid for Scientific Research from the Ministry of Education, Science, Sports, Culture, and Technology of Japan.

9. References

Aidinis, V., Plows, D., Haralambous, S., Armaka, M., Papadopoulos, P., Kanaki, M.Z., Koczan, D., Thiesen, H.J., & Kollias, G. (2003). Functional analysis of an arthritogenic synovial fibroblast. Arthritis Res Ther *5*, R140-157.

Aikawa, Y., Morimoto, K., Yamamoto, T., Chaki, H., Hashiramoto, A., Narita, H., Hirono, S., & Shiozawa, S. (2008). Treatment of arthritis with a selective inhibitor of c-Fos/activator protein-1. Nat Biotechnol *26*, 817-823.

Atsumi, T., Ishihara, K., Kamimura, D., Ikushima, H., Ohtani, T., Hirota, S., Kobayashi, H., Park, S.J., Saeki, Y., Kitamura, Y., *et al.* (2002). A point mutation of Tyr-759 in interleukin 6 family cytokine receptor subunit gp130 causes autoimmune arthritis. J Exp Med *196*, 979-990.

Babbage, G., Ottensmeier, C.H., Blaydes, J., Stevenson, F.K., & Sahota, S.S. (2006). Immunoglobulin heavy chain locus events and expression of activation-induced cytidine deaminase in epithelial breast cancer cell lines. Cancer Res *66*, 3996-4000.

Bartok, B., & Firestein, G.S. (2010). Fibroblast-like synoviocytes:key effector cells in rheumatoid arthritis. Immunol Rev *233*, 233-255.

Beekman, B., van El, B., Drijfhout, J.W., Ronday, H.K., & TeKoppele, J.M. (1997). Highly increased levels of active stromelysin in rheumatoid synovial fluid determined by a selective fluorogenic assay. FEBS Lett *418*, 305-309.

Wordsworth, B.P., Lanchbury, J.S., Sakkas, L.I., Welsh, K.I., Panayi, G.S., & Bell,J.I. (1989). HLA-DR4 subtype frequencies in rheumatoid arthritis indicate that DRB1 is the major susceptibility locus within the HLA class II region. Proc Natl Acad Sci U S A. *86*, 10049–10053.

Brennan, F.M., & McInnes, I.B. (2008). Evidence that cytokines play a role in rheumatoid arthritis. J Clin Invest *118*, 3537-3545.

Cha, H.S., Rosengren, S., Boyle, D.L., & Firestein, G.S. (2006). PUMA regulation and proapoptotic effects in fibroblast-like synoviocytes. Arthritis Rheum *54*, 587-592.

Chan-On, W., Kuwahara, K., Kobayashi, N., Ohta, K., Shimasaki, T., Sripa, B., Leelayuwat, C., & Sakaguchi, N. (2009). Cholangiocarcinomas associated with long-term inflammation express the activation-induced cytidine deaminase and germinal center-associated nuclear protein involved in immunoglobulin V-region diversification. Int J Oncol *35*, 287-295.

Cho, M.L., Cho, C.S., Min, S.Y., Kim, S.H., Lee, S.S., Kim, W.U., Min, D.J., Min, J.K., Youn, J., Hwang, S.Y., *et al.* (2002). Cyclosporine inhibition of vascular endothelial growth factor production in rheumatoid synovial fibroblasts. Arthritis Rheum *46*, 1202-1209.

Cui, J., Taylor, K.E., DeStefano, A.L., Criswell, L.A., Izmailova, E.S., Parker, A., Roubenoff, R., Plenge, R.M., Weinblatt, M.E., Shadick, N.A., *et al.* (2009). Genome-Wide

Association Study of Determinants of Anti-Cyclic Citrullinated Peptide Antibody Titer in Adults with Rheumatoid Arthritis. Molecular Medicine *15*, 136-143.

De Bari, C., Dell'Accio, F., Tylzanowski, P., & Luyten, F.P. (2001). Multipotent mesenchymal stem cells from adult human synovial membrane. Arthritis Rheum *44*, 1928-1942.

De Bari, C., Dell'Accio, F., Vanlauwe, J., Eyckmans, J., Khan, I.M., Archer, C.W., Jones, E.A., McGonagle, D., Mitsiadis, T.A., Pitzalis, C., *et al.* (2006). Mesenchymal multipotency of adult human periosteal cells demonstrated by single-cell lineage analysis. Arthritis Rheum *54*, 1209-1221.

Di Noia, J.M., & Neuberger, M.S. (2007). Molecular mechanisms of antibody somatic hypermutation. Annu Rev Biochem *76*, 1-22.

Dieguez-Gonzalez, R., Calaza, M., Perez-Pampin, E., Balsa, A., Blanco, F.J., Cañete, J.D., Caliz, R., Carreño, L., de la Serna, A.R., Fernandez-Gutierrez, B., *et al.* (2009). Analysis of TNFAIP3, a feedback inhibitor of nuclear factor-kappaB and the neighbor intergenic 6q23 region in rheumatoid arthritis susceptibility. Arthritis Res Ther *11*, R42.

Dixit, V.M., Green, S., Sarma, V., Holzman, L.B., Wolf, F.W., O'Rourke, K., Ward, P.A., Prochownik, E.V., & Marks, R.M. (1990). Tumor necrosis factor-alpha induction of novel gene products in human endothelial cells including a macrophage-specific chemotaxin. J Biol Chem *265*, 2973-2978.

Elsby, L. M., Orozco, G., Denton, J., Worthington, J., Ray, D. W., & Donn, R. P. (2010) Functional evaluation of TNFAIP3 (A20) in rheumatoid arthritis. Clin Exp Rheumatol *28*, 708-14.

Endo, H., Akahoshi, T., Nishimura, A., Tonegawa, M., Takagishi, K., Kashiwazaki, S., Matsushima, K., & Kondo, H. (1994). Experimental arthritis induced by continuous infusion of IL-8 into rabbit knee joints. Clin Exp Immunol *96*, 31-35.

Endo, Y., Marusawa, H., Kinoshita, K., Morisawa, T., Sakurai, T., Okazaki, I.M., Watashi, K., Shimotohno, K., Honjo, T., & Chiba, T. (2007). Expression of activation-induced cytidine deaminase in human hepatocytes via NF-kappaB signaling. Oncogene *26*, 5587-5595.

Endo, Y., Marusawa, H., Kou, T., Nakase, H., Fujii, S., Fujimori, T., Kinoshita, K., Honjo, T., & Chiba, T. (2008). Activation-induced cytidine deaminase links between inflammation and the development of colitis-associated colorectal cancers. Gastroenterology *135*, 889-898, 898 e881-883.

Firestein, G.S. (2009). 65, In: *Kelly's Textbook of Rheumatology,* Firestein,G.S, Budd, R.C., Harris, Jr. E.D., McInnes, I.B., Ruddy, S., Sergent, J.S., 1035-1086, SAUNDERS ELSEVIER, 978-1-4160-3285-4, Philadelphia

Firestein, G.S., Echeverri, F., Yeo, M., Zvaifler, N.J., & Green, D.R. (1997). Somatic mutations in the p53 tumor suppressor gene in rheumatoid arthritis synovium. Proc Natl Acad Sci U S A *94*, 10895-10900.

Firestein, G.S. (2007). Biomedicine. Every joint has a silver lining. Science *315*, 952-953.

Freudenberg, J., Lee, H.S., Han, B.G., Shin, H.D., Kang, Y.M., Sung, Y.K., Shim, S.C., Choi, C.B., Lee, A.T., Gregersen, P.K., *et al.* (2011). Genome-Wide Association Study of Rheumatoid Arthritis in Koreans. Arthritis and Rheumatism *63*, 884-893.

Galligan, C.L., Baig, E., Bykerk, V., Keystone, E.C., & Fish, E.N. (2007). Distinctive gene expression signatures in rheumatoid arthritis synovial tissue fibroblast cells: correlates with disease activity. Genes Immun *8*, 480-491.

Garcia-Vicuna, R., Gomez-Gaviro, M.V., Dominguez-Luis, M.J., Pec, M.K., Gonzalez-Alvaro, I., Alvaro-Gracia, J.M., & Diaz-Gonzalez, F. (2004). CC and CXC chemokine receptors mediate migration, proliferation, and matrix metalloproteinase production by fibroblast-like synoviocytes from rheumatoid arthritis patients. Arthritis Rheum *50*, 3866-3877.

Goila-Gaur, R., & Strebel, K. (2008). HIV-1 Vif, APOBEC, and intrinsic immunity. Retrovirology *5*, 51.

Gracie, J.A., Forsey, R.J., Chan, W.L., Gilmour, A., Leung, B.P., Greer, M.R., Kennedy, K., Carter, R., Wei, X.Q., Xu, D., *et al.* (1999). A proinflammatory role for IL-18 in rheumatoid arthritis. J Clin Invest *104*, 1393-1401.

Gudkov, A.V., & Komarova, E.A. (2010). Pathologies associated with the p53 response. Cold Spring Harb Perspect Biol 2:a001180

Han, Z., Boyle, D.L., Shi, Y., Green, D.R., & Firestein, G.S. (1999). Dominant-negative p53 mutations in rheumatoid arthritis. Arthritis Rheum *42*, 1088-1092.

Honjo, T., Muramatsu, M., & Fagarasan, S. (2004). AID: how does it aid antibody diversity? Immunity *20*, 659-668.

Horai, R., Saijo, S., Tanioka, H., Nakae, S., Sudo, K., Okahara, A., Ikuse, T., Asano, M., & Iwakura, Y. (2000). Development of chronic inflammatory arthropathy resembling rheumatoid arthritis in interleukin 1 receptor antagonist-deficient mice. J Exp Med *191*, 313-320.

Hosaka, S., Akahoshi, T., Wada, C., & Kondo, H. (1994). Expression of the chemokine superfamily in rheumatoid arthritis. Clin Exp Immunol *97*, 451-457.

Huet, G., Flipo, R.M., Colin, C., Janin, A., Hemon, B., Collyn-d'Hooghe, M., Lafyatis, R., Duquesnoy, B., & Degand, P. (1993). Stimulation of the secretion of latent cysteine proteinase activity by tumor necrosis factor alpha and interleukin-1. Arthritis Rheum *36*, 772-780.

Igarashi, H., Yahagi, A., Saika, T., Hashimoto, J., Tomita, T., Yoshikawa, H., & Ishihara, K. (2011). A pro-inflammatory role for A20 and ABIN family proteins in human fibroblast-like synoviocytes in rheumatoid arthritis. Immunol Lett., in press.

Igarashi, H., Hashimoto, J., Tomita, T., Yoshikawa, H., & Ishihara, K. (2010) TP53 mutations coincide with the ectopic expression of activation-induced cytidine deaminase in the fibroblast-like synoviocytes derived from a fraction of patients with rheumatoid arthritis. Clin Exp Immunol *161*, 71-80.

Inazuka, M., Tahira, T., Horiuchi, T., Harashima, S., Sawabe, T., Kondo, M., Miyahara, H., & Hayashi, K. (2000). Analysis of p53 tumor suppressor gene somatic mutations in rheumatoid arthritis synovium. Rheumatology *39*, 262-266.

Ishihara, K., Sawa, S., Ikushima, H., Hirota, S., Atsumi, T., Kamimura, D., Park, S.J., Murakami, M., Kitamura, Y., Iwakura, Y., & Hirano, T. (2004) The point mutation of tyrosine 759 of the IL-6 family cytokine receptor gp130 synergizes with HTLV-1 *pX* in promoting rheumatoid arthritis-like arthritis. Int Immunol *16*, 455-465.

Iwakura, Y., Tosu, M., Yoshida, E., Takiguchi, M., Sato, K., Kitajima, I., Nishioka, K., Yamamoto, K., Takeda, T., Hatanaka, M., *et al.* (1991). Induction of inflammatory arthropathy resembling rheumatoid arthritis in mice transgenic for HTLV-I. Science *253*, 1026-1028.

Iwamoto, T., Okamoto, H., Kobayashi, S., Ikari, K., Toyama, Y., Tomatsu, T., Kamatani, N., & Momohara, S. (2007). A role of monocyte chemoattractant protein-4 (MCP-4)/CCL13 from chondrocytes in rheumatoid arthritis. FEBS J *274,* 4904-4912.

Iwamoto, T., Okamoto, H., Toyama, Y., & Momohara, S. (2008). Molecular aspects of rheumatoid arhtiritis:chemokines in the joints of patients. FEBS J *275,* 4448-4455.

Jacob, R.A., Perrett, D., Axon, J.M., Herbert, K.E., Scott, D.L.(1995) Rheumatoid synovial cell proliferation, transformation and fibronectin secretion in culture. Clin Exp Rheumatol 13:717-723.

Jeong, J.G., Kim, J.M., Cho, H., Hahn, W., Yu, S.S., Kim, S.(2004) Effects of IL-1beta on gene expression in human rheumatoid synovial fibroblasts. Biochem Biophys Res Commun 324:3-7

Jones, E.A., English, A., Henshaw, K., Kinsey, S.E., Markham, A.F., Emery, P., & McGonagle, D. (2004). Enumeration and phenotypic characterization of synovial fluid multipotential mesenchymal progenitor cells in inflammatory and degenerative arthritis. Arthritis Rheum *50,* 817-827.

Joseph, L., Lapid, S., & Sukhatme, V. (1987). The major ras induced protein in NIH3T3 cells is cathepsin L. Nucleic Acids Res *15,* 3186.

Kasperkovitz, P.V., Timmer, T.C., Smeets, T.J., Verbeet, N.L., Tak, P.P., van Baarsen, L.G., Baltus, B., Huizinga, T.W., Pieterman, E., Fero, M., *et al.* (2005). Fibroblast-like synoviocytes derived from patients with rheumatoid arthritis show the imprint of synovial tissue heterogeneity: evidence of a link between an increased myofibroblast-like phenotype and high-inflammation synovitis. Arthritis Rheum *52,* 430-441.

Kawane, K., Ohtani, M., Miwa, K., Kizawa, T., Kanbara, Y., Yoshioka, Y., Yoshikawa, H., & Nagata, S. (2006). Chronic polyarthritis caused by mammalian DNA that escapes from degradation in macrophages. Nature *443,* 998-1002.

Kawane, K., Tanaka, H., Kitahara, Y., Shimaoka, S., & Nagata, S. (2010). Cytokine-dependent but acquired immunity- independent arthritis caused by DNA escaped from degradation. Proc Natl Acad Sci U S A *107,* 19432-19437.

Keffer, J., Probert, L., Cazlaris, H., Georgopoulos, S., Kaslaris, E., Kioussis, D., & Kollias, G. (1991). Transgenic mice expressing human tumour necrosis factor: a predictive genetic model of arthritis. EMBO J *10,* 4025-4031.

Kehlen, A., Thiele, K., Riemann, D., & Langner, J. (2002). Expression, modulation and signalling of IL-17 receptor in fibroblast-like synoviocytes of patients with rheumatoid arthritis. Clin Exp Immunol *127,* 539-546.

Keyszer, G.M., Heer, A.H., Kriegsmann, J., Geiler, T., Trabandt, A., Keysser, M., Gay, R.E., & Gay, S. (1995). Comparative analysis of cathepsin L, cathepsin D, and collagenase messenger RNA expression in synovial tissues of patients with rheumatoid arthritis and osteoarthritis, by in situ hybridization. Arthritis Rheum *38,* 976-984.

Keyszer, G., Redlich, A., Haupl, T., Zacher, J., Sparmann, M., Engethum, U., Gay, S., & Burmester, G.R. (1998). Differential expression of cathepsins B and L compared with matrix metalloproteinases and their respective inhibitors in rheumatoid arthritis and osteoarthritis: a parallel investigation by semiquantitative reverse transcriptase-polymerase chain reaction and immunohistochemistry. Arthritis Rheum *41,* 1378-1387.

Kitagawa, A., Miura, Y., Saura, R., Mitani, M., Ishikawa, H., Hashiramoto, A., Yoshiya, S., Shiozawa, S., & Kurosaka, M. (2006). Anchorage on fibronectin via VLA-5 (alpha5beta1 integrin) protects rheumatoid synovial cells from Fas-induced apoptosis. Ann Rheum Dis *65*, 721-727.

Ko, L. J., & Prives, C. (1996). p53: puzzle and paradigm. Genes Dev. *10*, 1054-1072.

Koch, A.E., Kunkel, S.L., Burrows, J.C., Evanoff, H.L., Haines, G.K., Pope, R.M., & Strieter, R.M. (1991). Synovial tissue macrophage as a source of the chemotactic cytokine IL-8. J Immunol *147*, 2187-2195.

Koch, A.E., Polverini, P.J., Kunkel, S.L., Harlow, L.A., DiPietro, L.A., Elner, V.M., Elner, S.G., & Strieter, R.M. (1992). Interleukin-8 as a macrophage-derived mediator of angiogenesis. Science *258*, 1798-1801.

Koch, A.E., Kunkel, S.L., Harlow, L.A., Mazarakis, D.D., Haines, G.K., Burdick, M.D., Pope, R.M., & Strieter, R.M. (1994). Macrophage inflammatory protein-1 alpha. A novel chemotactic cytokine for macrophages in rheumatoid arthritis. J Clin Invest *93*, 921-928.

Koch, A.E., Kunkel, S.L., Shah, M.R., Hosaka, S., Halloran, M.M., Haines, G.K., Burdick, M.D., Pope, R.M., & Strieter, R.M. (1995). Growth-related gene product alpha. A chemotactic cytokine for neutrophils in rheumatoid arthritis. J Immunol *155*, 3660-3666.

Kojima, F., Naraba, H., Sasaki, Y., Beppu, M., Aoki, H., & Kawai, S. (2003). Prostaglandin E2 is an enhancer of interleukin-1beta-induced expression of membrane-associated prostaglandin E synthase in rheumatoid synovial fibroblasts. Arthritis Rheum *48*, 2819-2828.

Komori, J., Marusawa, H., Machimoto, T., Endo, Y., Kinoshita, K., Kou, T., Haga, H., Ikai, I., Uemoto, S., & Chiba, T. (2008). Activation-induced cytidine deaminase links bile duct inflammation to human cholangiocarcinoma. Hepatology *47*, 888-896.

Kontoyiannis, D., Pasparakis, M., Pizarro, T.T., Cominelli, F., & Kollias, G. (1999). Impaired on/off regulation of TNF biosynthesis in mice lacking TNF AU-rich elements: implications for joint and gut-associated immunopathologies. Immunity *10*, 387-398.

Konttinen, Y.T., Ainola, M., Valleala, H., Ma, J., Ida, H., Mandelin, J., Kinne, R.W., Santavirta, S., Sorsa, T., Lopez-Otin, C., *et al.* (1999). Analysis of 16 different matrix metalloproteinases (MMP-1 to MMP-20) in the synovial membrane: different profiles in trauma and rheumatoid arthritis. Ann Rheum Dis *58*, 691-697.

Korb, A., Pavenstadt, H., & Pap, T. (2009). Cell death in rheumatoid arthritis. Apoptosis *14*, 447-454

Korganow, A.S., Ji, H., Mangialaio, S., Duchatelle, V., Pelanda, R., Martin, T., Degott, C., Kikutani, H., Rajewsky, K., Pasquali, J.L., *et al.* (1999). From systemic T cell self-reactivity to organ-specific autoimmune disease via immunoglobulins. Immunity *10*, 451-461.

Kou, T., Marusawa, H., Kinoshita, K., Endo, Y., Okazaki, I.M., Ueda, Y., Kodama, Y., Haga, H., Ikai, I., & Chiba, T. (2007). Expression of activation-induced cytidine deaminase in human hepatocytes during hepatocarcinogenesis. Int J Cancer *120*, 469-476.

Kullmann, F., Judex, M., Neudecker, I., Lechner, S., Justen, H.P., Green, D.R., Wessinghage, D., Firestein, G.S., Gay, S., Scholmerich, J., *et al.* (1999). Analysis of the p53 tumor suppressor gene in rheumatoid arthritis synovial fibroblasts. Arthritis Rheum *42*, 1594-1600.

Kuwana, M., Okazaki, Y., Kodama, H., Izumi, K., Yasuoka, H., Ogawa, Y., Kawakami Y., & Ikeda, Y. (2003). Human circulating CD14+ monocytes as a source of progenitors that exhibit mesenchymal cell differentiation. Leukoc Biol *74*, 833-845.

Lee, D.M., Kiener, H.P., Agarwal, S.K., Noss, E.H., Watts, G.F., Chisaka, O., Takeichi, M., Brenner, M.B. (2007). Cadherin-11 in synovial lining formation and pathology in arthritis. Science *315*, 1006-1010.

Lefevre, S., Knedla, A., Tennie, C., Kampmann, A., Wunrau, C., Dinser, R., Korb, A., Schnaker, E.M., Tarner, I.H., Robbins, P.D., *et al.* (2009). Synovial fibroblasts spread rheumatoid arthritis to unaffected joints. Nat Med *15*, 1414-1420.

Lemaire, R., Huet, G., Zerimech, F., Grard, G., Fontaine, C., Duquesnoy, B., & Flipo, R.M. (1997). Selective induction of the secretion of cathepsins B and L by cytokines in synovial fibroblast-like cells. Br J Rheumatol *36*, 735-743.

Li, X., Makarov, S. S. (2006). An essential role of NF-kappaB in the "tumor-like" phenotype of arthritic synoviocytes. Proc Natl Acad Sci U S A *103*, 17432-17437.

Lindberg, J., af Klint, E., Catrina, A. I., Nilsson, P., Klareskog, L., Ulfgren, A. K., & Lundeberg, J. (2006). Effect of infliximab on mRNA expression profiles in synovial tissue of rheumatoid arthritis patients. Arthritis Res Ther *8*, R179.

Lindy, O., Konttinen, Y.T., Sorsa, T., Ding, Y., Santavirta, S., Ceponis, A., & Lopez-Otin, C. (1997). Matrix metalloproteinase 13 (collagenase 3) in human rheumatoid synovium. Arthritis Rheum *40*, 1391-1399.

Liu, C.Y., Batliwalla, F., Li, W.T., Lee, A., Roubenoff, R., Beckman, E., Khalili, H., Damle, A., Kern, M., Furie, R., *et al.* (2008). Genome-wide association scan identifies candidate polymorphisms associated with differential response to anti-TNF treatment in rheumatoid arthritis. Molecular Medicine *14*, 575-581.

Maeda, S., Sawai, T., Uzuki, M., Takahashi, Y., Omoto, H., Seki, M., & Sakurai, M. (1995). Determination of interstitial collagenase (MMP-1) in patients with rheumatoid arthritis. Ann Rheum Dis *54*, 970-975.

Manicourt, D.H., Fujimoto, N., Obata, K., & Thonar, E.J. (1995). Levels of circulating collagenase, stromelysin-1, and tissue inhibitor of matrix metalloproteinases 1 in patients with rheumatoid arthritis. Relationship to serum levels of antigenic keratan sulfate and systemic parameters of inflammation. Arthritis Rheum *38*, 1031-1039.

Martin, J.E., Alizadeh, B.Z., Gonzalez-Gay, M.A., Balsa, A., Pascual-Salcedo, D., Fernandez-Gutierrez, B., Raya, E., Franke, L., van't Slot, R., Coenen, M.J.H., *et al.* (2010). Identification of the Oxidative Stress-Related Gene MSRA as a Rheumatoid Arthritis Susceptibility Locus by Genome-Wide Pathway Analysis. Arthritis and Rheumatism *62*, 3183-3190.

Min, D.J., Cho, M.L., Lee, S.H., Min, S.Y., Kim, W.U., Min, J.K., Park, S.H., Cho, C.S., & Kim, H.Y. (2004). Augmented production of chemokines by the interaction of type II collagen-reactive T cells with rheumatoid synovial fibroblasts. Arthritis Rheum *50*, 1146-1155.

Miranda-Carus, M.E., Balsa, A., Benito-Miguel, M., Perez de Ayala, C., & Martin-Mola, E. (2004). IL-15 and the initiation of cell contact-dependent synovial fibroblast-T lymphocyte cross-talk in rheumatoid arthritis: effect of methotrexate. J Immunol *173*, 1463-1476.

Mor, A., Abramson, S.B., & Pillimger, M.H. (2005). The fibroblast-like synovial cell in rheumatoid arthritis: a key player in inflammation and joint destruction. Clin Immunol *115*, 118-128.

Morisawa, T., Marusawa, H., Ueda, Y., Iwai, A., Okazaki, I.M., Honjo, T., & Chiba, T. (2008). Organ-specific profiles of genetic changes in cancers caused by activation-induced cytidine deaminase expression. Int J Cancer *123*, 2735-2740.

Muller-Ladner, U., Gay, R.E., & Gay, S. (2000). Activation of synoviocytes. Curr Opin Rheumatol *12*, 186-194.

Muller-Ladner, U., Kriegsmann, J., Franklin, B.N., Matsumoto, S., Geiler, T., Gay, R.E., & Gay, S. (1996). Synovial fibroblasts of patients with rheumatoid arthritis attach to and invade normal human cartilage when engrafted into SCID mice. Am J Pathol *149*, 1607-1615.

Murakami, M., Okuyama, Y., Ogura, H., Asano, S., Arima, Y., Tsuruoka, M., Harada, M., Kanamoto, M., Sawa, Y., Iwakura, Y., *et al.* (2011). Local microbleeding facilitates IL-6- and IL-17-dependent arthritis in the absence of tissue antigen recognition by activated T cells. J Exp Med *208*, 103-114.

Nanki, T., Hayashida, K., El-Gabalawy, H.S., Suson, S., Shi, K., Girschick, H.J., Yavuz, S., & Lipsky, P.E. (2000). Stromal cell-derived factor-1-CXC chemokine receptor 4 interactions play a central role in CD4+ T cell accumulation in rheumatoid arthritis synovium. J Immunol *165*, 6590-6598.

Niki, Y., Yamada, H., Seki, S., Kikuchi, T., Takaishi, H., Toyama, Y., Fujikawa, K., & Tada, N. (2001). Macrophage- and neutrophil-dominant arthritis in human IL-1 alpha transgenic mice. J Clin Invest *107*, 1127-1135.

Nishimoto, N., & Kishimoto, T. (2006). Interleukin 6: from bench to bedside. Nat Clin Pract Rheumatol 2, 619-626.

Ogura, H., Murakami, M., Okuyama, Y., Tsuruoka, M., Kitabayashi, C., Kanamoto, M., Nishihara, M., Iwakura, Y., & Hirano, T. (2008). Interleukin-17 promotes autoimmunity by triggering a positive-feedback loop via interleukin-6 induction. Immunity *29*, 628-636.

Ohshima, S., Mima, T., Sasai, M., Nishioka, K., Shimizu, M., Murata, N., Yoshikawa, H., Nakanishi, K., Suemura, M., McCloskey, R.V., *et al.* (2000). Tumour necrosis factor alpha (TNF-alpha) interferes with Fas-mediated apoptotic cell death on rheumatoid arthritis (RA) synovial cells: a possible mechanism of rheumatoid synovial hyperplasia and a clinical benefit of anti-TNF-alpha therapy for RA. Cytokine *12*, 281-288.

Ohtani, T., Ishihara, K., Atsumi, T., Nishida, K., Kaneko, Y., Miyata, T., Itoh, S., Narimatsu, M., Maeda, H., Fukada, T., *et al.* (2000). Dissection of signaling cascades through gp130 in vivo: reciprocal roles for STAT3- and SHP2-mediated signals in immune responses. Immunity *12*, 95-105.

Okada, Y.(2009). 7, In: *Kelly's Textbook of Rheumatology,* Firestein,G.S, Budd, R.C., Harris, Jr. E.D., McInnes, I.B., Ruddy, S., Sergent, J.S., 115-134, SAUNDERS ELSEVIER, 978-1-4160-3285-4, Philadelphia.

Orozco, G., Hinks, A., Eyre, S., Ke, X., Gibbons, L.J., Bowes, J., Flynn, E., Martin, P., Wilson, A.G., Bax, D.E., Morgan, A.W., Emery, P., Steer, S., Hocking, L., Reid, D.M., Wordsworth, P., Harrison, P., Thomson, W., Barton, A., Worthington, J. (2009).

Combined effects of three independent SNPs greatly increase the risk estimate for RA at 6q23. Hum Mol Genet *18*, 2693-2699.

Pap, T., Shigeyama, Y., Kuchen, S., Fernihough, J.K., Simmen, B., Gay, R.E., Billingham, M., Gay, S. (2000a). Differential expression pattern of membrane-type matrix metalloproteinases in rheumatoid arthritis. Arthritis Rheum *43*, 1226–1232.

Pap, T., Franz, J.K., Hummel, K.M., Jeisy, E., Gay, R., & Gay, S. (2000b). Activation of synovial fibroblasts in rheumatoid arthritis: lack of Expression of the tumour suppressor PTEN at sites of invasive growth and destruction. Arthritis Res *2*, 59-64.

Pap, T., Nawrath, M., Heinrich, J., Bosse, M., Baier, A., Hummel, K.M., Petrow, P., Kuchen, S., Michel, B.A., Gay, R.E., *et al.* (2004). Cooperation of Ras- and c-Myc-dependent pathways in regulating the growth and invasiveness of synovial fibroblasts in rheumatoid arthritis. Arthritis Rheum *50*, 2794-2802.

Pap,T., & Gay, S. (2009). 11, In: *Kelly's Textbook of Rheumatology,* Firestein,G.S, Budd, R.C., Harris, Jr. E.D., McInnes, I.B., Ruddy, S., Sergent, J.S., 201-214, SAUNDERS ELSEVIER, 978-1-4160-3285-4, Philadelphia.

Pauklin, S., Sernandez, I.V., Bachmann, G., Ramiro, A.R., & Petersen-Mahrt, S.K. (2009). Estrogen directly activates AID transcription and function. J Exp Med *206*, 99-111.

Pierer, M., Muller-Ladner, U., Pap, T., Neidhart, M., Gay, R.E., & Gay, S. (2003). The SCID mouse model: novel therapeutic targets - lessons from gene transfer. Springer Semin Immunopathol *25*, 65-78.

Plant, D., Bowes, J., Potter, C., Hyrich, K.L., Morgan, A.W., Wilson, A.G., Isaacs, J.D.,;Wellcome Trust Case Control Consortium; British Soc Rheumatology Biologics Register, & Barton, A.(2011). Genome-Wide Association Study of Genetic Predictors of Anti-Tumor Necrosis Factor Treatment Efficacy in Rheumatoid Arthritis Identifies Associations With Polymorphisms at Seven Loci. Arthritis and Rheumatism *63*, 645-653.

Pohlers, D., Beyer, A., Koczan, D., Wilhelm, T., Thiesen, H.J., & Kinne, R.W. (2007). Constitutive upregulation of the transforming growth factor-□ pathway in rheumatoid arthritis synovial fibroblasts. Arthritis Res Ther *9*, R59.

Pritchard, J., Tsui, S., Horst, N., Cruikshank, W.W., & Smith, T.J. (2004). Synovial fibroblasts from patients with rheumatoid arthritis, like fibroblasts from Graves' disease, express high levels of IL-16 when treated with Igs against insulin-like growth factor-1 receptor. J Immunol *173*, 3564-3569.

Rathanaswami, P., Hachicha, M., Sadick, M., Schall, T.J., & McColl, S.R. (1993). Expression of the cytokine RANTES in human rheumatoid synovial fibroblasts. Differential regulation of RANTES and interleukin-8 genes by inflammatory cytokines. J Biol Chem *268*, 5834-5839.

Reme, T., Travaglio, A., Gueydon, E., Adla, L., Jorgensen, C., & Sany, J. (1998). Mutations of the p53 tumour suppressor gene in erosive rheumatoid synovial tissue. Clin Exp Immunol *111*, 353-358.

Robinson, E., Keystone, E.C., Schall, T.J., Gillett, N., & Fish, E.N. (1995). Chemokine expression in rheumatoid arthritis (RA): evidence of RANTES and macrophage inflammatory protein (MIP)-1 beta production by synovial T cells. Clin Exp Immunol *101*, 398-407.

Roivainen, A., Pirila, L., Yli-Jama, T., Laaksonen, H., & Toivanen, P. (1999). Expression of the myc-family proto-oncogenes and related genes max and mad in synovial tissue. Scand J Rheumatol *28*, 314-318.

Sakaguchi, N., Takahashi, T., Hata, H., Nomura, T., Tagami, T., Yamazaki, S., Sakihama, T., Matsutani, T., Negishi, I., Nakatsuru, S., *et al.* (2003). Altered thymic T-cell selection due to a mutation of the ZAP-70 gene causes autoimmune arthritis in mice. Nature *426*, 454-460.

Salcedo, R., Wasserman, K., Young, H.A., Grimm, M.C., Howard, O.M., Anver, M.R., Kleinman, H.K., Murphy, W.J., & Oppenheim, J.J. (1999). Vascular endothelial growth factor and basic fibroblast growth factor induce expression of CXCR4 on human endothelial cells: In vivo neovascularization induced by stromal-derived factor-1alpha. Am J Pathol *154*, 1125-1135.

Salcedo, R., Ponce, M.L., Young, H.A., Wasserman, K., Ward, J.M., Kleinman, H.K., Oppenheim, J.J., & Murphy, W.J. (2000). Human endothelial cells express CCR2 and respond to MCP-1: direct role of MCP-1 in angiogenesis and tumor progression. Blood *96*, 34-40.

Sawa, S., Kamimura, D., Jin, G.H., Morikawa, H., Kamon, H., Nishihara, M., Ishihara, K., Murakami, M., & Hirano, T. (2006). Autoimmune arthritis associated with mutated interleukin (IL)-6 receptor gp130 is driven by STAT3/IL-7-dependent homeostatic proliferation of CD4+ T cells. J Exp Med *203*, 1459-1470.

Scott, B.B., Zaratin, P.F., Colombo, A., Hansbury, M.J., Winkler, J.D., & Jackson, J.R. (2002). Constitutive expression of angiopoietin-1 and -2 and modulation of their expression by inflammatory cytokines in rheumatoid arthritis synovial fibroblasts. J Rheumatol *29*, 230-239.

Szekanecz, Z., & Koch, A.E. (2007). Mechanisms of Disease: angiogenesis in inflammatory diseases. Nat Clin Pract Rheumatol *3*, 635-643.

Sorsa, T., Konttinen, Y.T., Lindy, O., Ritchlin, C., Saari, H., Suomalainen, K., Eklund, K.K., & Santavirta, S. (1992). Collagenase in synovitis of rheumatoid arthritis. Semin Arthritis Rheum *22*, 44-53.

Stahl, E.A., Raychaudhuri, S., Remmers, E.F., Xie, G., Eyre, S., Thomson, B.P., Li, Y.H., Kurreeman, F.A.S., Zhernakova, A., Hinks, A., *et al.* (2010). Genome-wide association study meta-analysis identifies seven new rheumatoid arthritis risk loci. Nature Genetics *42*, 508-U556.

Sugino, H., Lee, H.M., & Nishimoto, N. (2010). DNA microarray analysis of rheumatoid arthritis susceptibility genes identified by genome-wide association studies. Arthritis Res Ther *12*, 401.

Sun, Y., Zeng, X.R., Wenger, L., Firestein, G.S., & Cheung, H.S. (2004). P53 down-regulates matrix metalloproteinase-1 by targeting the communications between AP-1 and the basal transcription complex. J Cell Biochem *92*, 258-269.

Suzuki A, Yamada R, Chang X, Tokuhiro S, Sawada T, Suzuki M, Nagasaki M, Nakayama-Hamada M, Kawaida R, Ono M, *et al.* (2003). Functional haplotypes of PADI4, encoding citrullinating enzyme peptidylarginine deiminase 4, are associated with rheumatoid arthritis. Nat Genet *34*, 395-402.

Takai, A., Toyoshima, T., Uemura, M., Kitawaki, Y., Marusawa, H., Hiai, H., Yamada, S., Okazaki, I.M., Honjo, T., Chiba, T., *et al.* (2009). A novel mouse model of hepatocarcinogenesis triggered by AID causing deleterious p53 mutations. Oncogene *28*, 469-478.

Tamiya, G., Shinya, M., Imanishi, T., Ikuta, T., Makino, S., Okamoto, K., Furugaki, K., Matsumoto, T., Mano, S., Ando, S., *et al.* (2005). Whole genome association study of rheumatoid arthritis using 27 039 microsatellites. Human Molecular Genetics *14*, 2305-2321.

Taylor, D.J., Cheung, N.T., & Dawes, P.T. (1994). Increased serum proMMP-3 in inflammatory arthritides: a potential indicator of synovial inflammatory monokine activity. Ann Rheum Dis *53*, 768-772.

Tetlow, L.C., Lees, M., Ogata, Y., Nagase, H., and Woolley, D.E. (1993). Differential expression of gelatinase B (MMP-9) and stromelysin-1 (MMP-3) by rheumatoid synovial cells in vitro and in vivo. Rheumatol Int *13*, 53-59.

Thomas, J.W., Thieu, T.H., Byrd, V.M., & Miller, G.G. (2000). Acidic fibroblast growth factor in synovial cells. Arthritis Rheum *43*, 2152-2159.

Tolboom, T.C., Pieterman, E., van der Laan, W.H., Toes, R., Huidekoper, A., Nelissen, R., Breedveld, F., & Huizinga, T. (2002). Invasive properties of fibroblast-like synoviocytes: correlation with growth characteristics and expression of MMP-1, MMP-3, and MMP-10.Ann Rheum Dis 61:975-980.

van Baarsen, L.G., Wijbrandts, C.A., Timmer, T.C., van der Pouw Kraan, T.C., Tak, P.P., & Verweij, C.L. (2010). Synovial tissue heterogeneity in rheumatoid arthritis in relation to disease activity and biomarkers in peripheral blood. Arthritis Rheum *62*, 1602-1607.

van der Pouw Kraan, T.C., van Gaalen, F.A., Kasperkovitz, P.V., Verbeet, N.L., Smeets, T.J., Kraan, M.C., Fero, M., Tak, P.P., Huizinga, T.W., Pieterman, E., Breedveld, F.C., Alizadeh, A.A., & Verweij, C.L.(2003). Rheumatoid arthritis is a heterogeneous disease: evidence for differences in the activation of the STAT-1 pathway between rheumatoid tissues. Arthritis Rheum *48*, 2132-2145.

Vereecke, L., Beyaert, R., & van Loo, G. (2009). The ubiquitin-editing enzyme A20 (TNFAIP3) is a central regulator of immunopathology. Trend Immunol *30*, 383-391.

Volin, M.V., Woods, J.M., Amin, M.A., Connors, M.A., Harlow, L.A., & Koch, A.E. (2001). Fractalkine: a novel angiogenic chemokine in rheumatoid arthritis. Am J Pathol *159*, 1521-1530.

Wakisaka, S., Suzuki, N., Takeba, Y., Shimoyama, Y., Nagafuchi, H., Takeno, M., Saito, N., Yokoe, T., Kaneko, A., Asai, T., *et al.* (1998). Modulation by proinflammatory cytokines of Fas/Fas ligand-mediated apoptotic cell death of synovial cells in patients with rheumatoid arthritis (RA). Clin Exp Immunol *114*, 119-128.

Wang, C.R., Liu, M.F., Huang, Y.H., & Chen, H.C. (2004). Up-regulation of XCR1 expression in rheumatoid joints. Rheumatology *43*, 569-573.

Westhoff, C.S., Freudiger, D., Petrow, P., Seyfert, C., Zacher, J., Kriegsmann, J., Pap, T., Gay, S., Stiehl, P., Gromnica-Ihle, E., *et al.* (1999). Characterization of collagenase 3 (matrix metalloproteinase 13) messenger RNA expression in the synovial membrane and synovial fibroblasts of patients with rheumatoid arthritis. Arthritis Rheum *42*, 1517-1527.

Weyand, C.M., Hicok, K.C., Conn, D.L., Goronzy, J.J. (1992). The influence of HLA-DRB1 genes on disease severity in rheumatoid arthritis. Ann Intern Med *117*,801-6.

Wijbrandts, C.A., Dijkgraaf, M.G., Kraan, M.C., Vinkenoog, M., Smeets, T.J., Dinant, H., Vos, K., Lems, W.F., Wolbink, G.J., *et al.* (2008).The clinical response to infliximab in rheumatoid arthritis is in part dependent on pretreatment tumour necrosis factor alpha expression in the synovium. Ann Rheum Dis *67*, 1139-1144.

Yamanishi, Y., Boyle, D.L., Rosengren, S., Green, D.R., Zvaifler, N.J., & Firestein, G.S. (2002). Regional analysis of p53 mutations in rheumatoid arthritis synovium. Proc Natl Acad Sci U S A *99*, 10025-10030.

Yamanishi, Y., Boyle, D.L., Green, D.R., Keystone, E.C., Connor, A., Zollman, S., & Firestein, G.S. (2005). p53 tumor suppressor gene mutations in fibroblast-like synoviocytes from erosion synovium and non-erosion synovium in rheumatoid arthritis. Arthritis Res Ther *7*, R12-18.

Yoshihara, Y., Obata, K., Fujimoto, N., Yamashita, K., Hayakawa, T., & Shimmei, M. (1995). Increased levels of stromelysin-1 and tissue inhibitor of metalloproteinases-1 in sera from patients with rheumatoid arthritis. Arthritis Rheum *38*, 969-975.

Zhernakova, A., Stahl, E.A., Trynka, G., Raychaudhuri, S., Festen, E.A., Franke, L., Westra, H.J., Fehrmann, R.S.N., Kurreeman, F.A.S., Thomson, B., *et al.* (2011). Meta-Analysis of Genome-Wide Association Studies in Celiac Disease and Rheumatoid Arthritis Identifies Fourteen Non-HLA Shared Loci. Plos Genetics *7*.

Zimmermann, T., Kunisch, E., Pfeiffer, R., Hirth, A., Stahl, H. D., Sack, U., Laube, A., Liesaus, E., Roth, A., Palombo-Kinne, E., Emmrich, F., & Kinne, R. W. (2001).Isolation and characterization of rheumatoid arthritis synovial fibroblasts from primary culture--primary culture cells markedly differ from fourth-passage cells. Arthritis Res *3*, 72-76.

Zuk, P.A., Zhu, M., Ashjian, P., De Ugarte, D.A., Huang, J.I., Mizuno, H., Alfonso, Z.C., Fraser, J.K., Benhaim, P., & Hedrick, M.H. (2002). Human adipose tissue is a source of multipotent stem cells. Mol Biol Cell *13*, 4279-4295.

Zvaifler, N. J., Marinova-Mutafchieva, L., Adams, G., Edwards, C. J., Moss, J., Burger, J. A., & Maini, R. N. (2000). Mesenchymal precursor cells in the blood of normal individuals. Arthritis Res *2*, 477-488.

6

Lysosomal Glycosidases in Degradation of Human Articular Cartilage

Janusz Popko[1], Tomasz Guszczyn[1], Sławomir Olszewski[1], Krzysztof Zwierz[2]
[1]*Medical University, Białystok,*
[2]*Medical College of the Universal Education Society, Łomza,*
Poland

1. Introduction

Joint diseases cause serious medical problems for several million people world-wide and therefore the World Health Organization has designated years 2000-2010 as the Decade of the Bone and Joint (Popko et al.2011).

Osteoarthritis (OA) is the most common, and increasingly prevalent, human joint disorder (Dieppe, 2000). It has been estimated that in 1990 12 % of Americans, nearly 21 million people had clinical symptoms of osteoarthritis (Lawrence et al., 1998).

Rheumatoid arthritis (RA) affects about 0.3 to 1.5% of the world population(Chikanza et.al., 1998). Juvenile idiopatic arthritis (JIA) is one of the most common rheumatic diseases in children, which causes pain and functional disability. According to a 2008 study performed by the National Arthritis Data Workgroup, there were close to 3000,000 children in the U.S.A. with some form of juvenile arthritis (Giannini et al., 2010).

Lyme arthritis (LA) caused by spirochete Borrelia burgdorferi, is increasing in prevalence disease involving the musculoskeletal system, particularly affecting knee joints (Pancewicz et. al.2009).

RA and JIA are chronic autoimmune inflammatory diseases primarily affecting the synovial membrane, leading to joint damage and destruction. OA is the most common joint disorder and a major public health problem in western populations (Lawrence et al. 1998).

Clinical and epidemiological studies on OA have recognized a series of etiologic factors including local factors (such as malformations or joint injuries) and systemic factors (such as overweight, race, gender, or metabolic diseases). OA is associated with a loss of proper balance between synthesis and degradation of the macromolecules that gives articular cartilage its biomechanical and functional properties. Concomitantly in OA, changes occur in the structure and metabolism of the synovium and subchondral bone of the joint.

2. Degradation of human articular cartilage

Progressive destruction of articular cartilage is a common feature of OA, RA, and LA. The articular cartilage from patients with OA and RA has decreased concentrations of proteoglycans and glycosaminoglycans (GAGs), and the size of GAG molecules is also reduced (Inerot et al.1978). In established joint disease, loss of articular proteoglycans could be more significant than the collagen loss (Mankin & Lippiello, 1970; Popko et al. 1983). Destruction of articular cartilage is a multifactorial process, which is performed extracellularly by concerted action of matrix metalloproteinases (MMPs) and glycosidases (Fig.1).

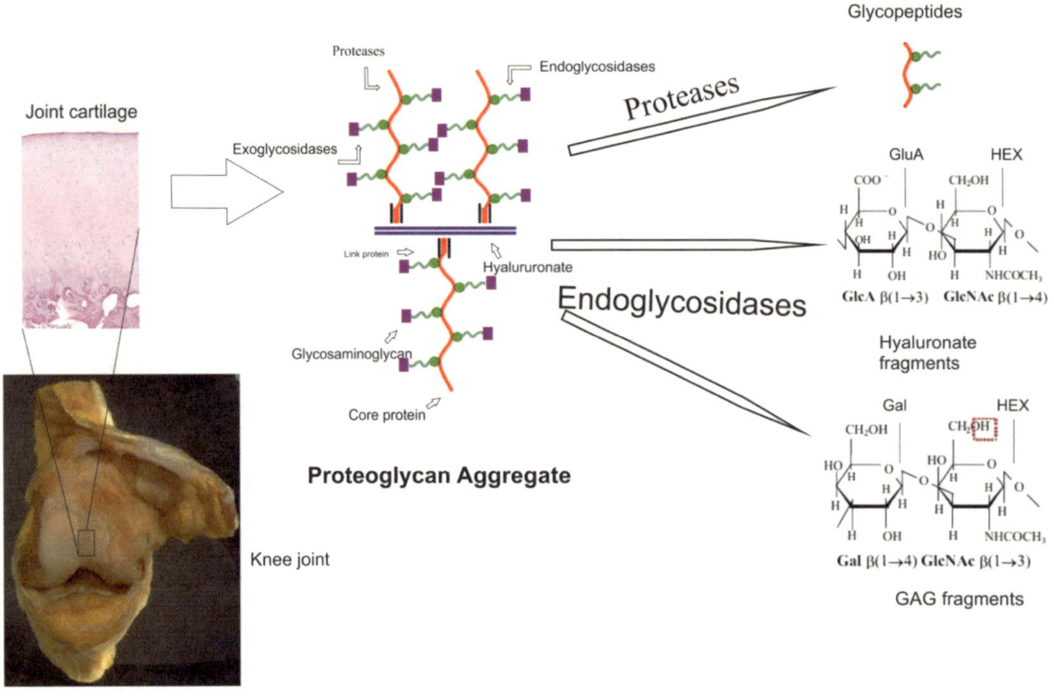

Fig. 1. Cartilage destruction by proteases and glycosidases.

Of the metalloproteinases, collagenase (MMP-1) in particular, appears to be responsible for the degradation of interstitial collagens. The gelatinases (MMP-2 and MMP-9) degrade the denatured forms of collagens, acting in synergy with MMP-1. The stromelysins (MMP-3) have broader substrate specificity for non-connective tissue proteins. Membrane-type MMPs (MT-MMP-1 and MT-MMP-3) have been detected at sites of destruction in rheumatoid arthritis (Pap et al., 2000).

Protease action increases the accessibility of cleavage sites for endo- and exoglycosidases (Ortutay et al. 2003) by production glycopeptides (Fig.1).

Endoglycosidases (hyaluronidases, chondroitinases, keratanases,etc.) cleave glycosidic linkages inside glycosaminoglycan or oligosaccharide chains of the proteoglycans or release oligosaccharide chains from protein cores (Stypułkowska et al. 2004).

In contrast to endoglycosidases, lysosomal exoglycosidases: N-acetyl-β-hexosaminidase (HEX), β-galactosidase (GAL), β-glucuronidase (GluA), α-mannosidase (MAN) and α-fucosidase (FUC), release monosaccharides from the non-reducing terminals of oligosaccharide chains of glycoproteins, glycolipids and proteoglycan glycosaminoglycans of synovial tissue, articular cartilage and synovial fluid. N-acetyl-β-hexosaminidase (HEX) is present as two isoenzymes HEX A and HEX B which both release terminal N-acetylhexosamines, whereas HEX A also hydrolyzes hexosamines in acidic oligosaccharides as in G_{M2} gangliosidases (Zwierz et al. 1999; Pennybacker et al. 1996; Sharma et al. 2003; Itakura et al. 2006). β-galactosidase (GAL) releases terminal galactose (Czartoryska 1977), from the non reducing terminal of oligosaccharide chains of glycoproteins, glycolipids and keratan sulfate. Mannose is liberated from N-linked sugar chains of glycoproteins, as well as a variety of synthetic and natural β-mannosides, by α-mannosidase (MAN) (Czartoryska 1977). Lysosomal α-fucosidase (FUC)) (Li,C.,Qian et al. 2006) is involved in the degradation a variety of fucose-containing oligosaccharide chains of glycoproteins and glycolipids and β-glucuronidase (GluA) cleaves glucuronic acid residues from the non-reducing terminal of glycosaminoglycans (GAGs) (Marciniak et al. 2006).

3. The characterization and function of lysosomal glycosidases

The main exoglycosidases in tissues, serum and synovial fluid of humans are:
N-acetyl-β-hexosaminidase (HEX), β-glucuronidase (GluA), β-galactosidase (GAL), α-mannosidase (α-MAN), and α-fucosidase (FUC). N-acetyl-β-hexosaminidase (EC 3.2.1.52, HEX, NAG) is the most active enzyme of the lysosomal exoglycosidases (Popko et al. 2006). HEX has several isoenzymes: A, B, S, C, I_1, I_2. HEX A and S are thermolabile and B, P, I_1, I_2, thermostable. In humans there are two major isoenzymes of hexosaminidase: HEX A (αβ), and HEX B (ββ). Both isoenzymes recognize terminal N-acetylglucosamine and N-acetylgalactosamine, but only HEX A recognizes 6-sulfated residues of these sugars. HEX A represents (an average) 48% of total HEX activity in serum, and 52% of total HEX activity in synovial fluid (Popko et. al.2006).
The hexosaminidase S (HEX S) is of minor importance, as it constitutes less than 0.02% of HEX activity (Ikonne et al. 1975)), and can be detected in patients with Sandhoff disease (Yamanak et al. 2001). The function of the HEX S is not well understood, but it is probably involved in the degradation of GAGs.
The protein moiety of lysosomal exoglycosidases is synthesized in the rough endoplasmic reticulum, and transported to lysosomes thought the endoplasmatic reticulum and Golgi apparatus (Zwierz et al.1999). Some of the lysosomal enzymes are secreted from the cell into the extracellular fluid. Another route for the secretion of lysosomal enzymes is from the lysosomes via the endosomes and Golgi compartment to the cell surface and extracellular fluid. The release of exoglycosidases is regulated by a small Ras-related GTP-binding protein Rho p21 (Rho proteins control the polymerization of actin into filaments and govern the organization of body filaments into specific types of structures). The release of exoglycosidases from mast cells has shown to be induced by an IgE mediated increase in intracellular Ca^{2+} (Zwierz et al. 1999).
Exoglycosidases activity of knee synovial fluid and serum of healthy humans is presented in Fig. 2.
The exoglycosidases activity, is higher in synovial fluid than in serum. Levels of the HEX activity are constant in serum of healthy humans up to 40 years of age, whereas in older people (more than 40 years of age) the level of HEX activity significantly increases.
The substrates for exoglycosidases in articular cartilage include cell surface and extracellular matrix glycoproteins as well as glycosaminoglycans: chondroitin 4-sulfate, chondroitin 6-sulfate, hyaluronic acid, keratin sulfate, and dermatan sulfate (Winchester 1996; Stypułkowska et al. 2004).

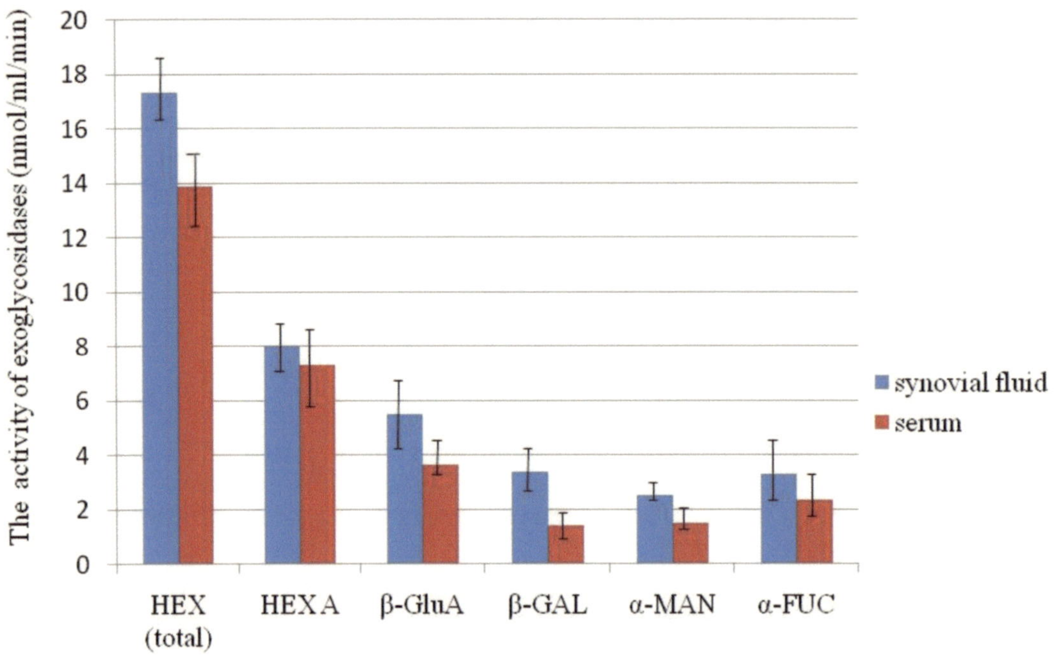

Fig. 2. Activity of exoglycosidases (nmol/ml/min) in synovial fluid and serum of healthy humans.

Exoglycosidases degrade glucoconjugates within the lysosome at an optimum pH ranging from 4.3 to 5.5 (Zwierz et. al. 1989; Marciniak et. al. 2006). Investigation of the pH dependence showed that HEX is active at pH 4.2 to 5.6 with optimum at pH 4.7, and β-glucuronidase is active between pH 3.4 and 5.6, with optimum activity at pH 4.5 (Marciniak et al. 2006).

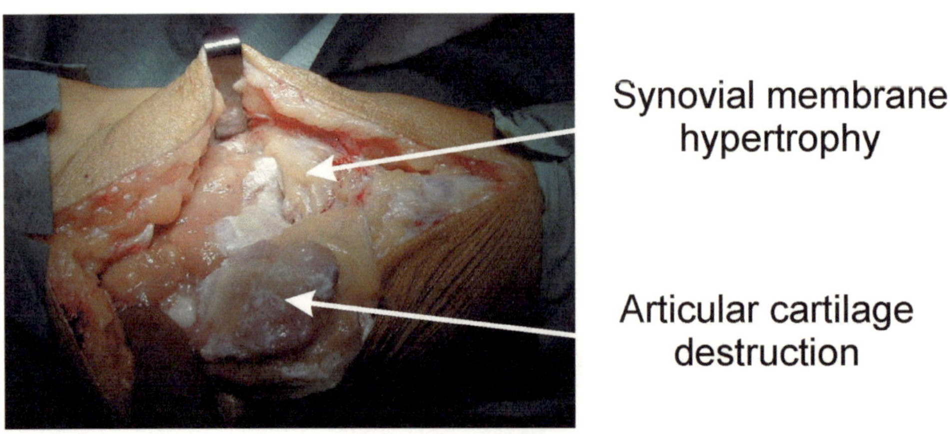

Fig. 3. Typical knee of a patient with RA. Showing destruction areas of articular cartilage and hypertrophy of synovial membrane.

4. The localization of exoglycosidases in joint tissues

Pugh and Walker (Pugh 1961), using histochemical techniques, reported that the source of HEX activity in synovial fluid is from cells of the synovial membrane. Others (Shikhman et al. 2000; Ortutay et. al. 2003) have suggested that chondrocytes of RA patients activated by IL 1β (interleukin-1β) may be a source of HEX activity in synovial fluid. Relating to this, it has been observed that damage to the joint reduces the volume of cartilage and increases a proliferation of synovial membrane (Fig. 3).
Profiles of the exoglycosidases in the synovial membrane of the knee joint of patients with RA, JIA and a control group are presented in Fig. 4.

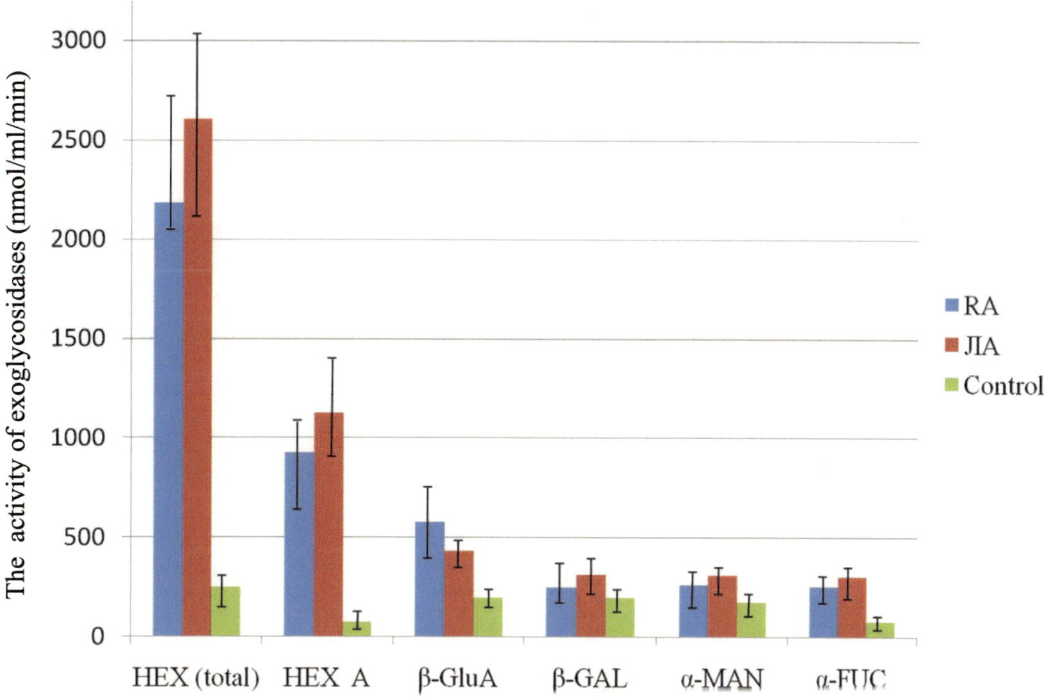

Fig. 4. The activity of exoglycosidases in the synovial tissue of the knee joint of patients with RA and JIA.

Normal and inflamed synovial tissues have similar patterns of exoglycosidases activity with a significant predominance of HEX activity (Popko et.al.2006). HEX activity in the synovial tissue of RA and JIA patients was approximately 10-fold higher than in the synovial tissue of the reference group. The increase in activity of GluA, GAL, MAN and FUC in synovial tissue of RA and JIA patients (in comparison with reference groups) was moderate, i.e. no more than doubled.
Synovial fibroblast-like cells and chondrocytes may be regarded as a source of mediators of joint destruction in RA and JIA. Synoviocytes and chondrocytes secrete proteolytic enzymes and exoglycosidases, especially HEX, that are crucial for the degradation of cartilage. The destructive phenotypes of the synovial fibroblasts-like cell and chondrocytes in RA are probably regulated by inflammatory cytokines released by the pannus connected to the cartilage.

The high activity of exoglycosidases in synovial tissue of RA and JIA patients (Popko et al.2006) suggest the value of synovectomy in treatment of rheumatoid diseases (Fig. 5).

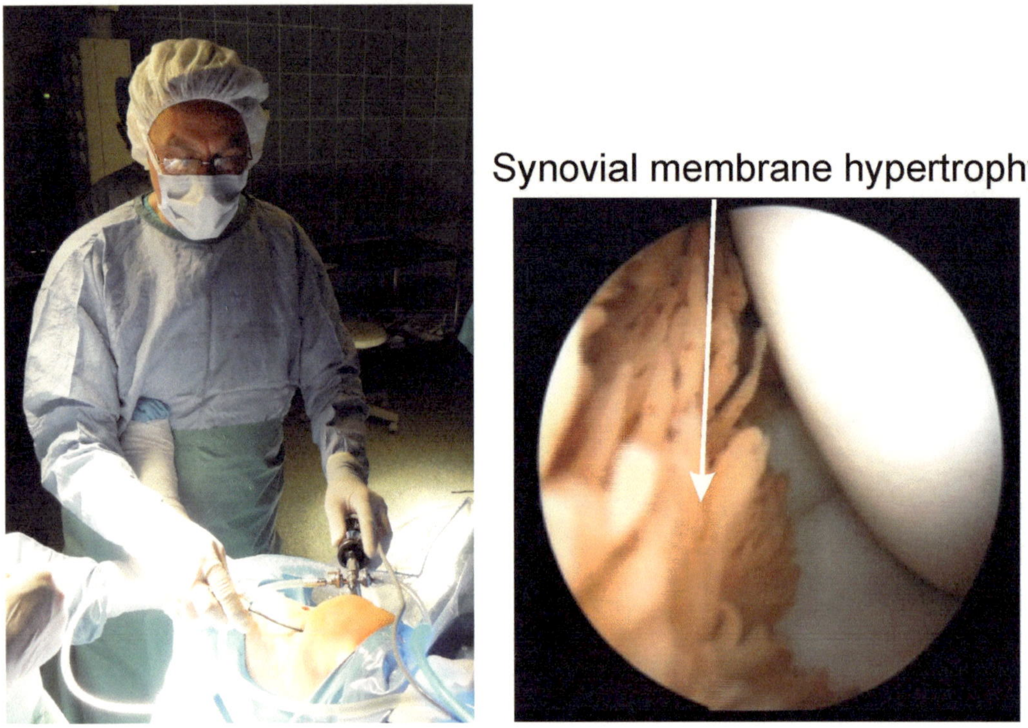

Fig. 5. Arthroscopic synovectomy a knee of patient with JIA.

We recommend the usefulness of synovectomy in patients with RA and JIA, as the removal of diseased synovial tissue (Fig. 5) could slow down the destructive process of the joint cartilage, and allow regeneration of a normal synovial membrane.

5. Exoglycosidases activity in cell cultured synoviocytes

The patterns of compartmental distribution of exoglycosidases activity in cultured synovial cells of RA and JIA patients are presented in Fig. 6.

The activity of HEX (total), HEX A, and Glu A in the intracellular compartment in cultured synoviocytes of RA and JIA patients is over 3-fold higher than in the extracellular compartment. In contrast, no activity of GAL, MAN and FUC in the extracellular compartments of these cultured synoviocytes was detectable. It is most likely that these exoglycosidases were released extracellularly in small quantities, i.e. below the limits of detection of our colorimetric procedure. Shikhman et al. (2000) have demonstrated similar results in cultured human articular chondrocytes. The high level of activity of exoglycosidases in the intracellular compartment of cultured synoviocytes indirectly confirms the suggestion that the degradation of glycosaminoglycans predominantly takes place in the intracellular compartment. However, Woynarowska et al. (1992) reported data indicating the contribution of extracellular HEX activity in glycosaminoglycan degradation.

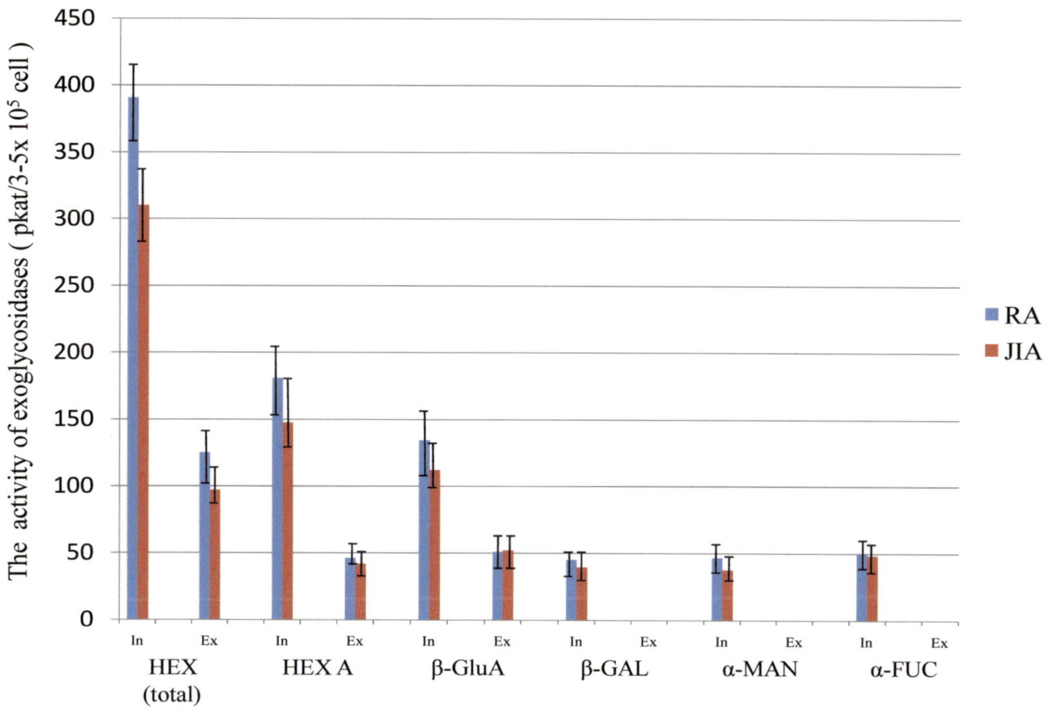

Fig. 6. Exoglycosidases activity of RA/JIA synovial fibroblast in the intra (In) / extracellular (Ex) compartment, expressed as pKat/3-5x10^5 cells.

IL-1 and TNF-α (tumor necrosis factor-α) are key proinflammatory cytokines whose concentration significantly increases in rheumatoid synovial fluid and joint tissues.

We have established a profile of exoglycosidases in cell cultures stimulated by IL-1β of inflamed (RA, JIA), and post-injury human synoviocytes (Popko et al. 2008) (Fig. 7).

Stimulation by IL-1β cultured synoviocytes taken from patients with ACL, JIA and RA causes much higher increases in activity of HEX and HEX A than remaining exoglycosidases (Fig. 7). On Fig. 7 one can see that the increase in HEX activity after IL-1β stimulation is more pronounced in the intracellular compartment of synoviocytes derived from rheumatoid patients than in ACL-injury, amounting 189.44 % increase (in comparison to untreated cultures) in synoviocytes from JIA, and 127.97 % in synoviocytes of RA patients. We noted a 201.18 % increase in HEX-A activity (in comparison to untreated cultures) in stimulated synoviocytes from JIA, and a 128.03 % increase in synoviocytes of patients with RA. In extracellular compartment of cultured rheumatoidal synoviocytes, stimulation by IL-1β cause only 33.4-72.44 % increases in HEX and HEX A activities. In extracellular compartment of cultured synoviocytes derived from injured knees of ACL patients, after stimulation by IL-1β the highest increase (121.80 %) was observed in HEX A activity. The mechanism of selective stimulation of HEX by IL-1β is not known. Shikhman et al. (2000) suggested that cytokines are involved in secretion of HEX from chondrocytes and stated that IL-1β could selectively up-regulate HEX synthesis and facilitate intra-compartmental transport of HEX from lysosomes/endosomes into the extracellular space, by modifying the mannose-6-phosphate receptor system.

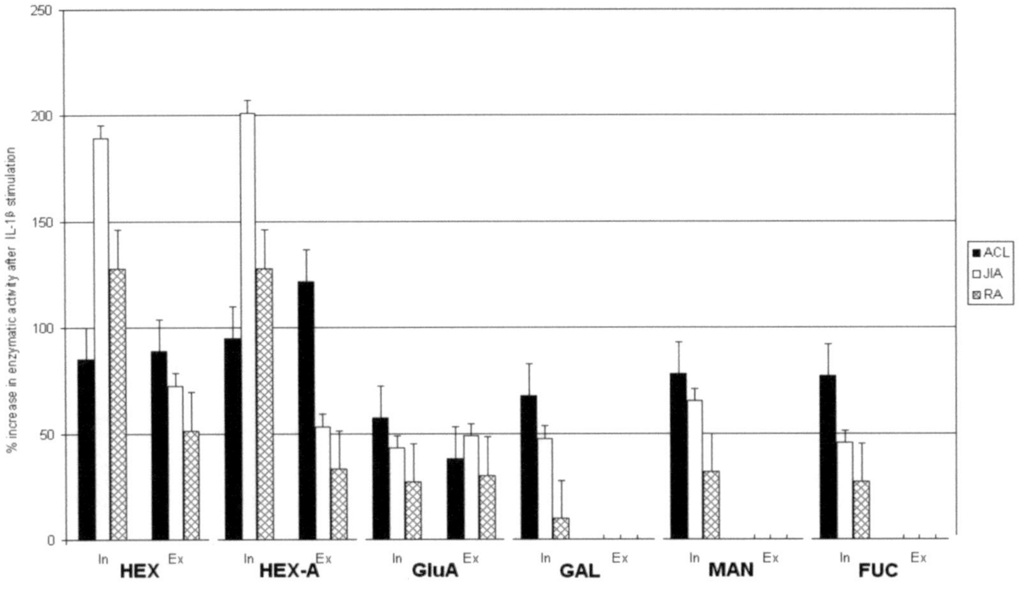

Fig. 7. Effect of interleukin 1β (IL-1β) on intra-(In) and extracellular (Ex) activity of lysosomal exoglycosidases in cultured human synovial cells from patients with anterior cruciate ligament (*ACL*) injuries, juvenile idiopathic arthritis (JIA), and rheumatoid arthritis (RA). Synoviocytes were stimulated with IL-1β for 24h at 37°C. After IL-1β stimulation, cultured cells and exracellular fluid were analyzed for exoglycosidase activities. The effect of IL-1β was expressed as the enzymatic activity in stimulated versus unstimulated cultures.

Rheumatoid synoviocytes exhibit altered morphology and show certain similarities to tumor cells (Mor et al. 2005). Our data confirmed the observation that synoviocytes obtained from patients with JIA and RA are more active in the synthesis and secretion of exoglycosidases than those obtained from patients with injured knees or healthy joints (Popko et. al.2008). (Popko et. al.2008).

6. Activity of lysosomal exoglycosidases in serum and synovial fluid of patients with RA and JIA

Information concerning the activity of exoglycosidases in patients with joint diseases is ambiguous and limited to a few, mostly old, publications (Bartholomew 1972; Stephens et al.1975; Ganguly et al. 1978; Berenbaum et al. 2000; Sohar et al. 2002). Serum HEX activity was higher in 35 % of the RA patients than in healthy controls (Berenbaum et al. 2000). Berenbaum et.al. (2000) found that the serum HEX concentration was significantly higher in destructive RA than in inflammatory RA. Since RA patients with high serum HEX activity have more erosions, than those with inflammatory RA, but have no differences in CRP levels, it is possible that HEX is a marker of erosions.

Lysosomal enzymes in human polymorphonuclear leukocytes are ubiquitous, biologically active molecules, that can degrade macromolecules such as proteins, glycosaminoglycans, nucleic acids, and lipids (Sohar et al.2002). Sohar et.al. (2002) have suggested that the increase of HEX activity in the serum of RA patients may be caused by an increase in HEX activity of RA leukocytes. Patients with long-standing RA had higher activity of lysosomal glycosidases in their leukocytes than those with disease of shorter duration.

We suggest that of the exoglycosidases, only HEX activity measurement in synovial fluid and serum has practical value (Popko et. al. 2006). The specific activity of HEX and its isoenzyme A in serum and synovial fluid from patients with different arthropathies is presented in Fig. 8.

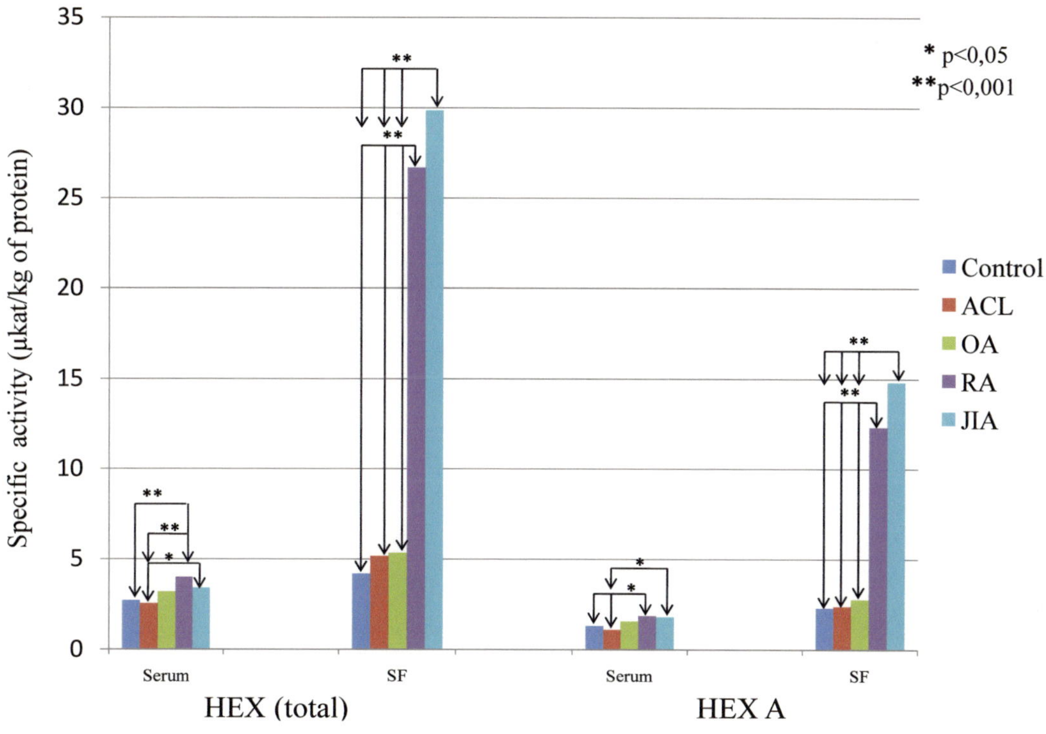

Fig. 8. Specific activity of N-acetyl-β-hexosaminidase and its isoenzyme A in serum and synovial fluid (µkat/kg of protein).

In the serum of RA patients, the specific activity of HEX was significantly increased in comparison to control (Fig. 8). This increase of HEX activity in the serum of RA patients may depend on the increase in HEX activity of RA leukocytes (Sohar et al. 2002). In the serum of patients with JIA and OA, we observed a moderate increase in HEX activity, i.e. 25.46% and 17.3 % respectively. In the case of patients with ACL injury, the specific activity of HEX and its isoenzymes in serum behaved similarly as in the control.

In the synovial fluid of JIA and RA patients, we found a significant increase in the specific activity of HEX and its isoenzymes, in comparison to HEX activity in synovial fluid from OA and ACL injuries. This suggests that release of HEX to synovial fluid is greatly enhanced by the autoimmunological inflammatory process in knee joint cavity.

The activity of HEX in synovial fluid of patients with JIA and RA was significantly higher than the activity in OA and ACL patients. Additionally, we have found that in JIA and RA patients, the specific activity of HEX in synovial fluid is 6-8 times higher than in serum from the same patients. This results suggest that HEX in synovial fluid derives mainly from articular tissues or articular leukocytes and not from serum. Therefore, activity of HEX in synovial fluid better reflects the situation in the joint cavity than activity of HEX in serum.

The differences between specific activities of HEX (activities calculated per 1 kg of protein) in synovial fluid of RA and JIA patients in comparison to OA and ACL patients (Fig. 9) are even more evident than differences in concentration of HEX (activities calculated per volume of synovial fluid) in the same situations.

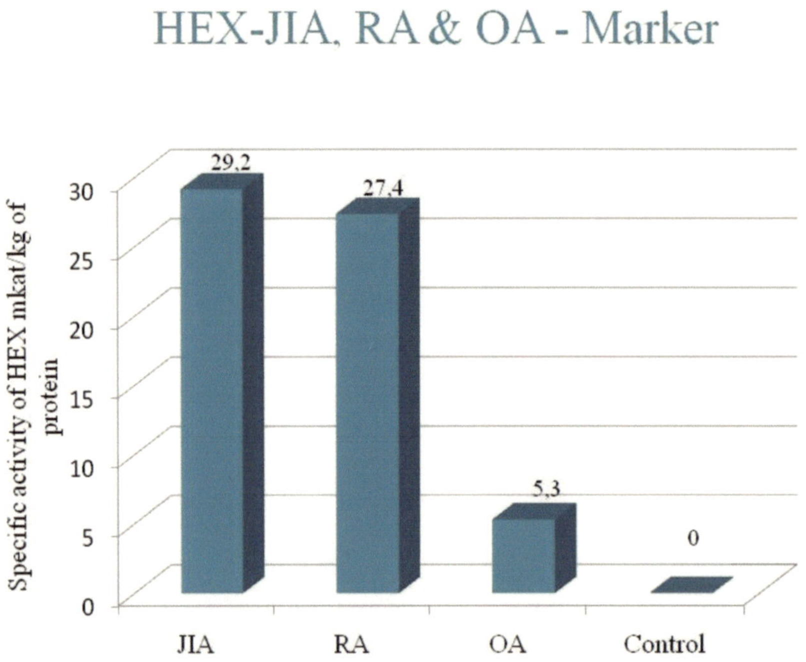

Fig. 9. The specific activity of HEX in synovial fluid of patients with rheumatoid arthritis.

Significant increase of specific HEX activity in synovial fluid of JIA patients (in comparison to OA and control) may be of diagnostic value in children with prolonged exudates in the knee joint, who are resistant to pharmacological and physiotherapeutical treatment. In these cases we advise determining specific activity of HEX in the synovial fluid, where values above 10-13 μkat/kg of protein suggest rheumatoid disease. It is worthy of note that specific activity of HEX in synovial fluid of patients with RA demonstrates a broad standard deviation which probably depends on destructive or inflammatory processes in the joint. However, significantly elevated HEX activity indicated an inflammatory or autoimmunological process within the joint.

7. Assay of exoglycosidase activity

Samples of the synovial fluid are easily taken from the knee joints during diagnostic or therapeutic arthrocentesis or at arthroscopy. Synovial fluid is aspirated from a lateral infrapatellar approach with a 21G needle (Fig. 10).

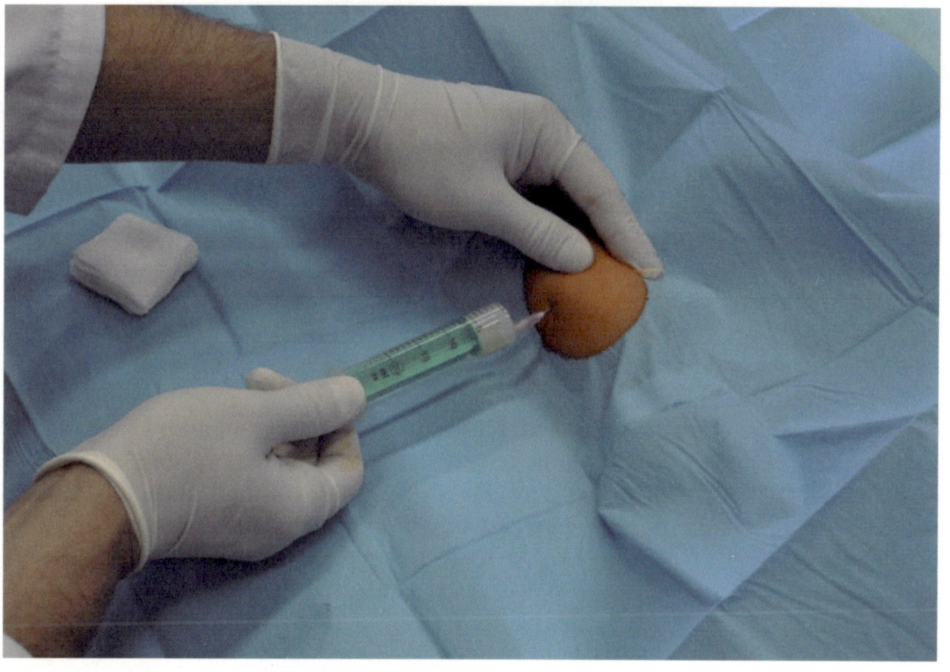

Fig. 10. Synovial fluid aspiration from the knee.

To obtain reliable results of exoglycosidase determinations, patients with inflammatory arthritis should avoid steroid drug treatment at the time of arthrocentesis, and for two days before arthrocentesis. About 1 ml of synovial fluid is sufficient for assays of exoglycosidase activity and protein concentration. Samples of synovial fluid are collected in plastic tubes and centrifuged at 10,000x g for 30 min, separated from the cell pellet, and stored at -70° C before use. As substrates for exoglycosidase activity we use p-nitrophenyl derivatives of appropriate sugars purchased from Sigma, St.Louis, Mo, USA (HEX, GAL, MAN, FUC), and Fluka Chemie GmbH (GluA).

The activities of HEX (E.C. 3.2.1.52), β-glucuronidase (E.C. 3.2.1.31), β-galactosidase (E.C. 3.2.1.23), α-mannosidase (E.C. 3.2.1.24), and α-fucosidase (E.C. 3.2.1.51) are determined by simple and inexpensive methods (Marciniak et. al. 2006). Before exoglycosidases determinations, the samples of synovial fluid are diluted with 0.1 M of the appropriate buffer and incubated with excess of substrate for 60 min at 37° C. The reaction is stopped by adding 0.2 M borate buffer, pH 9.8. HEX A activity is calculated as the difference between the total HEX activity and HEX B activity.

Spectrophotometric measurements of released 4-nitrophenol were carried out at 405 nm using a microplate reader Elx800™. The concentration of enzymatic activity of the appropriate exoglycosidase was expressed as nanomoles of p-nitrophenol released per minute per ml in synovial fluid and specific activity was expressed in µkat/kg of proteins of synovial fluid. The concentration of exoglycosidase activity indicates the ability of the specified volume of synovial fluid to release the quantity of monosaccharide indicated. The specific activity relates a particular exoglycosidase activity to total protein concentration, and shows the proportion of exoglycosidase protein to the total protein content of an articular sample of synovial fluid.

8. Conclusions

Although many publications (Shinmei et al. 1992; Lohmander et al. 1995; Saxne & Heinegard 1995; Myers 1999; Ortutay et al. 2003) have described increased release of markers of cartilage, bone, and synovial metabolism into joint fluid, serum, and urine in rheumatoid arthritis, the significance of several of these markers remains elusive. Up to now, no markers have yet been formally validated to monitor rheumatoid diseases of the joints. We hypothesize that determining HEX activity in the synovial fluid of patients with suspected idiopatic juvenile arthritis has diagnostic value. Elevation of HEX activity in synovial fluid to greater than 10 μkat/kg of protein, suggests rheumatoid disease.

Despite its huge public health impact, the conservative treatment of joint diseases, particularly of OA, is limited to a few types of medication which provide primarily symptomatic relief. Inhibition of hexosaminidase activity may represent a potentially novel strategy for treating RA and OA. Liu et al. (2001) have synthesized and investigated a series of iminocyclitols designed as transition-state analogue inhibitors of extracellular human hexosaminidase. Our team (Olszewski et al. 2010) is focusing on pyrimethamine which contributes to the regulation of HEX gene expression in synovial cells.

9. Acknowledgment

We are grateful to Dr Tony Merry from Manchester University for his critical reading of the manuscript before submission.

10. References

Bartholomew, BA.; (1972). Synovial fluid glycosidase activity. *Scand J Rheumatol*, 1, 69-74.

Berenbaum, F.; Le Gars, L.; Toussirot, E.; Sanon, A.; Bories, C.; Kaplan, G. & Loiseau, PM. (2000). Marked elevation of serum N-acetyl-β-D-hexosaminidase activity in rheumatoid arthritis. *Clin Exp Rheumatol*, 18, 63–66.

Czartoryska, B. (1977). Lysosomal glycosidases in heteropolysaccharide catabolism. *Post Bioch*, 23, 229-266.

Chikanza, IC.; Jawed, S.; Naughton, D. & Blade, DR. (1998). Why do we need new treatments for rheumatoid arthritis ? *J Pharm Pharmacol*, 50, 357–369.

Dieppe, P. (2000). The management of osteoarthritis in the third millennium. *Scand J Rheumatol*, 29, 279-281.

Ganguly, NK.; Kinghan, JG.; Lioyd, RS.; Price, CP.; Triger, DR. & Wright, R. (1978). Acid hydrolases in monocytes from patients with inflammatory bowel disease, chronic liver disease and rheumatoid arthritis. *Lancet*, 1, 1073-1075.

Giannini, EH.; Ilowite, NT.; Lovell, DJ.; Wallace, CA.; Rabinovich, CE.; Reiff, A.; Higgins, G. & Gottlieb, B. (2010). Effects of long-term etanercept treatment on growth in children with selected categories of juvenile idiopathic arthritis. Arthritis Rheum, 62, 11, 3250–3264.

Ikonne, IU.; Rattazzi, MC. & Desnik, RJ. (1975). Characterization of HEX S, the major residual β-hexosaminidase activity in type O Gm2 gangliosidosis (Sandhoff-Jatzkiewitz disease). *Am J Hum Genet*, 27, 639-650.

Inerot, S.; Heinegard, D.; Audell, L. & Olsson, S.-E. (1978). Articular-cartilage proteoglycans in aging and osteoarthritis. *Biochem J*, 169, 143–156.

Itakura, T.; Kuroki, A. & Ishibashi, Y. (2006). Inefficiency in GM2 ganglioside elimination by human lysosomal beta-hexosaminidase beta-subunit gene transfer to fibroblastic cell line derived from Sandhoff disease model mice. *Biol Pharm Bull, 29,* 1564-1569.

Lawrence, R.C.; Helmick, C.G.; Arnett, F.C.; Deyo, R.A.; Felson, D.T.; Giannimi, E.H.; Heyse, S.P.; Hirsch, R.; Hochberg, M.C.; Hunder, G.G.; Liang, M.H.; Pillemer, S.R.; Steen, V.D. & Wolfe, F. (1998). Estimates of the prevalence of arthritis and selected musculoskeletal disorders in the United States. *Arthritis Rheum*, 41, 778 -799.

Li, C.; Qian, J. & Lin, J S. (2006). Purification and characterization of alpha-L-fucosidase from human primary hepatocarcinoma tissue. *World J Gastroenterol, 12,* 3770-3775.

Liu, J.; Shikhman, AR.; Lotz, KM. & Wong, C-H. (2001). Hexosaminidase inhibitors as new drug candidates for the therapy of osteoarthritis. *Chem Biol*, 8, 701-711.

Lohmander, LS.; Roos, H.; Dahlberg, L. & Lark, MW. (1995). The role of molecular markers to monitor disease, intervention and cartilage breakdown in osteoarthritis. *Acta Orthop Scand Suppl*, 266, 84-87.

Mankin, HJ. & Lippiello, L. (1971). The glycosaminoglycans of normal and arthritic cartilage. *J Clin Invest*, 50, 1712–1719.

Marciniak, J.; Zalewska, A.; Popko, J. & Zwierz, K. (2006). Optimization of an enzymatic method for the determination of lysosomal N-acetyl-beta-D-hexosaminidase and beta-glucuronidase in synovial fluid. *Clin Chem Lab Med*, 44, 933-937.

Mor, A.; Abramson, SB. & Pillinger, MH. (2005). The fibroblast-like synovial cell in rheumatoid arthritis: a key player in inflammation and joint destruction. *Clin Immunol*, 115, 118-128.

Myers, SL. (1999). Synovial fluid markers in osteoarthritis. *Rheum Dis Clin North Am*, 25, 433-449.

Olszewski, S.; Rutkowska, J.; Popko, J.; Dąbrowska, K.; Bielawski, T. & Olszewska, E. (2010). The pirymethamine influence on hexosaminidase gene expression in synovial cell culture-preliminary report. *Pol Merkur Lekarski*, 164, 112-116.

Ortutay, Z.; Polgar, A.; Gömör, B.; Gěher, P.; Lakatos, T.; Glant, TT.; Gay, RE., Gay, S.; Pállinger, E.; Farkas, C.; Farkas, E.; Tóthfalusi, L.; Kocsis, K.; Falus, A. & Buzás, E. (2003). Synovial fluid exoglycosidases are predictors of rheumatoid arthritis and are effective in cartilage glycosaminoglycan depletion. *Arthritis Rheum*, 48, 2163–2172.

Pancewicz, S.; Popko, J.; Rutkowski, R.; Knaś, M.; Grygorczuk, S.; Guszczyn, T.; Bruczko, M.; Szajda, S.; Zajkowska, J.; Kondrusik, M.; Sierakowski, S. & Zwierz, K. (2009). Activity of lysosomal exoglycosidases in serum and synovial fluid in patients with chronic Lyme and rheumatoid arthritis. *Scand J Infect Dis*, 41, 584–589.

Pap, T.; Shigeyama, Y.; Kuchen, S.; Fernihough, JK.; Simmen, B. & Gay, RE. (2000). Differential expression pattern of membrane-type matrix metalloproteinases in rheumatoid arthritis. *Arthritis Rheum*, 43, 1226–1232.

Pennybacter, M.; Liessem, B.; Moczall, H.; Tifft, CJ.; Sandhoff, K. & Proia, RL. (1996). Identification of domains in human beta-hexosaminidase that determine substrate specificity. *J Biol Chem*, 271,17377-17382.

Popko, J.; Mnich, Z.; Kilczewska, D. & Trembaczowski, E. (1983). Topographical differences in the content and composition of glycosaminoglycans of patellar cartilage. *Reumatologia*, 21, 129–133.

Popko, J.; Marciniak, J.; Zalewska, A.; Górska, A.; Zwierz, K.; Sierakowski, S. & Urban, M. (2006). Activity of N-acetyl-β-hexosaminidase and its isoenzymes in serum and synovial fluid from patients with different arthropathies . *Clin Exp Rheumatol* 24, 690-693.

Popko, J.; Marciniak, J.; Zalewska, A.; Małdyk, P.; Rogalski, M.& Zwierz, K. (2006). The activity of exoglycosidases in the synovial membrane and knee fluid of patients with rheumatoid arthritis and juvenile idiopathic arthritis. *Scand J. Rheumat,* 35, 189-192.

Popko, J.; Marciniak, J.; Ilendo, E.; Knaś, M.; Guszczyn, T.; Stasiak-Barmuta, A.; Moniuszko, T.; Zwierz, K.& Wysocka, J. (2008). Profile of exoglycosidases in synovial cell cultures derived from human synovial membrane. *Cell Biochem Biophys,* 51, 89-95.

Popko, J.; Olszewski, S.; Guszczyn, T.; Zwierz, K. & Pancewicz, S. (2011). Glycoconjugate markers of joint diseases. *Biochem Soc Trans,* 39, 331-335.

Pugh, D. & Walker, PG. (1961). The localization of N-acetyl-β-glucosaminidase in tissues. *J Histochem Cytochem,* 9, 242-250.

Saxne, T. & Heinegard, D. (1995). Matrix proteins: potentials as body fluid markers of changes in the metabolism of cartilage and bone in arthritis. *J Rheumatol Suppl,* 22, 71-74.

Sharma, R.; Bukovac, S.; Callahan, J. & Mahuran, D. (2003). A single site in human beta-hexosaminidase A binds both 6-sulfate-groups on hexosamines and the sialic acid moiety of GM2 ganglioside. *Biochim Biophys Acta,* 1637, 113-118.

Shikhman, AR.; Brinson, DC. & Lotz, M. (2000). Profile of glycosaminoglycan-degrading glycosidases and glycoside sulfatases secreted by human articular chondrocytes in homeostasis and inflammation. *Arthritis Rheum,* 43, 1307–1314.

Shinmei , M.; Miyauchi, S.; Machida, A. & Iyazaki, K. (1992). Quantitation of chondroitin 4-sulfate and chondroitin 6-sulfate in pathologic joint fluid. *Arthritis Rheum*, 35, 1304-1308.

Sohar, N.; Hammer, H.& Sohar, I. (2002). Lysosomal peptidases and glycosidases in rheumatoid arthritis. *Biol Chem,* 383, 865–869.

Stephens, RM.; Ghosh, P.; Taylor, TK.; Gale, CA.; Swann, JC.; Robinson, RG.& Webb, J. (1975). The origins and relative distribution of polysaccharidases in rheumatoid and osteoarthritic fluids. *J Rheumatol,* 2, 393–400.

Stypułkowska, A.; Zwierz, P. & Zwierz, K. (2004). Endoglycosidases and glycoamidases. *Postepy Biochem,* 50, 82-88.

Winchester, BG. (1996). Lysosomal metabolism of glycoconjugates. *Subcell Biochem,* 27, 191–238.

Woynarowska, B.; Wikiel, H.; Sharma, M.; Carpenter, N.; Fleet, GWJ. & Bernacki, RJ. (1992). Inhibition of human ovarian carcinoma cell- and hexosaminidase -mediated degradation of extracellular matrix by sugar analogs. *Anticancer Res,* 12, 161-166.

Yamanak, S. (2001). Hexosaminidase system and mouse models of GM2 gangliosidoses (Tay-Sachs disease and Sandhoff disease) made by gene targeting. *Yokohama Med Bull,* 48, 65-71.

Zwierz, K.; Gindziński, A.; Ostrowska, L. & Stankiewicz-Choroszucha, B. (1989). Metabolism of glycoconjugates in human gastric mucosa a review. *Acta Med Hung,* 46, 275-288.

Zwierz, K.; Zalewska, A. & Zoch-Zwierz, W. (1999). Izoenzymes of N-acetyl-β-hexosaminidase. *Acta Biochim Pol,* 46, 739-751.

7

Innate Mechanisms of Synovitis – Fibrin Deposits Contribute to Invasion

Olga Sánchez-Pernaute[1] et al.*
[1]*Jiménez Díaz Foundation University Hospital, Madrid, Spain*

1. Introduction

1.1 Synovitis and the chicken or the egg dilemma

The studies approaching pathogenesis of rheumatoid arthritis shifted over the years to show that non-immune factors could precede activation of immune cells and were therefore targetable (Firestein & Zvaifler, 1990). In opposition to the classic model, in which an initial challenge to the immune system would over time lead to the autoimmune attack of joints, it was suggested that early mechanisms of disease induction were to be found inside joints. It was observed in vitro, that cells from the joints of patients with rheumatoid arthritis spontaneously produced several cytokines (Brennan et al., 1989a). Further studies would confirm the role of tumour necrosis factor alpha (TNFα) as a master cytokine, since its inhibition led to a drop in levels of the other soluble mediators (Brennan et al., 1989b), as well as reduction in the expression of HLA-DR molecules (Haworth et al., 1991). Interestingly, TNFα was not lymphocyte restricted, but rather pleiotropic. Moreover, it was shown that its principal sources in the arthritic joint were resident macrophages and fibroblast-like cells. This new paradigm was followed by the successful introduction of anti-cytokine therapies, which have totally changed the clinical picture of RA.

Indeed, the rheumatoid lesion at joints is quite unique, and probably sufficient to define the disease. It is characterized by the development of synovitis, a tumour-like transformation of the synovial tissue (Arend, 1997). On one hand, synovitis leads to joint destruction and disability, and on the other it provides a stronghold for spreading the inflammatory process.

1.2 Role of synovial fibroblasts in synovitis

1.2.1 Invasive features of synovial fibroblasts

There is not a uniform theory to explain how synovitis develops. However, one of the major features of synovitis is the acquisition of invasiveness of synovial fibroblasts. It could be said that rheumatoid synovial fibroblasts exhibit features of transformed cells, but unlike these, they do not show genetic aberrations. Rather, it seems that different activation processes are not correctly balanced by regulatory mechanisms in these cells. In this regard, it is typical of rheumatoid synovial fibroblasts to constitutively express growth factors, adhesion

---

* Antonio Gabucio[1], Astrid Jüngel[2], Michel Neidhart[2], María Comazzi[2], Gabriel Herrero-Beaumont[1], Renate E. Gay[2] and Steffen Gay[2]
[2]*Zürich University Hospital, Zürich, Switzerland*

molecules and proteases, which participate in inflammation and in the destruction of joint tissues (Pap et al., 2005).

One particularly altered regulatory mechanism in rheumatoid synovial fibroblasts is cell growth. In healthy individuals, the synovial membrane is formed by a limiting row of cells, the synovial intima, which overlays connective tissue in an epithelium-like fashion. In rheumatoid arthritis, the intimal layer is characteristically disarranged and hyperplastic (Tarner et al., 2005). Along with the infiltration by leukocytes, there is an increase in the density of synovial fibroblasts. However, the latter does not derive from a high proliferation rate, but from cell longevity. These cells are able to survive in adverse conditions, such as hypoxia and loss of matrix anchorage. Defective apoptosis might therefore be a critical process in acquisition of invasiveness, and different works have shed light on this, describing specific alterations in the regulation of death mechanisms in rheumatoid arthritis (Takami et al., 2003; Jüngel et al., 2006). But on the whole it could be said that the apoptotic machinery of rheumatoid synovial fibroblasts is not impaired, and most of its deregulation could be due to the influence of signals from the inflamed environment (Kammouni et al., 2007).

How rheumatoid synovial cells become invasive brings back the chicken or the egg dilemma. Are they mere effectors activated by immune cells or is it the activation of these cells by innate mechanisms what helps to trespass the barrier of peripheral tolerance, at the same time conferring them with aggressive features? Increasing evidence is rising supporting that local factors associated to inflammation can shape the phenotype of rheumatoid synovial fibroblasts. An intriguing feature of rheumatoid synovitis is local hypoxia (Stevens et al., 1991). The formation of new vessels is characteristic of synovitis, but still the density of blood vessels is insufficient to supply the overgrown tissue, so consequently there are focal areas of ischemia inside the inflamed joint. It has been shown that reduced oxygen leads to an activation of hypoxia sensitive elements, orchestrated by hypoxia induced transcription factor-1 (HIF-1). Apparently, there is a low threshold for the induction of the hypoxia program in rheumatoid arthritis, probably resulting from the stabilisation of HIF-1 by inflammatory cytokines. The vascular endothelium growth factor (VEGF) is one of the molecules induced by HIF-1 thought to play a prominent role in the acquisition of invasiveness by rheumatoid synovial fibroblasts (Distler et al., 2004).

1.2.2 Hurdles in the study of rheumatoid synovial fibroblasts' features

Synovitis is a non-conventional lesion, and it is difficult to put it into experimental coordinates in order to dissect its pathogenic mechanisms. Nonetheless, in primary cultures, rheumatoid synovial fibroblasts but not synovial fibroblasts from osteoarthritic or healthy joints, are able to maintain an activated phenotype after several passages. This rare feature suggests that cells carry with them a stable imprinting of the in vivo circumstances. However, in vitro studies have frequently failed to identify or consistently replicate mechanisms associated to acquisition of invasiveness by rheumatoid synovial fibroblasts. A possible explanation is that cells from the same joint can exhibit a heterogeneous spectrum of phenotypes (Kasperkovitz et al., 2005). In large synovial specimens, an alternation can be observed between overgrown sprouts of tissue (macroscopic villi) and normal-appearing areas, a finding that suggests that the aggressive transformation of synovial fibroblasts is focal. Studies based on primary cultures, as well as on high throughput techniques, can miss the features of small but critical subpopulations of cells.

In order to overcome these limitations, elegant strategies have been employed for the study of invasiveness of rheumatoid synovial fibroblasts. An interesting approach is to specifically look at areas where synovium invades cartilage and bone, the so-called cartilage-pannus junction (CPJ), looking for selective expression of molecules conferring invasiveness (Benito et al., 2004). From this type of study we have learned that cells located in the invasive fronts are mostly macrophages and fibroblasts. Both the up-regulation of anti-apoptotic factors, such as sentrin 1 and the Fas associated death domain-like interleukin 1 converting enzyme inhibitory protein (FLIP), and the expression of protooncogenes, have been found in these areas (Franz et al., 2000; Schedel et al., 2002). On the other hand, studies looking into CPJs are necessarily carried out in specimens obtained at the time of joint replacement surgery. Therefore, we need to be cautious at drawing conclusions, because these samples could reflect longstanding instead of active disease.

The invasive process has been studied in vitro in a transwell system with Matrigel, a method that was designed for the study of metastasis (Tolboom et al., 2002). More recently, a matrix-associated transepithelial resistance invasion (MATRIN) assay was developed to measure the rate of invasiveness from the breakdown of the electrical resistance generated by an epithelial monolayer (Wunrau et al., 2009). This system provides a means of directly assessing the participation of a particular factor in the ability of cells to scatter through the matrix. Also interesting are several three-dimensional co-culture systems in which minced, artificially generated, or native cartilage is put into contact with different subsets of cells that are present at the CPJ.

The experimental severe cellular immunodeficient (SCID) mouse co-implantation model allows the study of mechanisms of invasion in vivo. In this model, human cartilage and rheumatoid synovial fibroblasts are engrafted in nude mice, that is, in an immune independent environment. Several works using this model have shown the ability of rheumatoid synovial fibroblasts to migrate and to destroy cartilage in the absence of immune cell concurrence (Müller-Ladner et al., 1996). On the other hand, some mechanisms of destruction taking place in rheumatoid arthritis might not show up in the SCID mouse model, as the latter does not provide an inflammatory microenvironment comparable to synovitis (Jüngel et al, 2010).

1.2.3 The family of metalloproteinases and related molecules

There are probably several mechanisms accounting for cartilage and bone destruction in rheumatoid arthritis, and different cells and mediators can be involved. Activation of osteoclasts through the RANK ligand system stands as the principal pathway of bone erosion. In this sense, synovial fibroblasts, among other cell types, have an undeniable role as inductors of osteoclast differentiation and maturation in arthritic joints (Kim et al., 2007). But there is also much evidence of the direct ability of synovial fibroblasts to penetrate the adjacent joint structures as a result of their production of various proteases.

Metalloproteinases (MMPs) are a family of Zn^{2+} binding endoproteinases able to degrade the connective tissue. They are synthesized as precursors and cleaved at the N-terminus to their active forms. There is a considerable overlap of functions between them, and some of them are known to trigger the activation of others, as well as interact with additional proteases to generate proteolytic cascades in certain systems.

Of all MMPs, the interstitial collagenase, MMP-1, and stromelysin 1, or MMP-3, are the best characterized in the setting of synovitis. MMP-3 is able to degrade the most abundant extracellular components of the synovial tissue, including fibronectin and laminin, as well as collagens I and III. In addition, it activates MMP-1, which not only shares some of MMP-3 cleavage targets, but is also able to degrade collagen II, the principal component of articular cartilage. Plasma levels of both proteases have been found to be increased in patients with rheumatoid arthritis (Manicourt et al., 1995). Moreover, they correlated with disease activity, while intra-joint concentrations of the enzymes increased in parallel with the degree of joint inflammation (Ishiguro et al., 1996). Plasma levels of MMP-3 are currently regarded as a surrogate marker of severity, a fact that reflects its relevance as a mediator of joint destruction in rheumatoid arthritis. With immune-detection techniques, MMP-1 and -3 show a patchy distribution throughout the inflamed synovial tissue. Both molecules are consistently found at CPJs, where a diffuse immune-reactivity has been described (Tetlow & Woolley, 1995). Their pattern of distribution has confirmed synovial fibroblasts as the major source of these molecules in the joint.

Also of interest are the group of membrane-anchored (MT-) MMPs, which are bound to integrin chains, and, upon activation, digest pericellular matrix. Of this family, MT1-MMP (also MMP-14), which is over-expressed in rheumatoid synovial fibroblasts, is thought to confer to these cells some of their invasive potential (Yamanaka et al., 2000). In this regard, experiments carried out in the SCID mouse co-implantation model have shown the participation of MMP-1 and MT1-MMP in the degradation of cartilage by rheumatoid synovial fibroblasts (Rutkauskaite et al., 2004; Rutkauskaite et al., 2005). Based on this evidence, the pathway of MMPs has been for a while a promising area of research for therapeutics, not only in rheumatoid arthritis but also in metastatic tumours. The members of the family of tissue inhibitor of metalloproteinases (TIMPs), which act as natural regulators of MMPs, appeared as ideal candidates to develop anti-invasive compounds. In the SCID mouse model, TIMP-1 and -3 over-expressing mutants were able to slow the invasive process (van der Laan et al., 2003). However, less convincing results have been drawn so far in therapeutic experimental approaches and clinical trials.

In summary, it appears that synovial fibroblasts are the main effectors of destruction, a fact that could be considered natural. Fibroblasts are in charge of connective tissue remodelling, both under physiologic conditions and in disease. Production of proteases allows them to migrate through the matrix and restore the injured site in wound healing processes (Woessner, 1991). The same mechanisms take place during invasive processes. In this regard, rheumatoid synovial fibroblasts have been compared to tumour-associated stromal cells, which are non-neoplastic fibroblasts that contribute to metastatic growth by the production of MMPs (Hotary et al., 2003). Interestingly, the presence of MMPs at the synovial tissue is not related to the stage of the disease, and in fact the proteases can be abundant in early synovitis (Katrib et al., 2001). Therefore, fibroblast activation is not necessarily a consequence of longstanding disease, but could be one of the distinguishing processes between non-progressive disease and rheumatoid arthritis.

To help understand why rheumatoid and not other synovial fibroblasts turn invasive, a revealing study put in relationship the mRNA expression levels of MMPs with local hypoxia. Not only hypoxic cultures resulted in an increase in MMP-1 and MMP-3 transcripts, but also HIF-1α siRNA transfects yielded 50% lower mRNA levels of MMP-3 (Ahn et al., 2008).

Pulling the thread of research coming from invasive neoplasms and stromal cells, additional synovial fibroblast-dependent proteases were discovered at CPJs, showing potent in vitro capacity to destroy bone and cartilage. One of these molecules, that heralds the aggressive behaviour of tumours, is the urokinase type plasmin activator (uPA) (Duffy & Duggan,

2004). While uPA is able to degrade the extracellular matrix, it also activates MMPs and proteoglycanases through the cleavage of their precursors. Several studies have shown that uPA is over-expressed in joints from patients with rheumatoid arthritis, in correlation with disease severity (van der Laan et al., 2000). In spite of this role, uPA could be a double-edged therapeutic sword in rheumatoid arthritis, due to its activity in extra-vascular fibrinolysis, as we discuss in the next section. Interesting evidence was drawn in mice with antigen-induced arthritis, since uPA-deficient animals depicted a more severe phenotype as compared to wild type littermates (Busso et al., 1998). From subsequent studies, it can be concluded that aggressive features mediated by uPA are linked to its cell attachment activity, through the binding of its high affinity receptor, uPAR. New released work has found that the uPA-uPAR pair is a mediator of invasiveness in the SCID mouse co-implantation model (Serratì et al., 2011). In turn, uPAR is part of a larger complex, the urokinase plasminogen activating system (uPAS), formed by its assembly with 4 serin protease inhibitors at the cell surface. Triggering of uPAS is associated to proliferation, adhesion, migration and neoangiogenesis in tumours. These findings point to the complex as a better therapeutic target than the protease itself (Ulisse et al., 2009).

1.3 The role of fibrin in rheumatoid arthritis

1.3.1 Haemostasis activation overflows the fibrinolytic capacity in the joints with rheumatoid arthritis

Since the extra-vascular activation of haemostasis is a characteristic feature of inflammation, fibrin deposition in the inflamed synovial tissue is considered a non-specific event. During inflammation, the exudation of plasma into joints can result in coagulation factors achieving high concentrations at the synovial effusion. In fact, joints affected with osteoarthritis, infections, and trauma, often show fibrin deposits, albeit not as widespread as found in rheumatoid arthritis (Clemmensen et al., 1983). The striking abundance of fibrin in rheumatoid synovial tissues has been attributed to both an increased formation and a low clearance of the clots. As pointed out in different studies, rheumatoid arthritis flares provoke a status of extra-vascular thrombophilia, so that the influx of fibrinogen and its immobilization are high (Carmassi et al., 1996). Fibrin networks are thicker in patients with rheumatoid arthritis than in controls, and presumably more resistant to proteolysis as well (Kwasny-Krochin et al., 2010). This feature along with a reduced fibrinolytic activity can explain the accumulation of fibrin inside rheumatoid joints. Of the two regulatory systems that activate plasmin to degrade fibrin, the tissue plasminogen activator (tPA) is reduced in rheumatoid synovial tissues. Similarly, there is an increased production of the inhibitors of plasminogen activator, PAI-1 and PAI-2, which act by preventing fibrin dissolution through a constitutive pathway (Weinberg et al., 1991; Ronday, et al., 1996).

Local activation of complement is an inflammation-dependent mechanism that can help to stabilize fibrin clots thereby decreasing the fibrinolytic potential of the joint. In particular, we explored some years ago the local production of the regulatory factor C4b-binding protein (C4BP). The protein C-S anticoagulatory system is a principal mechanism for preventing the uncontrolled activation of haemostasis. The beta chain of C4BP binds protein S with high affinity in an equimolecular fashion (Dahlbäck, 1989). Only free protein S is active and the free fraction depends on the availability of C4BP beta. Reduced levels of free protein S are associated with an increased risk of thrombotic events. Interestingly, we showed local production of C4BP beta by rheumatoid synovial fibroblasts, as well as its co-localization with fibrin-rich areas at the synovial tissue (Sánchez-Pernaute et al., 2006). The

beta chain of C4BP has also been found in omen fibroblasts participating in the invasion and resorption of the corpus luteum, therefore indicating that besides its prothrombotic role, the molecule is important in fibroblast-dependent remodelling processes.
In the light of these experimental data, a potential participation of fibrin in synovitis has been argued by different groups including ourselves (Busso & Hamilton, 2002; So et al., 2003; Sánchez-Pernaute et al., 2003b), and several antithrombotic strategies have been tried, proving useful in attenuating the inflammatory process in experimental models of rheumatoid arthritis (Busso et al., 1998; Varisco et al., 2000).

1.3.2 Fibrin as an autoantigen

Fibrin is one of the major substrates for peptidyl deiminases (PAD) inside inflamed joints. These enzymes transform arginine residues into citrulline, and subsequently change the physical properties of the protein. This modification could alter binding sites of plasmin, making the polymer resistant to proteolytic degradation. Moreover, it can also turn the molecule antigenic (Schellekens et al., 1998). This fact was confirmed with the characterization of anti-citrullinated peptide antibodies (ACPA), since they were shown to target epitopes from fibrin in a specific association with rheumatoid arthritis (Masson-Bessiere et al., 2001). Thus, fibrin can been considered a key mediator in the loss of immune tolerance in the disease. Since ACPA antibodies reach higher concentrations inside joints than at the periphery, deposition of fibrin in joints and exposure of its citrullinated form to immune-competent cells should be an early pathogenic event. On the other hand, ACPA can be found in pre-clinical stages in at least half of patients. To explain this contradiction, it has been suggested that the immune system is primed for citrullinated epitopes outside joints, for example in the lung or the oral cavity, with arthritis coming on a second wave (Quirke et al, 2011). We propose a different mechanism. According to recent studies, synovitis can remain asymptomatic during the first stages of the disease. A first mild flare of arthritis could, therefore, be the event during which citrullinated fibrinopeptides are generated inside joints and presented to the central immune system (van de Sande et al., 2011).

1.3.3 Fibrin as a scaffold

We focused our studies on "a non-immune" participation of fibrin in the development of synovitis. Since fibrin networks provide binding sites for the migration of cells, in this way facilitating wound healing, we proposed that the synovial tissue might grow through the engulfing of fibrin deposits at the lining surface. In a time-dependent approach, we studied events taking place from the first stages of the disease in antigen induced arthritis, and were able to describe the transition from acute inflammation, to deposition of fibrin clots, and subsequent synovitis-like tissue modifications taking place at fibrin-synovium interfaces (Sánchez Pernaute et al., 2003a). We then proposed that the binding of the free-surface of the lining cells would alter their polarity, thereby changing their resting phenotype into a migrating one, a mechanism that would contribute to invasiveness.

1.3.3.1 Immobilization of fibrin affects cell binding

Soluble fibrinogen turns into solid fibrin through the release of fibrinopeptides A and B, with the rest of its alpha and beta chains remaining mostly unchanged. Therefore, most cell binding sites are shared by the two macromolecules. But it is in our opinion the insolubility of fibrin which accounts for an invasive response of synovial fibroblasts in rheumatoid arthritis. Experiments carried out in macrophages demonstrated that the binding affinity of cells increases with fibrinogen transformation into fibrin (Shainoff et al., 1990). Considering that blood cells express different alpha beta integrin chains that could bind circulating fibrinogen, the affinity of the soluble molecule needs to be low. In this regard, the shear forces elicited by fibrin networks may have an influence in the avidity towards cell receptors. This mechanism has been recently found to account for activation of colon tumour cells upon engagement of fibrin by the hyaluronate receptor, CD44 (Alves et a., 2009).

The cell binding activity of fibrin networks is further enriched by its cross-linking with different matrix proteins, including collagens, proteoglycans or fibronectin, which also bear a variety of cell binding sites.

Yet to be understood, is why rheumatoid but not non-rheumatoid hosts develop an invasive response to fibrin clots inside joints. It could be simply a matter of magnitude, as we discussed several years ago (Sanchez-Pernaute et al, 2003b). It could also rely on intrinsic features of rheumatoid synovial fibroblasts, that up to date have not been found. Alternatively, it is attractive to speculate that resistance of the clots to plasmin proteolysis in rheumatoid joints makes local macrophages and fibroblasts secrete additional proteases that degrade fibrin through a non-constitutive pathway (Bini et al., 1999). Between these potential fibrin-degrading proteases stands MMP-3, which is also one of the major mediators of joint destruction. In this way, the active process of digestion of the insoluble macromolecule could be regarded as a favourable environment for the destruction of structures nearby.

1.3.4 A potential role of fibrin in the architecture of synovitis

The early works focused on the histopathology of rheumatoid arthritis, described a gradient in fibrin deposition from more abundant and solid-like at the surface, to patchy and reticular in inner areas (Andersen & Gormsen, 1970). Working with specimens from patients undergoing joint replacement surgery we described that fibrin-rich areas of the synovium were organized differently than non-fibrinous regions (Sánchez-Pernaute et al., 2006). With immune-detection techniques we found that both cells and extracellular matrix elements had a differential distribution in fibrinous and non-fibrinous areas, and there were transition zones between them (Figure 1). In this regard, matrix deposition and fibroblast-like synovial cells, as well as vessels, increased in density in fibrin-rich areas, up to an interface with solid-like fibrin deposits at superficial areas, where cells were scant and there were no vessels. Macrophages were clustered in the vicinity of fibrin deposits, although they were also abundant in non-fibrinous regions; but lymphoid aggregates clearly stayed apart (unpublished observations). This particular organization has led us to focus on the interaction between fibrin and synovial fibroblasts aiming to find mechanisms of invasiveness induced by fibrin in these cells.

Studies conducted in synovial specimens are frequently based on small biopsies. These explants constitute a fine way to reflect events taking place in the whole synovial tissue, in particular as regards cell activation and the participation of subtypes of infiltrating leukocytes (Smith et al., 2006). Elegant studies have proved that the pathology of the synovial tissue from biopsies can be employed to measure response to therapy and even unveil specific molecular predictive markers. However, this kind of study rarely describes the features of fibrin-rich areas, probably because in these regions the architecture of the tissue is distorted and difficult to read (as illustrated in figure 1). We believe that these areas are routinely discarded and thus critical components of the synovial pathology might be underestimated.

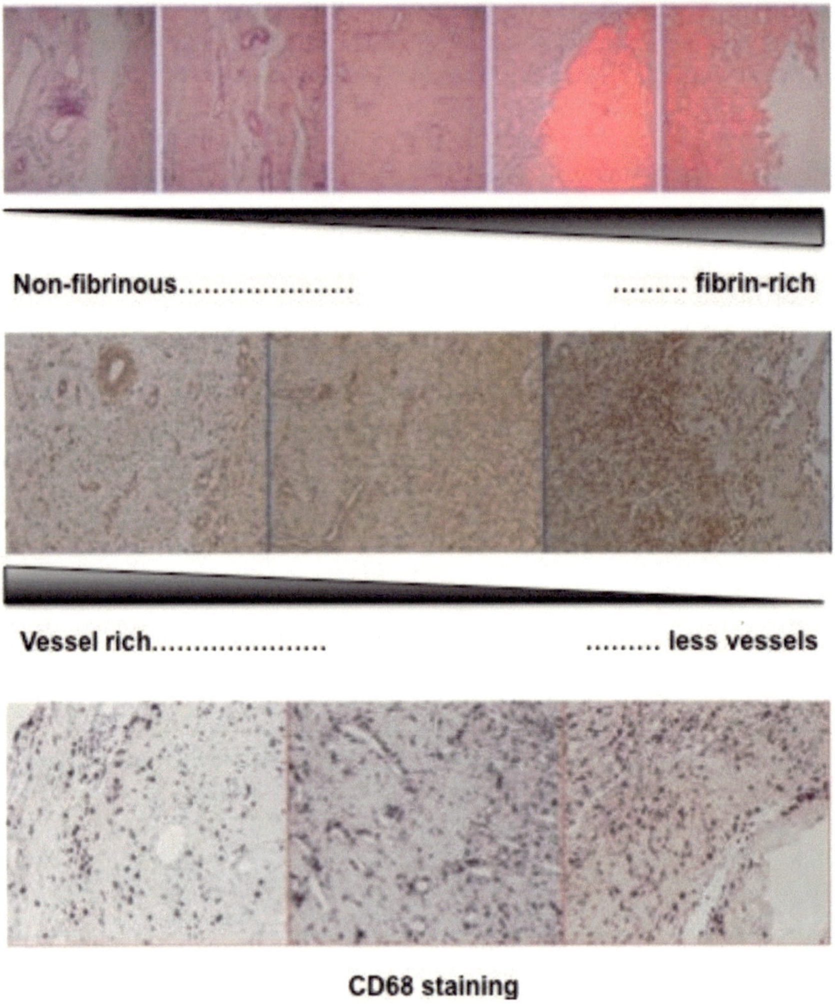

Fig. 1. Stratification of synovitis in relationship to fibrin deposits in a representative rheumatoid synovial tissue

Low-magnification microphotographs of a representative rheumatoid synovial tissue with an overlying fibrin deposit. Left column shows staining of the different tissue regions with haematoxylin-eosin. Middle column shows cell distribution with anti β actin antibodies. On the right side, immune-localization of macrophages with anti CD68 antibodies is shown.

2. Fibrin contributes to the production of MMP-1 and MMP-3 by rheumatoid synovial fibroblasts

In order to test whether deposition of fibrin might trigger the production of MMPs, we investigated the presence of fibrin in synovial tissues from patients with rheumatoid arthritis. We observed a similar pattern of distribution to those of MMP-1 and -3. These findings led us to explore in vitro whether fibrin could activate the production of MMPs by rheumatoid synovial fibroblasts. In these studies, which we next describe, we introduced an in vitro system that attempts to reproduce the interaction between fibrin and fibroblasts that takes place inside the joint. This model of cell stimulation had originally been developed to study leukocyte migration through vessel walls and is known as in situ fibrin polymerization (Qi & Kreutzer, 1995). In contrast to other types of cultures involving cells and matrix proteins, this approach conserves the shear forces of freshly clotted fibrin networks and exposes cells to the deposits by their apical surface.

2.1 Experimental methods

2.1.1 Obtention and handling of samples

Synovial tissues were obtained during joint replacement surgery from 8 patients with rheumatoid arthritis according to the American College of Rheumatology criteria (Arnett et al., 1988). For histologic studies, the synovial membrane was immediately fixed in formaldehyde, dehydrated in ethanol and embedded in paraffin. When tissues included bone edges, they were decalcified by a 48 hour incubation in formic acid. For in vitro studies, cells were isolated by disruption with 1.5 mg/ml dispase II at 37ºC for 1 hour in agitation, and cultured in 10% fetal calf serum (FCS) enriched Dulbecco's modified Eagle's medium (DMEM) supplemented with 2 mM L-glutamine, 50 UI/ml penicillin-streptomycin, 0.2% amphotericin B, and 10 mM HEPES.

2.1.2 Immune-detection techniques

We studied the distribution of fibrin, MMP-1 and MMP-3 with double labelling immune-detection methods. Tissues were rehydrated, blocked with 6% bovine albumin and 3% serum of second antibody hosts, and incubated with the specific antibodies at 10 μg/ml overnight, at 4ºC. Secondary antibodies were applied for 1 hour, at room temperature. As control, tissues were incubated with an isotype IgG from the species of primary antibodies. Development of fibrinogen immune-reactivity was done with peroxidase and Histogreen, using nuclear fast red for counterstaining. Diaminobenzidine was applied after a byotinilated secondary antibody to develop MMP-3, and counterstaining was done with hematoxylin. An alkaline phosphatase labelled antibody was employed to detect MMP-1, and nitroblue tetrazolium with 5-bromo 4-chloro 3-indolyl phosphate was used as substrate for development, plus nuclear fast red as counterstaining. Inhibition of endogenous peroxidase was done with 1% H_2O_2 methanol. Alkaline phosphatase activity was blocked with 5 mM levamisole.

2.1.3 Fibrin-cell cultures

Between passages 4th and 7th cells were grown to confluence at 37ºC in 5% CO_2, starved from serum during 48 hours and exposed to in situ clotted fibrin. Chilled fibrinogen was mixed in 0.5% foetal calf serum enriched DMEM at 1 mg/ml on ice, and 0.75 UI/ml thrombin was added. The mixture was immediately spread on top of the cell monolayers and the cultures were transferred to the incubator to allow formation of fibrin clots.

2.1.4 Gene expression studies

Four different cell cultures were employed. Cells were incubated with fibrin or medium alone for 12 hours. At the end of the incubation period, the clots and supernatants were removed, cells were washed and total RNA was isolated. Following retrotranscription, gene expression studies were done with quantitative PCR (qPCR) using cDNA as templates and

TaqMan primer-probe reagents (MMPs) or SYBR Green techniques (urokinase). Results were analysed following the ΔΔCt method, using the expression of ribosomal 18s as house keeping gene and an untreated culture as reference.

2.1.5 Immunoblot techniques

Confluent cells were incubated with or without fibrin and protein levels of MMPs were measured at several time points. The protein levels of MMP-1 were determined in cells lysates as obtained with Laemmli's solution. Supernatants and fibrin were mixed with 150 mM NaCl, 10 mM Tris, pH 7.2, 0.1% sodium dodecyl sulphate, 1% Triton X-100, 1% sodium deoxycholate and 5 mM ethylenediamine tetraacetic actid, with 1 μg/ml aprotinin, 1 μg/ml leupeptin, 1 mM Na_3VO_4, and 1 mM phenylmethylsulfonylfluoride, at 4°C and homogenised. One hundred μl of the homogenates were incubated with the anti MMP-3 antibody for 1 hour at 4°C. Then, protein A/G plus-agarose immunoprecipitation reagent (20 μl) was added, and samples were incubated overnight on a rocking platform at 4°C. Finally, samples were washed and centrifuged to pellet beads with the complexed MMP-3, supernatants were discarded and precipitates were mixed in loading buffer. Protein extracts and immuno-precipitates were resolved in 10% SDS-polyacrylamide gel electrophoresis and transferred onto nitrocellulose filters. The filters were then blocked with 5% skimmed milk and 0.03% Tween and blotted overnight with the specific antibodies. Horseradish peroxidase-labelled secondary antibodies were applied for 1 hour, at room temperature, and the binding was developed with enhanced chemi-luminescence. Results were expressed as relative increase with regard to baseline. Beta-tubulin levels were used as control of cell protein content, and the Coomassie blue staining method was used in supernatants.

2.1.6 Statistics

Data are expressed as median (range); comparison between conditions was done with the non-parametric Wilcoxon rank test, using SPSS software.

2.1.7 Reagents and probes

Mouse anti human MMP-1 and goat anti human MMP-3 (R&D systems, Basel, Switzerland), goat anti human Fibrinogen (Abcam, Cambridge, UK), donkey anti goat-HRP, goat anti mouse-HRP, rabbit anti goat biotinylated antibodies, 1:500 in IHC, 1:10000 in WB (Jackson ImmunoResearch, LaRoche, Switzerland), goat anti mouse-alkaline phosphatase antibodies 1:40, Histogreen, nuclear fast red, DAB, peroxidase ABComplex (Dako, Zug, Switzerland), NBT-BCIP (Roche), Protein A/G Plus Agarose Immunoprecipitation Reagent (Santa Cruz Biotechnology Inc., CA), ECL chemoluminiscence (Amersham Pharmacia Biotech, Little Chalfont, UK) Fetal calf serum, DMEM, penicillin, streptomycin, HEPES, fungizone (Life Technologies, Basel, Switzerland), dispase (Roche, Reinach, Switzerland), fibrinogen (American Diagnostica inc., Stamford, CT), mouse anti human tubulin, thrombin (Sigma Aldrich, Buchs, Switzerland) MiniRNeasy spin column purification kit, RNase-free DNase set (Qiagen, Basel, Switzerland), SYBR green master mix, ABI Prism 7500 Sequence Detector (Applied Biosystems, Rotkreuz, Switzerland). Primer pairs and probes: MMP 1: 5′-tgtggaccatgccattgaga-3′ (fwd), 5′-tctgcttgaccctcagagacc-3′ (rev), FAM5′-ccaactctggagtaatgtcacacctctgacattcacc-3′TAMRA (probe); MMP 3: 5′-gggccatcagaggaaatgag-

3′ (fwd), 5′-cacggttggagggaaaccta-3′ (rev), FAM5′-agctggatacccaagaggcatccacac-3′TAMRA (probe); MMP 9: 5′-ggccactactgtgcctttgag-3′ (fwd), 5′-gatggcgtcgaagatgttcac-3′ (rev), FAM5′-ttgcaggcatcgtccaccgg-3′TAMRA (probe); MMP 13: 5′-tcctacaaatctcgcgggaat-3′ (fwd), gcatttctcggagcctctca-3′ (rev), FAM5′-catggagcttgctgcattctccttcag-3′TAMRA (probe); MMP 14: 5′-tggaggagacacccactttga-3′ (fwd), 5′-gccaccaggaagatgtcatttc-3′ (rev), FAM5′-cctgacagtccaaggctcggcaga-3′TAMRA (probe); urokinase: 5′-tgtcagcagccccactactac-3′ (fwd), 5′-cacagcattttggtggtgac-3′ (rev).

2.2 Results

2.2.1 Fibrin and MMPs co-localized in the synovial tissues from patients with rheumatoid arthritis

We studied the distribution of fibrin(ogen) in synovial tissues from 8 patients with rheumatoid arthritis. Three of them included areas of invasion into cartilage and bone. The binding was strong and abundant in all samples, showing either an amorphous or a reticular pattern, as has been described (Andersen & Gormsen, 1970; Clemmensen et al., 1983). Fibrin predominated in the vicinity of the lining layer. Solid-looking deposits were mostly acellular, while more organized material was found in interstitial areas, with cells inside also capturing the antibody. Fibrin immune-reactivity was strong at areas of interface with bone and cartilage.

Next, we studied the distribution of MMP-1 and MMP-3 in serial cuts of the same tissues, alone and in combination with fibrin, using double-staining methods. Immune-reactivity to both MMPs was high in the rheumatoid synovial tissues. Interestingly, MMP-1 predominated inside cells, and MMP-3 was mostly secreted. The binding of both antibodies was high at erosive fronts.

In double-staining studies, interstitial immune-reactivity to both MMP-1 and MMP-3 was associated with fibrin deposits. Furthermore, both proteases co-localized with fibrin at the invasive fronts. Fibroblast-like cells in fibrin-rich areas depicted a strong immune-reactivity to MMP-1 and MMP-3. These findings indicated that fibrin-rich areas were at the same time active sites of protease production.

2.2.2 Gene expression of proteases in rheumatoid synovial fibroblasts exposed to fibrin clots

In view of these observations, we carried out in vitro studies to look into a possible effect of fibrin on the production of proteases by rheumatoid synovial fibroblasts.

Thus, we studied five members of the MMP family that are prominent effectors of cartilage and bone destruction in rheumatoid arthritis. This revealed that exposure to in situ clotted fibrin resulted in the up-regulation of the gene expression of MMP-1, MMP-3, and MMP-9 to a variable extent in all cell cultures (Figure 3). The mRNA levels of MMP-1 were 26-fold increased (range: 1,5 to 71; $p < 0.07$), and those of MMP-3 were 27-fold increased (range: 2 to 126; $p < 0.07$). MMP-9 gene expression was increased 7-fold the presence of fibrin (range: 3 to 39; $p < 0.07$), while no differences were found in the gene expression of MMP-13 and MMP-14. Additionally, we studied urokinase gene expression, since it is the constitutive fibrin-degrading molecule, and a potential mediator of tissue injury in rheumatoid synovial tissues. In our conditions, fibrin did not elicit any changes in urokinase mRNA levels compared to baseline.

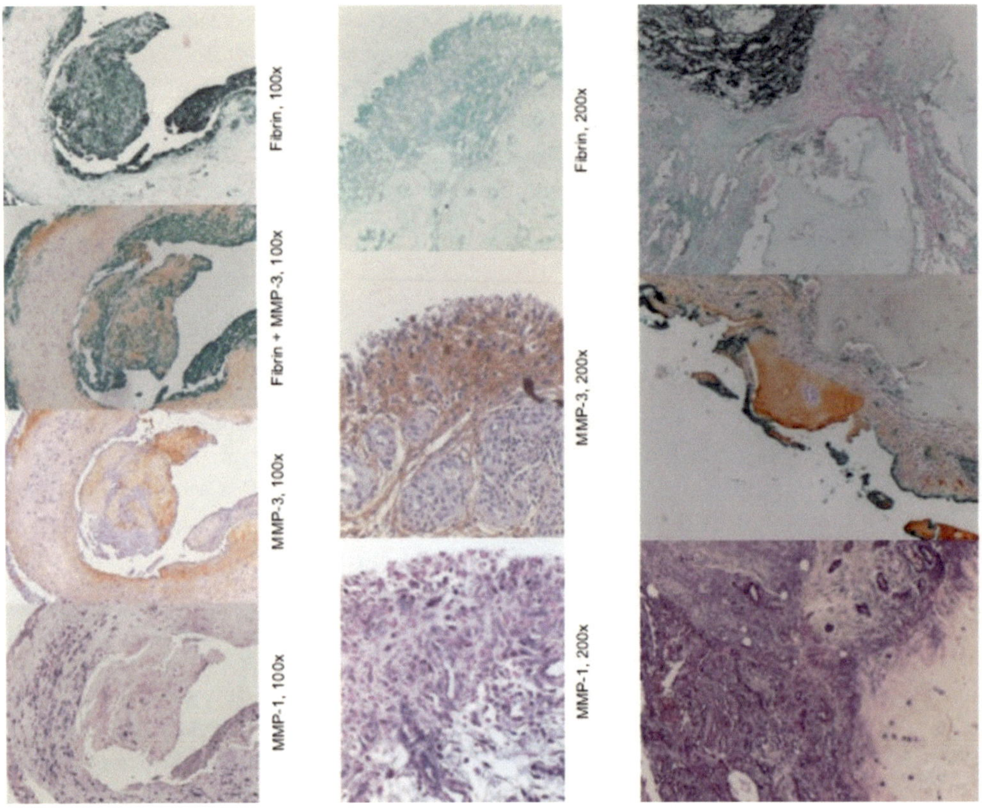

Fig. 2. Immune-staining of fibrin and MMPs in the rheumatoid synovial tissues

Left column shows a low-magnification view of a fibrin-rich area of the synovial tissue, with the different staining techniques. Middle column shows the intimal layer of a fibrin-rich area in detail. Right column depicts the staining of the molecules at areas of invasion into bone and cartilage. Fibrin is shown in green (with red counterstaining), MMP-3 is shown in brown (and counterstained in blue), and MMP-1 is shown in blue (with red counterstaining).

2.2.3 Fibrin increased the production of MMP-1 by rheumatoid synovial fibroblasts

Six different cell cultures were employed in immunoblot experiments. In all cases, treatment with fibrin increased MMP-1 production. In our conditions, both the proenzime and the active form of MMP-1 increased between 18 h and 24 h in rheumatoid synovial fibroblasts treated with fibrin (Figure 3). At 24 h, the active enzyme increased to 4-fold as compared to untreated cells (range: 1,5 to 6; $p < 0.03$). On the other hand, we could not detect MMP-3 in cell lysates, but it was abundantly found in supernatants from cell cultures. Upon stimulation with fibrin, baseline levels of MMP-3 in supernatants were found increased only in half of the cell lines tested (ns) (Figure 3).

2.3 Discussion and future research

Our studies illustrate how deposition of fibrin can contribute to the invasive process in rheumatoid arthritis. Previous works had described the distribution of MMP-1 and MMP-3 in the rheumatoid synovial tissue. In the same way, fibrin distribution in rheumatoid joints was well known. A novel finding is that all three followed a similar pattern of distribution. We could also confirm their abundance at CPJs, although we cannot draw conclusions as regards the impact of these finding in the erosive tendency.

Our studies suggest that fibrin triggers the transcription of several MMPs and the production of MMP-1. However, the study of MMPs is complex. These molecules are secreted in the form of zymogens, and need in situ activation through the cleavage of an N-terminus peptide. This post-translational modification probably constitutes a major check-point for the regulation of MMPs. Additionally, to find out what the global matrix turn-over could be, it would have been desirable to assess levels of TIMPs. TIMPs are the natural regulators of MMPs, an effect carried out through an equimolecular binding and inactivation. Both chondrocytes and synovial fibroblasts can produce TIMPs. In this regard, the balance between TIMPs and MMPs is decisive for the outcome (Martel-Pelletier et al., 1994). Functional studies, such as substrate-based zymography, are usually performed to demonstrate active proteolysis.

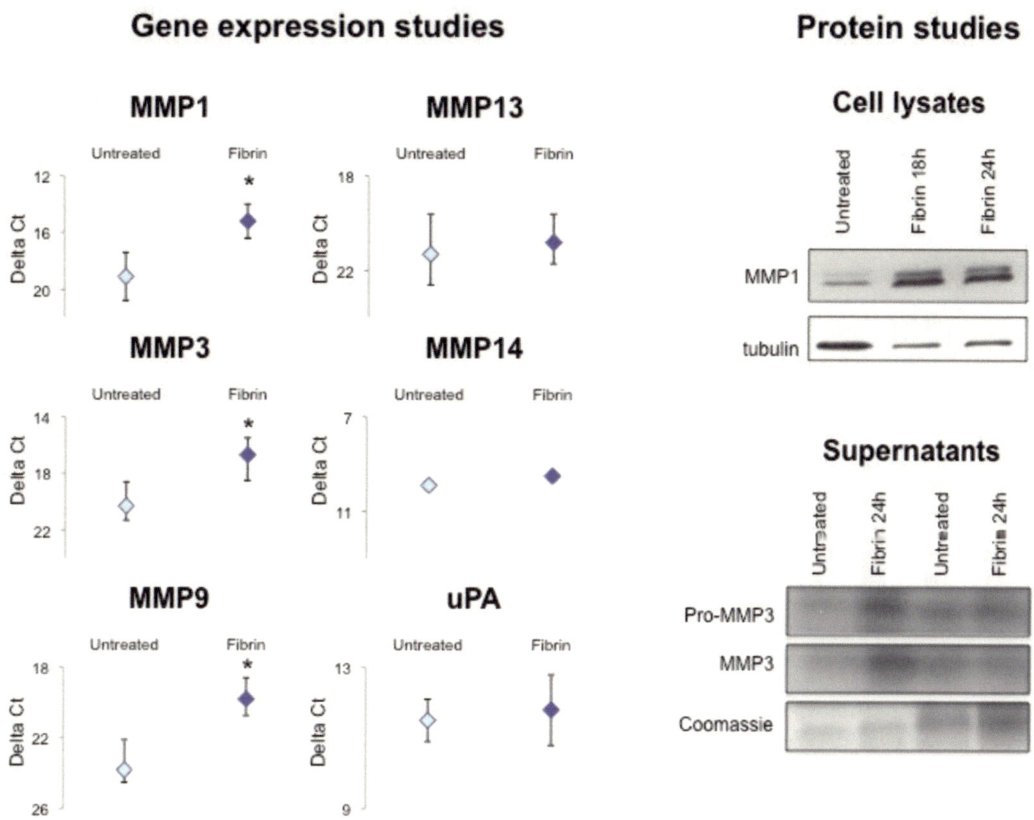

Fig. 3. Expression of MMPs in rheumatoid synovial fibroblasts exposed to fibrin

Graphs on the left show changes in baseline level expression of the mentioned genes (median ± SEM), in ΔCt values using 18s as house keeping gene (the lower ΔCt values, the higher gene levels are). On the right, representative immunoblots from different experiments are shown. Detection of MMP-1 was done in cell lysates and MMP-3 was

studied in the extracellular fraction. Both antibodies detected both the zymogen (upper band) and the active protease (lower band).
Nevetheless, it was interesting to find that three MMPs previously correlated to the invasive potential of rheumatoid synovial fibroblasts, were up-regulated by fibrin at the mRNA level (Tolboom et al., 2002). Due to its insolubility, fibrin might be degraded in a non-constitutive way by MMP-3 secreted by surrounding cells (Bini et al., 1999). On the balance of the evidence, we believe that fibrin-rich regions should not be considered a result of long-standing inflammation, but a site for active destruction.
In agreement with previous studies, most of the synovial fibroblast cultures that we employed in our studies did not constitutively express MMP-13 as assessed with qPCR techniques, and only in some was it induced after exposure to fibrin (Moore et al., 2000). In the production of this, as well as the other proteases tested, there seemed to be a high variability between patients. In fact, our studies suggested the existence of two subsets according to their response to fibrin. Approximately half of the cultures strongly reacted with the up-regulation of MMPs, while the other half showed mild or absent response. We believe that this is another example of the heterogeneous character of rheumatoid arthritis.
Although there was no regulation of MT1-MMP at the mRNA level by fibrin, an interesting finding drawn by our experiments was the high expression of MT1-MMP by unstimulated rheumatoid synovial cells, pointing to the prominent role of the protease in the activity of synovial fibroblasts as already suggested (Miller et al., 2009).
In summary, using a novel culture system for the study of fibrin interaction with synovial cells, we could show induction of proteases putatively associated to invasiveness, that were further localized at fibrin-rich areas in the synovial tissues.

3. Conclusion

In this chapter, we give an overview of the role of fibrin in the pathogenesis of synovitis. In doing so, we have neither solved the paradigm about what starts first nor discovered what triggers the invasive behaviour of rheumatoid synovial fibroblasts. Instead we provide some lines of thinking supporting the "inside - out pathway" as it has recently been named (Schett & Firestein, 2010).
The "fibrin pathway" has been little explored in rheumatoid arthritis therapeutics. The balance between clotting and dissolution of fibrin is a candidate process to target that could help to retard joint destruction.

4. Acknowledgements

We thank Conchita Rábago Foundation (FCR) and the Foundation of the Spanish Society for Rheumatology (FER) for their financial support.

5. References

Ahn, J.K.; Koh, E.M., Cha, H.S., Lee, Y.S., Kim, J., Bae, E.K. & Ahn, K.S. (2008). Role of hypoxia-inducible factor-1alpha in hypoxia-induced expression of IL-8, MMP-1 and MMP-3 in rheumatoid fibroblast-like synoviocytes. *Rheumatology (Oxford)*, Vol.47, No.6, pp. 834-839, ISSN: 1462-0324

Alves, C.S.; Yakovlev, S., Medved, L. & Konstantopoulos, K. (2009). Biomolecular characterization of CD44-fibrin(ogen) binding: distinct molecular requirements mediate binding of standard and variant isoforms of CD44 to immobilized fibrin(ogen). *J Biol Chem,* Vol.284, No.2, pp. 1177-1189, ISSN: 0021-9258

Andersen, R.B. & Gormsen, J. (1970). Fibrinolytic and fibrin stabilizing activity of synovial membranes. *Ann Rheum Dis,* Vol.29, No.3, pp. 287-293, ISSN: 0003-4967

Arend, W.P. (1997). The pathophysiology and treatment of rheumatoid arthritis. *Arthritis Rheum,* Vol.40, No.4, pp. 595-597, ISSN: 0004-3591

Arnett, F.C.; Edworthy, S.M, Bloch, D.A., McShane. D,J., Fries, J.F., Cooper, N.S. et al. (1988). The American Rheumatism Association 1987 revised criteria for the classification of rheumatoid arthritis. *Arthritis Rheum,* Vol.31, No.3, pp. 315-324, ISSN: 0004-3591

Benito, M.J.; Murphy, E., Murphy, E.P., van den Berg, W.B., FitzGerald, O. & Bresnihan, B. (2004). Increased synovial tissue NF-kappa B1 expression at sites adjacent to the cartilage-pannus junction in rheumatoid arthritis. *Arthritis Rheum,* Vol.50, No.6, pp. 1781-1787, ISSN: 0004-3591

Bini, A.; Wu, D., Schnuer, J. & Kudryk, B.J. (1999). Characterization of stromelysin 1 (MMP-3), matrilysin (MMP-7), and membrane type 1 matrix metalloproteinase (MT1-MMP) derived fibrin(ogen) fragments D-dimer and D-like monomer: NH2-terminal sequences of late-stage digest fragments. *Biochemistry,* Vol.38, No.42, pp. 13928-13936, ISSN: 0006-2960

Brennan, F.M.; Chantry, D., Jacksin, AM., Maini, R.N. & Feldmann, M. (1989). Cytokine production in culture by cells isolated from the synovial membrane. *J Autoimmun,* Vol.2 Suppl, pp. 177-186, ISSN: 0896-8411

Brennan, F.M.; Chantry. D., Jackson, A., Maini, R. & Feldmann, M. (1989). Inhibitory effect of TNF alpha antibodies on synovial cell interleukin-1 production in rheumatoid arthritis. *Lancet,* Vol.2, No.8657, pp. 244-247, ISSN: 0140-6736

Busso, N.; Peclat, V., Van Ness, K., Kolodziesczyk, E., Degen, J., Bugge, T. & So, A. (1998). Exacerbation of antigen-induced arthritis in urokinase-deficient mice. *J Clin Invest,* Vol.102, No.1, pp. 41–50, ISSN: 0021-9738

Busso, N. & Hamilton, J.A. (2002). Extravascular coagulation and the plasminogen activator/plasmin system in rheumatoid arthritis. *Arthritis Rheum,* Vol.46, No.9, pp. 2268-2279, ISSN:

Carmassi, F.; de Negri, F., Morale, M., Song, K.Y. & Chung, S.I. (1996). Fibrin degradation in the synovial fluid of rheumatoid arthritis patients: a model for extravascular fibrinolysis. *Semin Thromb Hemost,* Vol.22, No. 6, pp. 489–496, ISSN: 0094-6176

Clemmensen, I.; Holund, B. & Andersen, R.B. (1983). Fibrin and fibronectin in rheumatoid synovial membrane and rheumatoid synovial fluid. *Arthritis Rheum,* Vol.26, No.4, pp. 479-485, ISSN: 0004-3591

Dahlbäck, B. (1986). Inhibition of protein Ca cofactor function of human and bovine protein S by C4b-binding protein. *J Biol Chem,* Vol.261, No.26, pp. 12022-12027, ISSN: 0021-9258

Distler, J.H.W.; Wenger, R.H., Gassmann, M., Kurowska, M., Hirth, A., Gay, S. & Distler, O. (2004). Physiologic responses to hypoxia and implications for hypoxia-inducible factors in the pathogenesis of rheumatoid arthritis. *Arthritis Rheum,* Vol.50, No.1, pp. 10-23, ISSN: 0004-3591

Duffy, M.J. & Duggan, C. (2004). The urokinase plasminogen activator system: a rich source of tumour markers for the individualised management of patients with cancer. *Clin Biochem,* Vol.37, No.7, pp. 541-548, ISSN: 0009-9120

Firestein, G.S. & Zvaifler, N.J. (2002). How important are T cells in chronic rheumatoid synovitis? II. T cell-independent mechanisms from beginning to end. *Arthritis Rheum,* Vol.46, No.2, pp 298-308, ISSN: 0004-3591

Franz, J.K.; Pap, T., Hummel, K.M., Nawrath, M., Aicher, W.K., Shigeyama, Y. et al. (2000). Expression of sentrin, a novel antiapoptotic molecule, at sites of synovial invasion in rheumatoid arthritis. *Arthritis Rheum,* Vol.43, No.3, pp. 599-607, ISSN: 0004-3591

Haworth, C.; Brennan, F.M., Chantry, D., Turner, M., Maini, R.N. & Feldmann, M. (1991). Expression of granulocyte-macrophage colony-stimulating factor in rheumatoid arthritis: regulation by tumor necrosis factor-alpha. *Eur J Immunol,* Vol.21, No.10, pp. 2575-2579, ISSN: 1521-4141

Hotary, K.B.; Allen, E.D., Brooks, P.C., Datta, N.S., Long, M.W. & Weiss, S.J. (2003). Membrane type I matrix metalloproteinase usurps tumor growth control imposed by the three-dimensional extracellular matrix. *Cell,* Vol.114, No.1, pp. 33-45, ISSN: 0092-8674

Ishiguro, N.; Ito, T., Obata, K., Fujimoto, N. & Iwata, H. (1996). Determination of stromelysin-1, 72 and 92 kDa type IV collagenase, tissue inhibitor of metalloproteinase-1 (TIMP-1), and TIMP-2 in synovial fluid and serum from patients with rheumatoid arthritis. *J Rheumatol,* Vol.23, No.9, pp. 1599-1604, ISSN: 0315-162X

Jüngel, A.; Baresova, V., Ospelt, C., Simmen, B.R., Michel, B.A., Gay, R.E. et al. (2006). Trichostatin A sensitises rheumatoid arthritis synovial fibroblasts for TRAIL-induced apoptosis. *Ann Rheum Dis,* Vol.65, No.7, pp. 910–912, ISSN: 0003-4967

Jüngel, A.; Ospelt, C., Lesch, M., Thiel, M., Sunyer, T., Schorr, O. et al. (2010). Effect of the oral application of a highly selective MMP-13 inhibitor in three different animal models of rheumatoid arthritis. *Ann Rheum Dis,* Vol.69, No.5, pp. 898-902, ISSN: 0003-4967

Kammouni, W.; Wong, K, Ma, G., Firestein, G.S., Gibson, S.B. & El-Gabalawy, H.S. (2007). Regulation of apoptosis in fibroblast-like synoviocytes by the hypoxia-induced Bcl-2 family member Bcl-2/Adenovirus E1B 19-kd protein-intercting protein 3. *Arthritis Rheum,* Vol.56, No.9, pp. 2854-2863, ISSN: 0004-3591

Kasperkovitz, P.V.; Timmer, T.C., Smeets, T.J., Verbeet, N.L., Tak, P.P., van Baarsen, L.G. et al. (2005). Fibroblast-like synoviocytes derived from patients with rheumatoid arthritis show the imprint of synovial tissue heterogeneity: evidence of a link between an increased myofibroblast-like phenotype and high-inflammation synovitis. *Arthritis Rheum,* Vol.52, No.2, pp. 430-441, ISSN: 0004-3591

Katrib, A.; Tak, P.P., Bertouch, J.V., Cuello, C., McNeil, H.P., Smeets, T.J. et al. (2001). Expression of chemokines and matrix metalloproteinases in early rheumatoid arthritis. *Rheumatology (Oxford),* Vol.40, No.9, pp. 988-994, ISSN: 1462-0324

Kim, K.W.; Cho, M.L., Lee, S.H., Oh, H.J., Kang, C.M., Ju, J.H. et al. (2007). Human rheumatoid synovial fibroblasts promote osteoclastogenic activity by activating RANKL via TLR-2 and TLR-4 activation. *Immunol Lett,* Vol.110, No.1, pp. 54–64, ISSN: 0165-2478

Kwasny-Krochin, B.; Gluszko, P. & Undas, A. (2010). Unfavorably altered fibrin clot properties in patients with active rheumatoid arthritis. Thromb Res, Vol.126, No.1:e11-6, ISSN: 1879-2472

Manicourt, D.H.; Fujimoto N., Obata, K. & Thornal E.J. (1995). Levels of circulating collagenase, stromelysin-1, and tissue inhibitor of matrix metalloproteinases 1 in patients with rheumatoid arthritis. Relationship to serum levels of antigenic keratan sulfate and systemic parameters of inflammation. *Arthritis Rheum,* Vol.38, No.8, pp. 1031-1039, ISSN: 0004-3591

Martel-Pelletier, J.; McCollum, R., Fujimoto, N., Obata, K., Cloutier, J.M. & Pelletier- J.P. (1994). Excess of metalloproteases over tissue inhibitor of metalloprotease may contribute to cartilage degradation in osteoarthritis and rheumatoid arthritis. *Lav Invest,* Vol.70, No.6, pp. 807-815, ISSN: 0023-6837

Masson-Bessière, C.; Sebbag, M., Girbal-Neuhauser, E., Nogueira, L., Vincent, C., Senshu, T. & Serre, G. (2001). The major synovial tiargets of the rheumatoid arthritis-specific antifilaggrin autoantibodies are deiminated forms of the alpha- and beta-chains of fibrin. *J Immunol,* Vol.166, No.6, pp. 4177-4184, ISSN: 0022-1767

Moore, B.A.; Aznavoorian, S., Engler, J.A. & Windsor, L.J. (2000). Induction of collagenase-3 (MMP-13) in rheumatoid synovial fibroblasts. *Biochim Biophys Acta,* Vol.1502, No.2, pp. 307-318, ISSN: 0006-3002

Müller-Ladner, U.; Kriegsmann, J., Franklin, B.N., Matsumoto, S., Geiler, T., Gay, R.E. & Gay, S. (1996). Synovial fibroblasts of patients with rheumatoid arthritis attach to and invade normal human cartilage when engrafted into SCID mice. *Am J Pathol,* Vol.149, No.5, pp. 1607–1615, ISSN: 0002-9440

Pap, T.; Shigeyama, Y., Kuchen, S., Fernihough, J.K., Simmen, B., Gay R.E. & et al. (2000). Differential expression pattern of membrane-type matrix metalloproteinases in rheumatoid arthritis. *Arthritis Rheum,* Vol.43, pp. 1226-1232, ISSN: 0004-3591

Pap, T.; Nawrath, M., Heinrich, J., Bosse, M., Baier, A. & Hummel, K.M. (2004). Cooperation of Ras- and c-Myc-dependent pathways in regulating the growth and invasiveness of synovial fibroblasts in rheumatoid arthritis. *Arthritis Rheum,* Vol.50, No.9, pp. 2794-2802, ISSN: 0004-3591

Pap, T.; Meinecke, I., Müller-Ladner, U. & Gay, S. (2005). Are fibroblasts involved in joint destruction? *Ann Rheum Dis,* Vol.64, Suppl4, pp. iv52-54, ISSN: 0003-4967

Qi, J. & Kreutzer, D.L. (1995). Fibrin activation of vascular endothelial cells. Induction of IL-8 expression. *J Immunol,* Vol.155, No.2, pp. 867-876, ISSN: 0022-1767

Quirke, A.M.; Fisher, B.A., Kinloch, A.J. & Venables, P.J. (2011). Citrullination of autoantigens: Upstream of TNFα in the pathogenesis of rheumatoid arthritis. *FEBS Lett,* Jun 23, [Epub ahead of print], ISSN: 1873-3468

Ronday, H.K.; Smits, H.H., Van Muijen, G.N., Pruszczynski, M.S., Dolhain, R.J. et al. (1996). Difference in expression of the plasminogen activation system in synovial tissue of patients with rheumatoid arthritis and osteoarthritis. *Br J Rheumatol,* Vol. 35, No.5, pp. 416-423, ISSN: 0263-7103

Rutkauskaite, E., Zacharias, W., Schedel, J., Müller-Ladner, U., Mawrin, C., Seemayer, C.A., et al. (2004). Ribozymes that inhibit the production of matrix metalloproteinase 1 reduce the invasiveness of rheumatoid arthritis synovial fibroblasts. *Arthritis Rheum,* Vol.50, 1448-1456, ISSN: 0004-3591

Rutkauskaite, E.; Volkmer, D., Shigeyama, Y., Schedel, J., Pap, G., Müller-Ladner, U. et al. (2005). Retroviral gene transfer of an antisense construct against membrane type 1 matrix metalloproteinase reduces the invasiveness of rheumatoid arthritis synovial fibroblasts. *Arthritis Rheum,* Vol.52, No.7, pp. 2010-2014, ISSN: 0004-3591

Sánchez-Pernaute, O.; López-Armada, M.J., Calvo, E., Díez-Ortego, I., Largo, R., Egido, J. & Herrero-Beaumont, G. (2003). Fibrin generated in the synovial fluid activates intimal cells from their apical surface: a sequential morpholocial study in antigen-induced arthritis. *Rheumatology (Oxford),* Vol.42, No.1, pp. 19-25, ISSN: 1462-0324

Sánchez-Pernaute, O.; Largo, R., Calvo, E., Alvarez-Soria, M.A., Egido, J. & Herrero-Beaumont, G. (2003). A fibrin based model for rheumatoid synovitis. *Ann Rheum Dis,* Vol.62, No.12, pp. 1135-1138, ISSN: 0003-4967

Sánchez-Pernaute, O.; Esparza-Gordillo, J., Largo, R., Calvo, E., Alvarez-Soria, M.A., Marcos, M.E. et al. (2006). Expression of the peptide C4b-binding protein beta in the arthritic joint. *Ann Rheum Dis,* Vol.65, No.10, pp. 1279-1285, ISSN: 0003-4967

Schedel, J.; Gay, R.E., Kuenzler, P., Seemayer, C., Simmen, B., Michel, B.A. & Gay, S. (2002). FLICE-inhibitory protein expression in synovial fibroblasts and at sites of cartilage and bone erosion in rheumatoid arthritis. *Arthritis Rheum,* Vol.46, No.6, pp. 1512-1518, ISSN: 0004-3591

Schellekens, G.A.; de Jong, B.A.W., van den Hoogen, F.H.J., van de Putte, L.B.A. & van Venrooij, W.J. (1998). Citrulline is an essential constituent of antigenic determinants recognized by rheumatoid arthritis-specific autoantibodies. *J Clin Invest,* Vol.101, No.1, pp. 273-281, ISSN: 0021-9738

Schett, G. & Firestein, G.S. (2010). Mr Outside and Mr Inside: classic and alternative views on the pathogenesis of rheumatoid arthritis. *Ann Rheum Dis,* Vol.69, No.5, pp. 787-789, ISSN: 0003-4967

Serratì, S.; Margheri, F., Chillà, A., Neumann, E., Müller-Ladner, U., Benucci, M. et al. (2011). Reduction of in vitro invasion and in vivo cartilage degradation in a SCID mouse model by loss of function of the fibrinolytic system of rheumatoid arthritis synovial fibroblasts. *Arthritis Rheum,* May 5, doi: 10.1002/art.30439, ISSN: 1529-0131

Shainoff, J.R.; Stearns, D.J., DiBello, P.M. & Hishikawa-Itoh, Y. (1990). Characterization of a mode of specific binding of fibrin monomer thorugh ist amino-terminal domain by macrophages and macrophage cell-lines. *Thromb Haemost,* Vol.63, No.2, pp. 193-203, ISSN: 0340-6245

Smeets, T.J.; Kraan, M.C., Galjaard, S., Youssef, P.P., Smith, M.D. & Tak, P.P. (2001). Analysis of the cell infiltrat and expression of matrix metalloproteinases and granzyme B in paired synovial biopsy specimens from the cartilage-pannus junction in patients with RA. *Ann Rheum Dis,* Vol.60, pp. 561-565, ISSN: 0003-4967

Smith, M.D.; Baeten, D., Ulfgren, A.K., McInnes, I.B., Fitzgerald, O., Bresnihan, B. et al. (2006). Standarisation of synovial tissue infiltrate analysis: how far have we come? How muc further do we need to go? *Ann Rheum Dis,* Vol.65, No.1, pp. 93-100, ISSN: 0003-4967

So, A.K.; Varisco, P.A., Kemkes-Matthes, B., Herkenne-Morard, C., Chobaz-Péclat, V., Gerster, J.C. & Busso, N. (2003). Arthritis is linked to local and systemic activation of coagulation and fibrinolysis pathways. *J Thromb Haemost,* Vol.1, No.12, pp. 2510-2515, ISSN: 1538-7933

Stevens, C.R.; Blake, D.R., Merry, P., Revell, P.A. & Levick, J.R. (1991). A comparative study by morphometry of the microvasculature in normal and rheumatoid synovium. *Arthritis Rheum,* Vol.34, No.12, pp. 1508-1513, ISSN: 0004-3591

Takami, N.; Osawa, K., Miura, Y., Komai, K., Taniguchi, M., Shiraishi, M. et al. (2006). Hypermethylated promoter region of DR3, the death receptor 3 gene, in rheumatoid arthritis synovial cells. *Arthritis Rheum,* Vol.54, No.3, pp. 779–787, ISSN: 0004-3591

Tarner, I.H.; Härle, P., Müller-Ladner, U., Gay, R.E. & Gay, S. (2005). The different stages of synovitis: acute vs chronic, eary vs late and non-erosive vs erosive. *Best Pract Res Clin Rheumatol,* Vol.19, No.1 pp. 19-35, ISSN: 1521-6942

Tetlow, L.C. & Woolley, D.E. (1995). Mast cells, cytokines, and metalloproteinases at the rheumatoid lesion: dual immunolocalisation studies. *Ann Rheum Dis,* Vol.54, No.11, pp. 896-903, ISSN: 0003-4967

Tolboom, T.C.; Pieterman, E., van der Laan, W.H., Toes, R.E., Huidekoper, A.L., Nelissen, R.G. et al. (2002). Invasive properties of fibroblast-like synoviocytes: correlation with growth characteristics and expression of MMP-1, MMP-3, and MMP-10. *Ann Rheum Dis,* Vol.61, No.11, pp. 975-980, ISSN: 0003-4967

Ulisse, S.; Baldini, E., Sorrenti, S. & D'Armiento, M. (2009). The urokinase plasminogen activator system: a target for anti-cancer therapy. *Curr Cancer Drug Targets,* Vol.9, No.1, pp. 32-71, ISSN: 1568-0096

van de Sande, M.G.; de Hair, M.J., van der Leij, C., Klarenbeek, P.L., Bos, W.H., Smith, M.D. et al. (2011). *Ann Rheum Dis,* Vol.70, No.5, pp. 77-777, ISSN: 0003-4967

van der Laan, W.H.; Pap, T., Ronday, H.K., Grimbergen, J.M., Huisman, L.G., TeKoppele, J.M. et al. (2000). Cartilage degradation and invasion by rheumatoid synovial fibrobalsts is inhibited by gene transfer of a cell surface-targeted plasmin inhibitor. *Arthritis Rheum,* Vol.43, No.8, pp. 1710-1718, ISSN: 0004-3591

van der Laan, W.H.; Quax, P.H., Seemayer, C.A., Huisman, L.G., Pieterman, E.J., Grimbergen, J.M. et al. (2003). Cartilage degradation and invasion by rheumatoid synovial fibroblasts is inhibited by gene transfer of TIMP-1 and TIMP-3. *Gene Ther,* Vol.10, No.3, pp. 234-242, ISSN: 0969-7128

Varisco, P. A.; Péclat, V., van Ness, K., Bischof-Delaloye, A., So, A. & Busso, N. (2000). Effect of thrombin inhibition on synovial inflammation in antigen induced arthritis. *Ann Rheum Dis,* Vol.59, No.10, pp. 781-787, ISSN: 0003-4967

Weinberg, J.B.; Pippen, A.M. & Greenberg, C.S. (1991). Extravascular fibrin formation and dissolution in synovial tissues of patients with osteoarthritis and rheumatoid arthritis. *Arthritis Rheum,* Vol.34, No.8, pp. 996-1005, ISSN: 0004-3591

Wernicke, D.; Schulze-Westhoff, C., Bräuer, R., Petrow, P., Zacher, J., Gay, S. & Gromnica-Ihle, E. (2002). Stimulation of collagenase 3 expression in synovial fibroblasts of patients with rheumatoid arthritis by contact with a three.dimensional collagen matrix or with normal cartilage when coimplanted in NOD/SCID mice. *Arthritis Rheum,* Vol.46, No.1, pp. 64-74, ISSN: 0004-3591

Wunrau, C.; Schnaeker, E.M., Freyth, K., Pundt, N., Wendholt, D., Neugebauer, K. & et al. (2009). *Arthritis Rheum,* Vol.60, No.9, pp. 2606-2611, ISSN: 0004-3591

Woessner, J.F.Jr. (1991). Matrix metalloproteinases and their inhibitors in connective tissue remodeling. *FASEB J,* Vol.5, No.8, pp. 2145-2154, ISSN: 0892-6638

Yamanaka, H.; Makino, K., Takizawa, H., Fujimoto, N., Moriya, H. et al. (2000). Expression and tissue localization of membrane-types 1, 2, and 3 matrix metralloproteinases in rheumatoid synovium. *Lab Invest,* Vol.80, No.5, pp. 677-687, ISSN: 0023-6837

Yoshihara, Y.; Nakamura, H., Obata, K., Yamada, H., Hayakawa, T., Fujikawa, K. & Okada, Y. (2000). Matrix metalloproteinases and tissue inhibitors of metalloproteinases in synovial fluids from patients with rheumatoid arthritis or osteoarthritis. *Ann Rheum Dis,* Vol.59, No.6, pp. 455-461, ISSN: 0003-4967

8

Glycoproteomics of Lubricin-Implication of Important Biological Glyco- and Peptide-Epitopes in Synovial Fluid

Liaqat Ali, Chunsheng Jin and Niclas G. Karlsson*
Medical Biochemistry, University of Gothenburg
Sweden

1. Introduction

The dynamic milieu of synovial fluid is of particular interest for biomarker discovery of joint related diseases as it is composed not only of ultra-filtrated proteins originating in serum, but also proteins exclusively expressed and secreted by cells localized within the synovial membrane, fluid or cartilage. Lubricin (proteoglycan 4, prg4) is an abundant mucinous and secretory glycoprotein (~227 to 345 kDa) in synovial fluid (SF) and one of the factors considered responsible for boundary lubrication of diarthrodial joints (Swann et al., 1981; Swann et al., 1985; Jay, 1992). Lubricin is encoded by gene *PRG4* and synthesized in synovial fibroblasts (synoviocytes) and superficial zone chondrocytes. Different transcripts of *PRG4* have been referred to as superficial zone protein (SZP), megakaryocyte stimulating factor (MSF) precursor, camptodactyly arthropathy coxa vara pericarditis (CACP) protein, and hemangiopoietin (HAPO), which has recently been reviewed by Bao et al (Bao et al., 2011). As a primarily lubricating glycoprotein, lubricin has been found in SF, superficial layer of articular cartilage, tendons, and menisci (Schumacher et al., 1994; Schumacher et al., 1999; Rees et al., 2002; Rhee et al., 2005b; Schumacher et al., 2005; Sun et al., 2006). This tissue-specific distribution makes lubricin a potential biomarker during the exacerbation of chronic articular inflammation.

Human synovial lubricin (1404 amino acids) has a large and central mucin-like domain characterized with 59 imperfect repeating units of EPAPTTPK which is subject to extensive *O*-linked glycosylation. The abundance of negatively charged sugars in this domain contributes to the protein's boundary lubrication of the cartilage surface due to strong repulsive hydration forces (Jay, 1992). The mucin domain is flanked by a *C*-terminal hemopexin (PEX)-like domain and two somatomedin B (SMB)-like domains at its *N*-terminus (Flannery et al., 1999; Schumacher et al., 1999; Ikegawa et al., 2000). The two *N*-terminal SMB-like domains have 60% similarity to that of vitronectin, while *C*-terminal PEX-like domain also shows similarity to domains in vitronectin (40-50%) as well as to the matrix metalloproteinase (MMPs) family. Purified serum hemopexin has been showed to interact with hyaluronan, suggesting that the PEX-like domain in lubricin may also medicate the binding of lubricin to hyaluronan at or near cartilage surface (Hrkal et al., 1996). In addition to boundary lubrication, lubricin protects cartilage surfaces from protein deposition and cell adhesion (Rhee et al., 2005b).

* Corresponding author

During inflammation, glycosylation properties such as sialylation, sulfation, and fucosylation, are regulated to manipulate cell adhesion, differentiation, maturation, and activation in the case of immune cells. Bone and cartilage cells like osteoblasts, synovial fibroblasts and chondrocytes have been shown to possess the enzymes necessary for the synthesis of *N*- and *O*-glycans of glycoproteins, among which some activities are regulated by cytokines found in inflamed joints (Brockhausen & Anastassiades, 2008). Based on the established biosynthetic pathways, it was reported that human joint glycoproteins mainly had complex bi-antennary *N*-glycans and *O*-glycans with core 1 and the branched core 2 structures (Brockhausen & Anastassiades, 2008). In our previous study, the *O*-linked oligosaccharides of lubricin were characterized (Estrella et al., 2010). On lubricin, core 1 *O*-linked oligosaccharides are the predominant structures. Removal of sialic acid and core 1 oligosaccharides caused loss of boundary lubrication (Jay, 1992; Jay et al., 2001), showing that these structural elements are sufficient for providing lubricating property of lubricin. With aid of liquid-chromatography-mass spectrometry (LC-MS), small proportion of sialylated core 2 oligosaccharides were also found on lubricin both with and without sulfation. This indicates that lubricin glycosylation also have other task requiring complex *O*-glycosylation. In summary, both core 1 and core 2 glyco-epitopes on lubricin have the potential of excessive interactions with glyco-binding proteins, such as selectins and galectins, to facilitate inflammation.

Degenerative joint disease and joint injury are associated with increased turnover of articular cartilage proteins, inflammation, and alterations to other joint tissue proteins (Goldring & Goldring, 2007). So far, several synovial joint-specific biomarkers have been identified in adults, such as calgranulin A, B, and C (Sinz et al., 2002; Liao et al., 2004), fibrinogen β-chain, fructose bisphosphonate aldolase A, alpha-enolase (Tilleman et al., 2005), tenascin-C (Hasegawa et al., 2004), serum amyloid A (SAA), and broader inflammatory biomarkers, such as C-reactive protein (Kuhn et al., 2004) and haptoglobin (Sinz et al., 2002; Kantor et al., 2004). Lubricin as one important synovial component to monitor the state of a joint is less investigated, despite its highly relevant function as a biolubricant. Because of the size and posttranslational modifications of lubricin, it is not readily detectable by traditional two-dimensional electrophoresis (2-DE). However, a decreased expression of lubricin together with increased degradation of lubricin have been associated with more aggressive rheumatoid arthritis (RA) and osteoarthritis (OA). This strongly indicates that lubricin may be a good joint-specific biomarker. For example, *in vitro* boundary lubricating test indicated that SF from chronic inflammatory RA patients had decreased lubricating ability in comparison with SF from acute knee joint synovitis patients and cartilage transplant donors (Elsaid et al., 2005). According to the expression level of lubricin in synovium, RA patients could be classified into two groups, of where lower expression level of lubricin was associated with a more aggressive disease stage (Ungethuem et al., 2010). As for OA, animal models of OA also feature reduced levels of lubricin, particularly in the early stage of the disorder (Young et al., 2006; Elsaid et al., 2007). Also, when applied exogenous lubricin in an animal model of OA, it appears to be chondroprotective and to reduce structural damage (Flannery et al., 2009; Teeple et al., 2011). It has been demonstrated that lubricin expression is down-regulated by proinflammatory cytokines (e.g., interleukin (IL)-1β, tumor necrosis factor α (TNFα), and IL-6) (Flannery et al., 1999; Rhee et al., 2005b; Young et al., 2006; Schmidt et al., 2008). Decreased synovial lubricin level may be caused by degradation with neutrophil elastase, cathepsin B, and MMPs (Jones et al., 2003; Elsaid et al., 2005). MMPs are an enzyme family of calcium-dependent zinc-containing endopeptidase which is known to play important roles in tissue remodeling during physiological as well as pathological processes. In cartilage, MMPs are the principal proteases capable of degrading a wide variety of the extracellular matrix components (Nagase & Woessner, 1999). The released fragment of lubricin together with other synovial residual proteins and cartilage matrices floating in synovial fluid may be detected by biochemical or immunochemical assay. The profile of proteins or fragments within SF may represent diagnostic or prognostic biomarker for degenerative joint diseases.

Defect of lubricin function leads to CACP syndrome in human, which is a rare and Mendelian genetic arthropathy causing juvenile-onset, inflammatory, precocious joint failure (Marcelino et al., 1999). Although *Prg4*$^{-/-}$ mice did not have noticeably reduced fertility or life span, with aging knockout mice underwent synovial hyperplasia, subintimal fibrosis, proteinaceous deposits on the cartilage surface, irregular cartilage surface and endochondral growth plates, and ultimate invasion of the cartilage surface by synoviocytes reminiscent of human CACP and the cartilage invasion of RA joints by the inflammatory pannus (Rhee et al., 2005b).

As all these studies indicate, it is reasonable to speculate that inflammation-induced alterations of both the level, degradation and glycosylation of lubricin that occur in the joints of patients with RA and OA may accelerate the destruction of joints and exacerbate the disease. Monitoring new glyco-epitopes and/or proteolytic fragments of lubricin may serve as a potential biomarker for advanced diagnosis of early stage. To perform this, it is necessary to fully characterize the lubricin molecule by glycoproteomics. In this study, we used various biotinylated lectins or anti-carbohydrate antibodies together with MS to characterize glyco-epitopes on lubricin. The results confirm that lubricin contains immunologically important *O*-linked oligosaccharide epitopes that are capable of binding selectins and galectins. Proteomic analysis indicated that not all repeat units are occupied with *O*-linked oligosaccharides and also revealed several fragments of lubricin in synovial fluid.

It is known that joint damage may progress despite decreased inflammatory activity and erosions may develop in patients with few signs of inflammation by conventional assessments (Flato et al., 2003). Therefore, predicting the progression and consequences of inflammatory pathology are essential for optimal clinical management. The ideal biomarker of persistent inflammation in arthritis should fulfill a number of criteria including: detectable levels in early disease, expression which coincides with each inflammatory episode and expression that is restricted to the inflamed joint. The identification of differentially expressed proteins contributes to understanding the molecular factors of the disease better and paves the way for new diagnostic and prognostic markers, and eventually to novel targets in the development of therapeutic strategies.

2. Glycoproteomic characterization of synovial lubricin

2.1 Materials and methods

2.1.1 Enrichments of lubricin from synovial fluid

Synovial fluid samples from RA patients were collected during therapeutic joint aspiration at the Rheumatology Clinic, Sahlgrenska University Hospital (Gothenburg, Sweden). All patients gave informed consent and the procedure was approved by the Ethics Committee of Sahlgrenska University Hospital. All patients fulfilled the American College of Rheumatology 1987 revised criteria for RA (Arnett et al., 1988). The samples were clarified by centrifugation at 10,000 g for 10 minutes and stored at -80°C before use. The acidic proteins were purified as previously described (Estrella et al., 2010). In brief, synovial fluid sample was diluted with washing buffer (250 mM NaCl, 20 mM Tris-HCl, 10 mM EDTA, pH 7.5) before applying to 1 mL DEAE FF Hi-Trap column (GE Healthcare, Uppsala, Sweden). Enriched glycoproteins were eluted with 1 M NaCl in washing buffer. Lubricin containing fractions were precipitated with 80% ethanol for 16 hours at -20°C. The precipitate was collected by centrifugation at 12,100 g for 20 minutes and re-suspended in phosphate buffered saline (PBS) at pH 7.4 after air-dry. Protein concentration was determined by BCA protein assay kit (Thermo Scientific, San Jose, CA, USA) using bovine serum albumin (BSA) as standard.

For sandwich ELISA, 96-well microtiter plates (Nunc, Roskilde, Denmark) were coated with rabbit anti-lubricin polyclonal antibody (Thermo Scientific) in 0.1 M carbonate buffer, pH 9.5, at a concentration of 2 ng/mL and 4°C overnight. The plates were then blocked with 1% BSA in TBS-T buffer (Tris-buffered saline with 0.01% Tween 20) at 37°C for 1 hour. Fractions were diluted with 1% BSA in TBS-T buffer, added to each well, and incubated at 37°C for 1 hour. After washing with TBS-T buffer, diluted anti-lubricin mouse monoclonal antibody (Pfizer Research, Cambridge, MA, USA) was added to each well and incubated at 37°C for 1 hour. After extensive wash, horseradish peroxidase (HRP)-labeled goat anti-rabbit immunoglobulin antibody (DakoCytomation, Glostrup, Denmark) was added. Color was developed by using tetramethyl benzidine (TMB) buffer (Sigma-Aldrich, St. Louis, MO, USA) as substrate for 10 minutes at room temperature; and reaction was stopped by adding 1 M H_2SO_4. The optical density was measured at 450 nm wavelength.

2.1.2 Western blot and lectin immunoblot

Samples were reduced with 10 mM dithiothreitol (Sigma-Aldrich) and denatured by heating at 95°C for 20 minutes, and then alkylated with 25 mM iodoacetamide (Sigma-Aldrich) for 1 hour at room temperature in the dark. As for non-reduced samples, protein samples were mixed with SDS loading buffer and heated at 95°C for 20 minutes. The samples were then applied to a 3-8% Tris/acetate NuPAGE gel (Invitrogen AB, Stockholm, Sweden) or agarose-polyacrylamide gel (AgPAGE) which was made as described previously (Schulz et al., 2002). The samples were blotted onto PVDF membrane (Immobilon P, Millipore, Billerica, MA, USA) using a semi-dry blotter (Bio-Rad, Hercules, CA, USA).

PVDF membranes were blocked for 1-2 hour at room temperature in TBS-T buffer containing 1% BSA at room temperature on a shaker, and then incubated with primary antibodies or biotinylated lectins at the appropriate concentration diluted in TBS-T buffer with 1% BSA for 1 hour at room temperature on a shaker. After washing the blots three times with TBS-T, blots were incubated with secondary antibodies or streptavidin labeled with HRP for 1 hour at room temperature. After wash, bound antibodies and lectins were detected by using SuperSignal West Femto maximum sensitivity substrate (Thermo Scientific).

Anti-carbohydrate antibodies used in study including anti-T antigen (mAb 3C9), anti-Tn antigen (mAb 5F4 and 1E3), and anti-sialyl Tn (mAb TKH2 and 3F1), which were kindly provided by Prof. Henrick Clausen and Prof. Ola Blixt (University of Copenhagen,

Denmark). Mouse anti-3′-sulfo-Le^a was kindly provided by Dr. Antoon J Ligtenberg (Department of Oral Biochemistry, University of Amsterdam, The Netherlands). The other anti-carbohydrate antibodies tested in this study were mouse anti- sialyl Lewis x (sLe^x , CD15s, or mAb CSLEX1, BD Biosciences, Franklin Lakes, NJ, USA), MECA-79 (CD62L, BD Biosciences), mouse anti-chondroitin sulfate (mAb CS56, Sigma-Aldrich), mouse anti-sLe^a (mAb CA19-9, Abcam, Cambridge, MA, USA), and mouse anti-Le^b (mAb 2-25LE, Abcam). Biotinylated lectins were also used in this study including ConA (concanavalin A), MAA-I (*Maackia amurensis* lectin I), WGA (succinylated wheat germ agglutinin), and AAL (*Aleuria aurantia* lectin), all from Vector (Vector Laboratories, Burlingame, CA, USA). Biotinylated PNA (*Arachis hypogaea* lectin) and HAA (*Helix aspersa* agglutinin) were from Sigma-Aldrich. Secondary antibodies used were HRP conjugated rabbit anti-mouse IgG, HRP conjugated rabbit anti-rat IgG+IgM (Jackson ImmunoResearch, Suffolk, UK). For biotin labeled lectin, HRP conjugated streptavidin (Vector Laboratories) was used. The immunoassay was validated and optimized with human salivary mucin as described previously (Issa et al., 2010) and bovine fetuin (Sigma-Aldrich).

2.1.3 Glycomic analysis of lubricin *O*-glycan structures

O-linked oligosaccharides were released by reductive β-elimination (Schulz et al., 2002). In brief, membrane strips were incubated with 50 µL of 1.0 M $NaBH_4$ in 100 mM NaOH for 16 hours at 50°C. Reactions were quenched with 1 µL of glacial acetic acid. Samples were then desalted and dried for capillary graphitized carbon LC-MS and LC-MS^2 in negative ion mode using an LTQ Ion Trap (Thermo Scientific). Oligosaccharides were identified from their MS^2 spectra using the UniCarb-DB (2011 version) (Hayes et al., 2011) and validated manually.

For deglycosylation, the reduced and alkylated samples (20 µg) were incubated with 5 mU of sialidase A (Prozyme Inc., Oxford, UK) to remove sialic acids at 37°C for 16 hours. An aliquot of sample was also treated with 2.5 mU *O*-glycanase (endo-α-*N*-acetylgalactosaminidase, Prozyme Inc.), which cleaves core 1 type *O*-linked glycan on glycoproteins and glycopeptides, at 37°C for 16 hours. The reaction was stopped by heating at 95°C for 10 minutes in SDS-loading buffer, and enzymes were removed by electrophoresis.

2.1.4 Proteomic characterization of lubricin

Coomassie blue-stained protein bands in Tris/acetate NuPAGE gels were excised and digested with trypsin as described (Kuster et al., 1997). The resultant peptides were subjected to nano-LC-MS^2 using LTQ-Orbitrap XL mass spectrometer (Thermo Scientific). Peptide MS/MS spectra were searched against UniProt and NCBI human protein databases using GPM (Zhang et al., 2011) and Mascot software (v.2.2.04, Matrix Science Inc., MA, USA). Only peptides with a mass deviation lower than 10 ppm were accepted and two peptide sequences with manual inspection were used for positive protein identification.

Enriched synovial lubricin sample was also treated with *O*-sialoglycoprotein endopeptidase from *Pasteurella haemolytica* (Cedarlane Laboratories, Ontario, Canada). 5 µg of samples were incubated with endopeptidase in PBS (pH 7.4) at 37°C; and small aliquots were taken out at 0, 3, 6, and 16 hours. The reaction was stopped by adding SDS-loading buffer with boiling.

2.2 Result

2.2.1 Enrichment of synovial lubricin

Synovial lubricin is a heavily negatively charged glycoprotein that can be enriched by ion-exchange chromatography (Fig. 1A). Lubricin containing fractions which were determined by sandwich ELISA were pooled and precipitated by 80% ethanol. The amount of protein in these fractions corresponded to 1.38 mg/mL synovial fluid (mean, n=5). Considering that lubricin has been shown to be in the range of 0.2-0.5 mg/mL(Marcelino et al., 1999; Schmid et al., 2001; Elsaid et al., 2005), this indicates that additional proteins (*e.g.*, albumin) and glycoproteins (*e.g.*, fibronectin, aggrecan) are co-purified (See proteomic section).

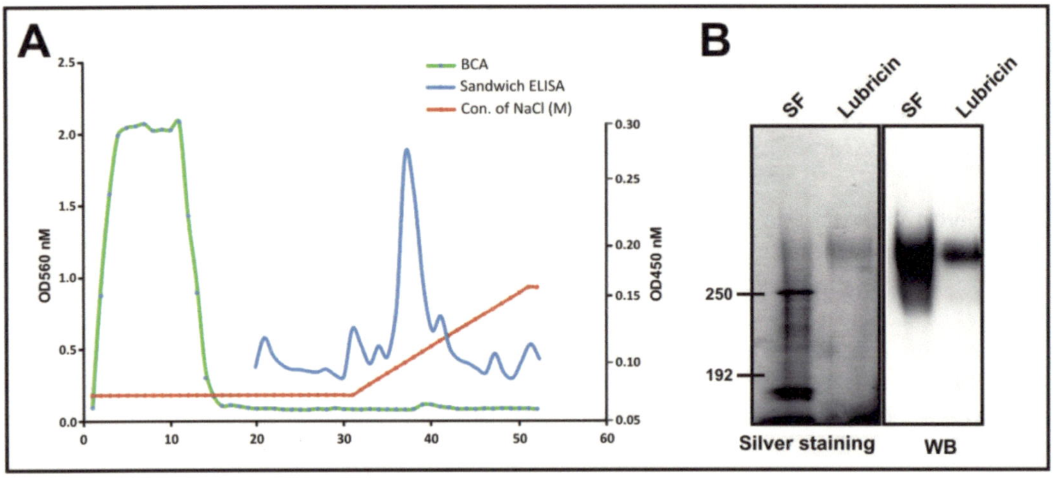

Fig. 1. Enrichment of human lubricin from synovial fluid. (A) Representative elution profile of DEAE ion-exchange chromatography. Protein levels in each fraction were determined by BCA method, while lubricin-containing fractions (Fr. 35-41) were pooled and precipitated with 80% ethanol. (B) Reduced and alkylated synovial fluid (SF, 1 μL) and enriched sample (Lubricin, 2 μg) were separated by Ag-PAGE. Protein bands were visualized by silver nitrate or detected by Western blot (WB).

As shown in Fig. 1B, silver staining of Ag-PAGE showed one major band around 300 kDa indicating that the majority of synovial proteins were removed during enrichment. When more samples were loaded, additional faint bands were also detected (Fig. 4B-2). Both mouse monoclonal (Fig. 1B) and rabbit polyclonal antibody (not shown) specifically react to prepared lubricin, respectively. Though there are few bands smaller than lubricin, none of them reacted with lubricin-specific antibodies.

2.2.2 Glyco-epitope on synovial lubricin verified by immunoassay

To examine the glycan profile on lubricin, purified samples were primarily analyzed by immunoassay with lectins or anti-carbohydrate antibodies (Fig. 2). Synovial lubricin was positive to the lectins specific to sialic acid and T antigen, such as WGA (sialic acid and terminal GlcNAcβ1,4), MAA-I (specific to α2,3-linked sialic acid), and PNA (T antigen, Galβ1,3GalNAcα1-*O*-Ser/Thr). Lubricin also reacted with HAA, a lectin specific to terminal GalNAcα1- including Tn antigen (GalNAcα1-*O*-Ser/Thr). Lectin immunoblot of synovial lubricin was also negative to ConA, which binds to branched Manα1- on high-mannose and hybrid type *N*-glycans, suggesting *N*-glycans were absent on lubricin or in very low amounts. The same negative results were obtained with *Aleuria aurantia* lectin (AAL), which recognized both peripheral and core fucosylated glycans.

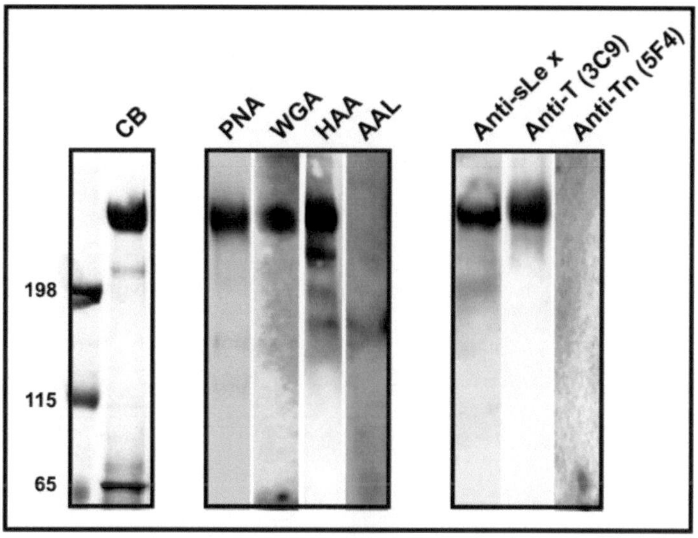

Fig. 2. Glyco-epitope on lubricin analyzed by immunoblot. Reduced and alkylated enriched lubricin sample (6 µg/lane) was separated by 3-8% Tris/acetate NuPAGE and blotted to PVDF membrane. Strips were incubated with various lectins or anti-carbohydrate antibodies after blocking with 1% BSA in TBS-T buffer. After incubating with HRP conjugated corresponding secondary antibodies and streptavidin, bands were developed by SuperSignal West Femto maximum sensitivity substrate. CB, Coomassie blue stained gel; PNA, peanut agglutinin; WGA, wheat germ agglutinin; AAL, *Aleuria aurantia* lectin; HAA, *Helix aspersa* agglutinin; Anti-sLe^x, sialyl Lewis x-specific antibody; T, T antigen, Galβ1,3GalNAc-*O*-Ser/Thr; Tn, Tn antigen, GalNAc-*O*-Ser/Thr.

When synovial lubricin was investigated by anti-carbohydrate antibodies (Fig. 2), lubricin was suggested to have T antigen and sialyl Lewis x (sLe^x, structure in Fig. 3C). Western blot showed (data not presented) that lubricin was negative for anti-carbohydrate antibodies specific to chondroitin sulfate (mAb CS56), sLe^a [NeuAcα2,3Galβ1,3(Fucα1,4)GlcNAcβ1-], (mAb CA19-9), 3′-sulfo-Le^a [NeuAcα2,3Gal(3S)β1,3(Fucα1,4)GlcNAc-], Le^b [Fucα1,2Galβ1,3(Fucα1,4)GlcNAcβ1-], (mAb 2-25LE], MECA-79 epitopes, Tn antigen (mAb 5F4 and 1E3), and sialyl Tn antigen [NeuAcα2,6GalNAc-*O*-Ser/Thr], (mAb TKH2 and 3F1). Results obtained from anti-carbohydrate antibodies agree with results from the lectin immunoblot except for lectin HAA. Together with the lectin immunoblot, these results demonstrated synovial lubricin had sialylated glycans, core 1 *O*-glycan and peripheral sLe^x epitope. In order to reveal the identity of the sLe^x containing *O*-glycans and identify other glycan epitopes not recognized by the antibodies and lectin used, additional experiments were carried out.

2.2.3 Glyco-epitope on synovial lubricin verified by LC-MS

Though immunoassay with lectins and anti-carbohydrate antibodies is convenient to detect glyco-epitopes, inner structural information is commonly scant. Furthermore, some glyco-epitopes may not be detectable because of hindrance in space or detect limitations. In addition, certain glyco-epitopes are short of specific antibodies. For example, there is currently no antibody available that could distinguish 3-*O*-sulfation from 6-*O*- sulfation. Therefore, to scrutinize the result obtained by Western blot/lectin blot of *O*-linked oligosaccharides on lubricin, purified samples were also subjected to β-elimination with mild base. Released oligosaccharides were then analyzed by LC-MS equipped with online graphitized carbon column as previously described (Estrella et al., 2010).

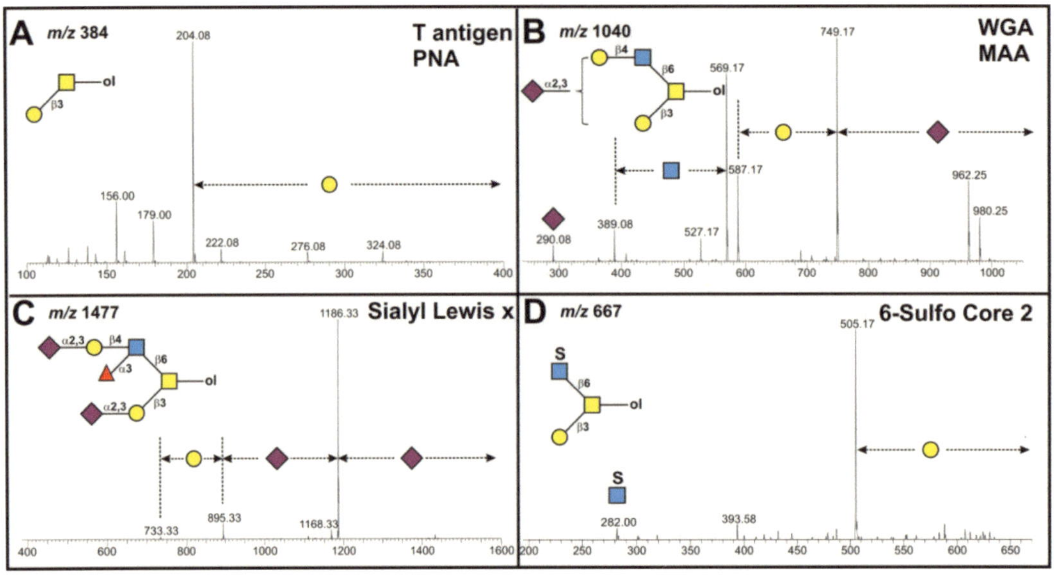

Fig. 3. Examples of core 1 and 2 *O*-linked oligosaccharides found on synovial lubricin determined by LC-MS using the $[M\text{-}H]^-$-ions as precursors. (A) MS^2 spectra of core 1 *O*-glycan (T antigen) at *m/z* 384; (B) MS^2 spectra of mono-sialylated core 2 *O*-glycan with one α2,3-linked NeuAc at *m/z* 1040; (C) MS^2 spectra of ion at *m/z* 1477 indicating a terminal sLe^x [NeuAcα2,3Galβ1,4(Fucα1,3)GlcNAc] epitope; (D) MS^2 spectra of ion at *m/z* 667, in which produced ion at *m/z* 282 indicate a sulfate group linked to GlcNAc. Purple diamond stands for sialic acid (NeuAc); yellow circle for galactose (Gal); blue square for *N*-acetylglucosamine (GlcNAc); yellow square for *N*-acetylgalactosamine (GalNAc); red triangle for fucose (Fuc); S for sulfate.

Consistent with findings from a previous study of lubricin (Estrella et al., 2010), core 1 *O*-linked oligosaccharides including T antigen (Galβ1,3GalNAc-*O*-Ser/Thr) and sialyl T antigen were the predominant *O*-linked oligosaccharides. As illustrated in Fig. 3A, MS^2 of ion at *m/z* 384 ($[M\text{-}H]^-$) indicates a composition of $Hex_1HexNAc_1$, corresponding to a T antigen. The presence of the Z ion fragment at *m/z* 204.1 is consistent with a composition of reduced HexNAc, while C ion fragment at *m/z* 179.0 indicates a terminal Hex. In comparison with MS^2 spectra in the database of UniCarb-DB (2011 version) (Hayes et al., 2011), the structure is consistent with Galβ1,3GalNAc, and its amount approximately accounts for 10% of total *O*-glycans on lubricin. Together with mono-sialylated [NeuAcα2,3Galβ1,3GalNAc] and [Galβ1,3(NeuAcα2,6)GalNAc] and di-sialylated [NeuAcα2,3Galβ1,3(NeuAcα2,6)GalNAc] structures, core 1-based structures accounted for up to 82% of total *O*-glycan, based on the total ion count. A small proportion of core 2 oligosaccharides, which account for the remaining 18% of the total *O*-glycans detected, were found in this and a previous study (Estrella et al., 2010). Three representative MS^2 spectra of core 2 *O*-linked oligosaccharide is shown, with ions at *m/z* 1040, 1477 and 667 (Fig. 3B, C and D). The $[M-H]^-$-ion at *m/z* 1040 ($NeuAc_1Hex_2HexNAc_2$) demonstrates a mono-sialylated core 2 *O*-linked oligosaccharide, while ion at *m/z* 1477 ($[M-H]^-$, $NeuAc_2Hex_2deHex_1HexNAc_2$) is the same core with one additional sialic acid and one fucose. This structure has a sequence indicative of a sialyl Lewis-type terminal glyco-epitope. These types of sialylated structures together with sialylated core 1 *O*-glycan are consistent with the positive WGA and MAA lectin blots. The Western blot results showed that lubricin were only positive to sLe^x-specific antibody but negative to sLe^a. This suggests that synovial lubricin carries sLe^x [NeuAcα2,3Galβ1,4(Fucα1,3)GlcNAc] epitope (spectrum in Fig. 3C) on core 2 structures. Sulfated core 2 *O*-glycans were also found in this study (Fig. 3D) and previous study (Estrella et al., 2010). Due to lack of good antibodies and lectins, this epitope could only be identified by MS but not by lectin analysis. This argues for LC-MS and lectin as complementary techniques that need to be applied in glycomics studies.

2.2.4 Identification of synovial lubricin fragment by proteomic analysis

Though several proteomic analyses using synovial fluid samples have been carried out (Ruiz-Romero & Blanco, 2010), lubricin (or its fragments) appeared in only a few reports (Gobezie et al., 2007; Kamphorst et al., 2007; Estrella et al., 2010). To fully characterize synovial lubricin, the enriched samples were also subjected to proteomic analysis.

When the dominating band (area 2, Fig. 4B-2) was analyzed, 28.5% of the lubricin sequence could be identified and believed to represent the fully glycosylated full-length secreted lubricin. The unidentified portion was mostly located to the mucin-like domain of lubricin (Fig. 4C). Lubricin was also detected in all other pieces of the gel indicating that lubricin existed as fragments or splice variants. Sequences of all exons could be detected except exon 1, consisting of the *N*-terminal 24 amino acid-signal sequence. In addition to the area 2 (Fig. 4B-2) where full-length lubricin was detected, remarkably high sequence recovery of lubricin was also found in the low mass region below 65 kDa (Fig. 4B-5). Identified peptides were from both *N*- and *C*-terminal implying these fragments were generated by proteolytic cleavage close to or within mucin-like domain. Examples of LC-MS^2 spectra of tryptic peptides from *N*-and *C*-terminal region of lubricin is shown in Fig. 5. Both *N*- and *C*-terminal fragments of lubricin have been found in other studies (Flannery et al., 1999; Rhee et al., 2005b). These data together with our presented data suggest that lubricin is present in synovial fluid as both full-length and degraded proteins. Few peptides (7.7%) were recovered from the area higher than lubricin area (Fig. 4B-1). This is probably caused by inefficient reduction and trace amount of multimer of lubricin which has been found in synovial fluid recently (Schmidt et al., 2009). The dominating bands in area 3 and 5 are fibronectin and the *C*-terminal fragment of lubricin, respectively (Fig. 4B, Jin et al., unpublished results).

In addition to detection of lubricin, co-purified proteins were also identified by the proteomic approach. Table 1 listed top 3 proteins identified in each gel area, which consisted of 7 unique proteins and their fragments. Except serum albumin, other proteins are glycoproteins. The presence of the lower molecular weight fibronectin in high molecular area (area 1) confirmed inefficient reduction and suggest the presence of fibronectin dimers or oligomers. Alternatively, both serum albumin and fibronectin have both been reported to bind to lubricin *in vitro* (Schmid et al., 2002) and may have been attached to lubricin during the purification. The possible association of lubricin with these proteins or their fragments is under investigation by our group.

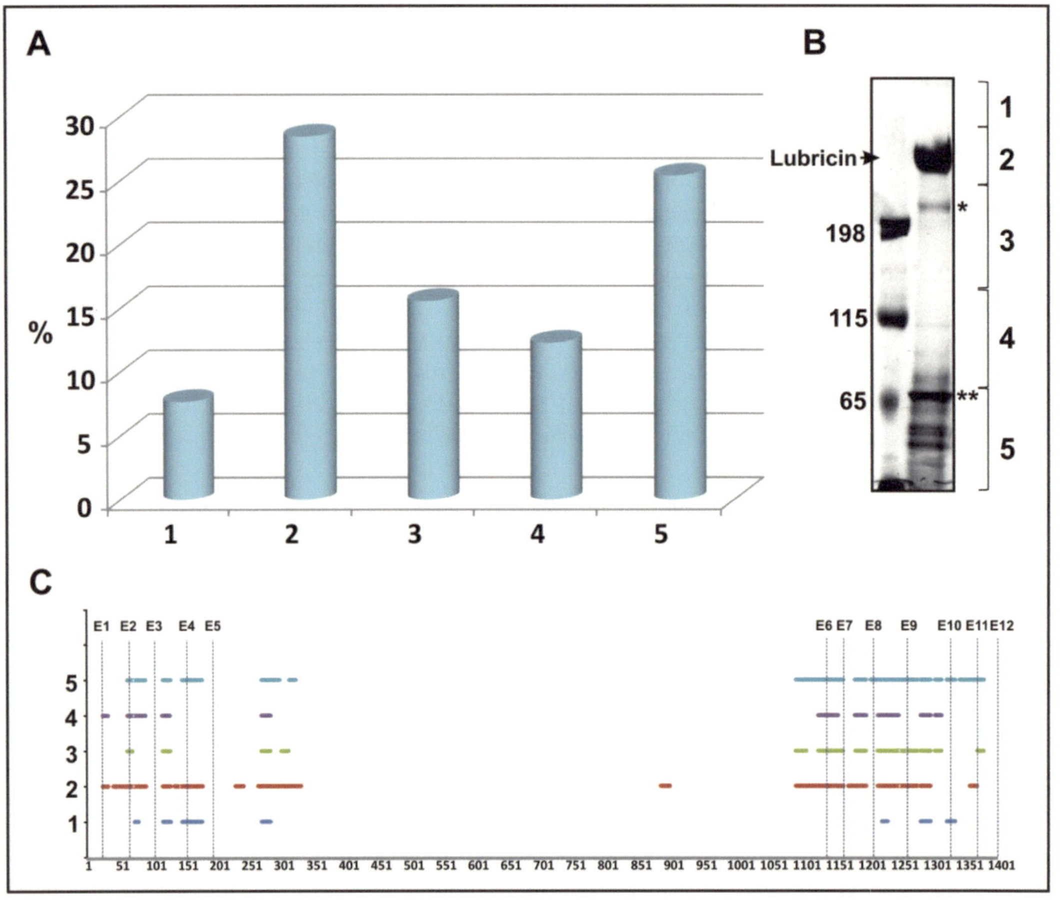

Fig. 4. Proteomic analysis of enriched synovial lubricin. (A and B) Reduced and alkylated lubricin sample was separated by 3-8% Tris/acetate NuPAGE. Protein bands were visualized by Coomassie blue. Gel slab was cut into five pieces (1 to 5) and subjected to LC-MS/MS analysis after trypsin digestion. The graph (A) shows the recoveries (%) of lubricin sequence from different cut areas. (C) Peptide map of lubricin recovered from different gel areas. The horizontal axis stands for the lubricin amino acid sequence (in total 1404 amino acids). E1 to E12 indicates the end of exon. *fibronectin; **C-terminus of lubricin

2.2.5 Characterization of lubricin mucin-like domain

Because the sequence in mucin-like domain is still largely unknown, several ways were tried to characterize this heavily *O*-glycosylated domain. As shown in Fig. 4C, resolved peptides from lubricin contain both *N*- and *C*-terminus (Fig. 5). Sequenced *N*-terminus spanned from residue 25 to 334, while *C*-terminus spanned from residue 1094 to 1383 (1404 amino acids in full-length). Only one peptide (A^{888}LENSPKEPGVPTTK^{902}) within mucin-like domain (348-855) containing 59 imperfect/perfect 8-amino acid repeats (KxPxPTTx) was found in area 2. It is believed that because of heavy *O*-glycosylation, the protein domain with this modification is normally not accessible to proteases and hence the low recovery obtained. In the case of synovial lubricin, however, it could be completely digested with trypsin in both reducing and non-reducing condition (Fig. 6A). The digestion was so complete that lubricin-

Gel area	Protein identified	MW (kDa)*	Peptide identified	Protein ID	Coverage (%)
1	Fibronectin	262.4	42	P02751	24.9
	Basement membrane-specific heparan sulfate proteoglycan core protein	468.5	14	P98160	4.0
	Apolipoprotein B-100	515.2	13	P04114	4.0
2	Lubricin	151.0	69	Q92954	28.5
	Alpha-2-macroglobulin	163.2	15	P01023	15.0
	Aggrecan core protein	250.0	15	P16112	6.9
3	Apolipoprotein B-100	515.2	111	P04114	30.9
	Fibronectin	262.4	85	P02751	44.9
	Alpha-2-macroglobulin	163.2	36	P01023	36.2
4	Fibronectin	262.4	51	P02751	30.9
	Serum albumin (HSA)	69.2	50	P02768	75.5
	Apolipoprotein B-100	515.2	52	P04114	16.9
5	Lubricin	151.0	39	Q92954	25.4
	Fibronectin	262.4	38	P02751	23.1
	Serum albumin	69.3	33	P02768	60.4

* Molecular weight of apoprotein obtained from protein database.

Table 1. Proteins identified in enriched synovial fluid sample. Reduced and alkylated lubricin sample was separated by 3-8% Tris/acetate NuPAGE. The entire gel line (Fig. 4B) was cut into five pieces (1 to 5). Gel pieces were subjected to in-gel digestion with trypsin. The resultant peptides were applied to nano-LC-MS^2. The proteins were identified from peptide MS/MS spectra, searched against Uniprot human protein database using GPM software. The 3 top ranked proteins from 1-5 cut areas with their molecular weight in kDa and with the number of unique peptides for each protein are listed in the table 1. The recoveries (%) of the 3 top ranked proteins sequence and their UniProt identification numbers are also listed.

specific antibodies showed negative in Western blot (data not shown). This data suggests that the mucin domain of lubricin is different from mucin domains of traditional mucous mucins which are not susceptible to trypsin. Difference in glycosylation between lubricin and traditional mucins was also suggested by the treatment with *O*-sialoglycoprotein endopeptidase from *Pasteurella haemolytica* which cleaves heavily sialylated mucin-domain, but only had minor effect on lubricin. As shown in Fig. 6B, after overnight incubation, the density of Coomassie blue stained band was significantly diminished. However, when the digested same samples were probed with mouse monoclonal antibody, Western blot showed that epitope of the antibody, recognizing part of the unglycosylated *N*-terminal region, was still attached to the large mucin domain. Only a small shift in the migration in SDS-PAGE was observed after the endopeptidase treatment.

In order to show that the reason for low recovery of the mucin domain was due to glycosylation, sialidase A and *O*-glycanase were used to remove the majority of *O*-linked oligosaccharides (Fig. 6C and 7). Desialylation with sialidase A decreased the size of lubricin on Ag-PAGE verified that synovial lubricin contained sialic acid (Fig. 6C). When further treated with *O*-glycanase, which cleaves core 1 type *O*-linked glycan (Galβ1,3GalNAcα1-*O*-Ser/Thr) on glycoproteins and glycopeptides, the size of lubricin decreased dramatically and was close to the calculated molecular weight of lubricin without posttranslational modification, i.e. 148 kDa. These results suggested that lubricin is heavily glycosylated and core 1 type *O*-linked oligosaccharides are the predominant *O*-glycans on lubricin. Bands after sialidase A treatment with or without subsequent *O*-glycanase treatment were subjected to LC-MS/MS analysis after trypsin digestion. Sialidase A alone recover 19.1% of lubricin sequence (Fig. 7), most of the peptides were located in the mucin-like domain including 18 random repeats of EPAPTTPK. In contrast, removal of glycosylation using both sialidase and *O*-glycanase gave up to 48% recovery of the lubricin sequence (Fig. 7). By removal of core 1 *O*-glycans, more protein core was revealed and made accessible for digestion providing peptides from the mucin domain repeated to be recovered and detected by LC-MS. Resolved sequence covered almost entire mucin-like domain of lubricin and repeat region without glycosylation could be identified (Fig. 8).

2.3 Discussion

Though several biomarkers in SF and serum have been associated with RA and OA, no single biomarker has sufficient discriminating power to clearly indicate prognosis. Hence, the quest to find new, more efficient single biomarker for cartilage degrading diseases remains. On the other hand, measurement of multiple biomarkers at the time of diagnosis would improve diagnosis accuracy and even early diagnosis. As a candidate biomarker, SF lubricin has been found to be an important lubricant in SF, but expression level is also associated with inflammation. Lubricin has not been characterized fully because of its size and heavily *O*-glycosylation. In this study, SF lubricin was characterized by both glycomic and proteomic means, indicating that in addition to the level of lubricin in SF, both the glycosylation and its degradation are potential marker for disease progression and inflammation.

In combination with our previous study (Estrella et al., 2010) and this study (Fig. 2 and 3), synovial lubricin was shown to possess predominantly core 1 *O*-linked oligosaccharides. Even in a low amounts, with the aid of liquid chromatography-mass spectrometry (LC-MS), small proportions of core 2 oligosaccharides were found to carry sulfate group. In addition,

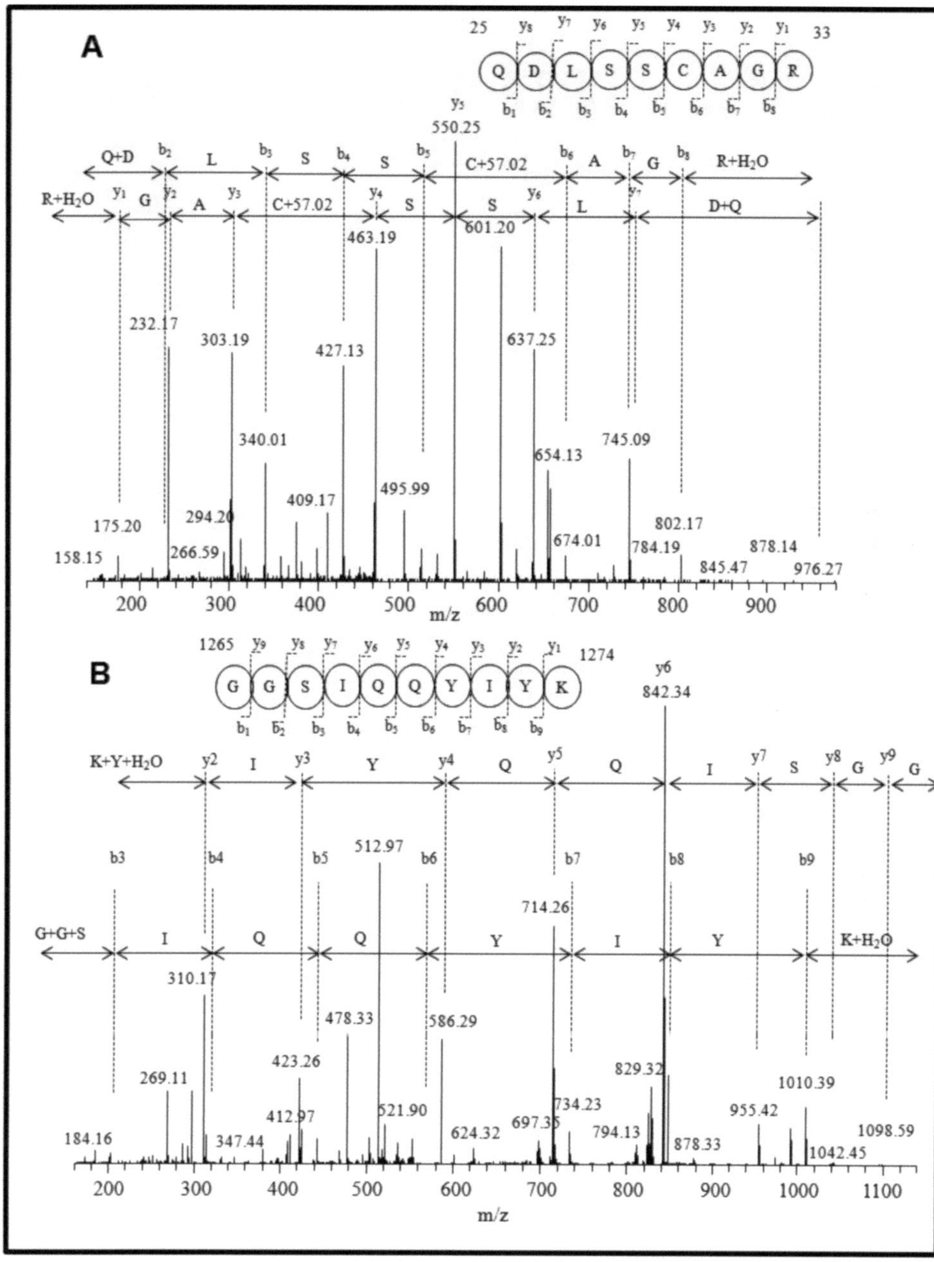

Fig. 5. MS2 spectra of one *N*-terminal (A) and one *C*-terminal (B) peptide derived from reduced and alkylated lubricin that was searched against UniProt and NCBI human protein database using GPM software. The position of the *N*-terminal peptide in the protein sequence starts from amino acid 25 and ends at 33. The *m/z* 976.41 is the $[M+H]^+$ precursor ion and *m/z* 488.71 is the $[M+H]^{2+}$. The assigned ID number for this peptide in the GPM database is 1193. The position of the *C*-terminal peptide starts from amino acid 1265 and ends at 1274. The *m/z* 1156.59 is the $[M+H]^+$ precursor ion and *m/z* 578.80 is the $[M+H]^{2+}$.The assigned ID number for this peptide in the GPM is 2538.

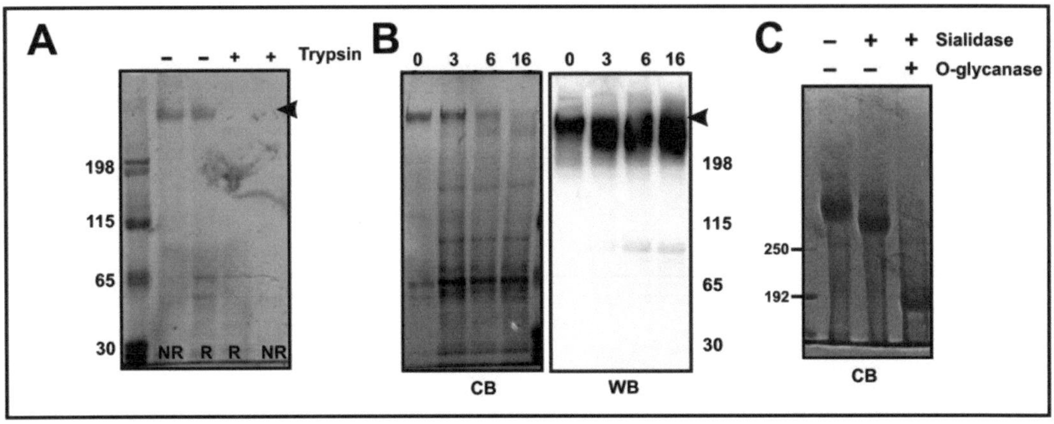

Fig. 6. Proteomic analysis of lubricin under various conditions. All purified samples were reduced and alkylated before separation by 3-8% Tris/acetate NuPAGE gel. (A) Samples (5 μg) were incubated with trypsin. Aliquots were taken out at different time (0 to 16 hours). SDS-PAGE gel was stained with Coomassie blue. (B) Samples (5 μg) were treated with *O*-sialoglycoprotein endopeptidase from *Pasteurella haemolytica*. A duplicated gel was blotted to PVDF membrane and probed with moue monoclonal anti-lubricin antibody. (C) Enriched lubricin sample (8 μg/lane) was treated with sialidase in absence or presence of *O*-glycanase at 37°C overnight. The resultant products were separated by Ag-PAGE under reducing condition.

a sLe^{x} epitope was also found present on a small proportion of the core 2 oligosaccharides. However, unlike sulfation, the level of fucosylation on lubricin was very low. Though in comparison with LC-MS, immunoassay seems less efficient but very specific to certain glyco-epitopes. For example, MS^{2} spectra of ion at *m/z* 1477 suggested a Lewis type epitope. Without further fragmentation and known retention time on LC, it is not easy to define this structure of sLe^{a} or sLe^{x}. With sLe^{a}- and sLe^{x}-specific antibody, immunoblot demonstrated lubricin was modified with sLe^{x}. HAA is a lectin specific to terminal GalNAcα1- on *N*- or *O*-glycans. The lack of antibody recognition to Tn-antigen despite HAA reactivity indicated that exposed GalNAcα1- to protein backbone was only sparingly found. Additionally, synovial lubricin was shown to contain PNA binding epitopes (Fig. 2B). This is consistent with that PNA can been used as an affinity ligand to enrich synovial lubricin (Jay et al., 2001; Teeple et al., 2011). The result from the glycomic study using both LC-MS^{n} and antibody/lectins showed the presence of a trace amount of Tn antigen, high abundant sialylated and unsialylated core 1 and several sialylated, fucosylated and sulfated core 2 oligosaccharides to be present on lubricin.

Suggestions of lubricin involvement in disease and inflammation can be identified from its glycosylation. Glycomic analysis showed that approximately 50% of the lubricin *O*-glycans contain terminal galactose, such as the T antigen. It makes lubricin a potential ligand for galectins, which are a mammalian lectin family recognizing terminal galactose. Increased expression of galectin-3 has been reported in synovial fluid from RA patients (Ohshima et al., 2003). Galectin-3 is believed to play a pro-inflammation role in joint diseases in which galectin-3 together with soluble fibrinogen was found to regulate neutrophil activation, degranulation and survival (Fernandez et al., 2005). Another attractive glyco-epitope on lubricin, sLe^{x}, is reminiscent of selectin ligands which are involved in leukocyte trafficking. For instance, although it is in a low amount, L-selectin on the surface of synovial neutrophils as well as soluble L-selectin are reported in synovial fluid (Humbria et al., 1994; De Clerck et al., 1995).

mawktlpiyllllsvfviqqvssqdlsscagrcgegysrdatcncdyncqhymeccpdfkrvctaelsckgrcfesfergrecdcdaqckkydkc
cpdyesfcaevhnptsppsskkapppsgasqtiksttkrspkppnkkktkkvieseeiteehsvsenqesssssssssstirkikssknsaanr
elqkklkVKDNKKNRTKKKPTPKPPVVDEAGSGLDNGDFKVTTPDTSTTQHNKVSTSPKITTAKPINPRPSLPPNSDTSK
ETSLTVNKETTVETKETTTTNKQTSTDGKEKTTSAKETQSIEKTSAKDLAPTSKVLAKPTPKAETTTKGPALTTPKEPTPT
TPKEPASTTPKEPTPTTIKSAPTTPKEPAPTTTKSAPTTPKEPAPTTTKEPAPTTPKEPAPTTTKEPAPTTTKSAPTTPKEP
APTTPKKPAPTTPKEPAPTTPKEPTPTTPKEPAPTTKEPAPTTPKEPAPTAPKKPAPTTPKEPAPTTPKEPAPTTTKEPSP
TTPKEPAPTTTKSAPTTTKEPAPTTTKSAPTTPKEPSPTTTKEPAPTTPKEPAPTTPKKPAPTTPKEPAPTTPKEPAPTTTK
KPAPTTPKEPAPTTPKETAPTTPKKLTPTTPEKLAPTTPEKPAPTTPEELAPTTPEEPTPTTPEEPAPTTPKAAAPNTPKEP
APTTPKEPAPTTPKEPAPTTPKETAPTTPKGTAPTTLKEPAPTTPKKPAPKELAPTTTKEPTSTTCDKPAPTTPKGTAPTT
PKEPAPTTPKEPAPTTPKGTAPTTLKEPAPTTPKKPAPKELAPTTTKGPTSTTSDKPAPTTPKETAPTTPKEPAPTTPKKP
APTTPETPPPTTSEVSTPTTTKEPTTIHKSPDESTPELSAEPTPKALENSPKEPGVPTTKTPAATKPEMTTTAKDKTTERD
LRTTPETTTAAPKMTKETATTTEKTTESKITATTTQVTSTTTQDTTPFKITTLKTTTLAPKVTTTKKTITTTEIMNKPEETA
KPKDRATNSKATTPKPQKPTKAPKKPTSTKKPKTMPRVRKPKTTPTPRKMTSTMPELNPTSRIAEAMLQTTTRPNQT
PNSKLVEVNPKSEDAGGAEGETPHMLLRPHVFMPEVTPDMDYLPRVPNQGIIINPMLSdetnicngkpvdglttlrngtlva
frghyfwmlspfsppsparritevwgipspidtvftrcncegktfffkdsqywrftndikdagypkpifkgfggltgqivaalstakyknwpesvyf
fkrggsiqqyiykqepvqkcpgrrpalnypvygettqvrrrrferaigpsqthtiriqysparlayqdkgvlhnevkvsilwrglpnvvtsaislpnir
kpdgydyyafskdqyynidvpsrtaraittrsgqtlskvwyncp

Fig. 7. Peptides recovery of bands excised from sialidase A and *O*-glycanase (Fig. 6C). The mucin-like domain is in capital (encoded by exon 6). Sequences recovered after sialidase A treatment were underlined, while sequences recovered after sialidase A and *O*-glycanase treatment were in blue.

With increased mechanical stress and protease activity associated with OA and RA, the fragmentation of lubricin shown here opens up a new possibility for disease-specific biomarkers. A few fragments of lubricin were detected in synovial fluid, which were enriched together with intact protein. The *O*-glycosylation domain is supposed to protect against proteolytic cleavage. In the case of lubricin, however, it was extensively degraded by trypsin but resistant to *O*-sialoglycoprotein endopeptidase (Fig . 5A). Similarly, lubricin has been found to be extensively degraded by papain, trypsin and pronase and to a lesser extent by pepsin (Flannery et al., 1999). Other proteases, such as neutrophil elastase (a serine protease) and cathepsin B (a cysteine protease), are also able to degrade lubricin *in vitro* (Jones et al., 2003; Elsaid et al., 2005). Interestingly, lubricin tryptic peptides were detected as low as the 30-65 kDa region (Table 1 and Fig. 1). These fragments are unlikely to contain the full mucin-like domain, but more likely an *N*- or *C*-terminal domain with a portion of mucin-like domain (non-glycosylated *N*-terminus has a mass of 33.8 kDa and the *C*-terminus 35.4 kDa). So far, it is not clear whether they were from unique cleavages along lubricin sequence or just randomly excised *in vivo*. Evidence has indicated *N*-terminus of lubricin is more sensitive to neutrophil elastase (Elsaid et al., 2005). Purified neutrophil elastase has been shown to damage cartilage explants *in vitro* (Burkhardt et al., 1988). Also neutrophil elastase, and not MMPs, can destroy the superficial layer of cartilage where lubricin locates. Consequently, MMPs have better access to cartilage molecules in less superficial layers of cartilage (Jasin & Taurog, 1991).

Are lubricin fragments associated with inflammation or pathophysiology of degenerative joint disease? Or does lubricin fragmentation patterns in OA or RA differ from those in healthy individuals? Recent studies reported the fragment of lubricin in SF (Gobezie et al., 2007; Kamphorst et al., 2007). In the work of Kamphorst et al., they found two lubricin *C*-terminal fragments (R^{1285}PALNYPVYGETTQV^{1299} and D^{1373}QYYNIDVPSRTA^{1385}) in OA SF but not in healthy SF (Kamphorst et al., 2007). In the current study with enriched RA synovial lubricin, the first sequence (1285-1300) was found distributed throughout the gel; while the second sequence (1373-1385) was only detected in area 3 and 5, areas lower than the lubricin area (Fig. 4B and C). Additionally, several new peptides derived from both *N*-terminus and *C*-termini were found in this study. These fragments could be solely by-products of degenerative joint. Alternatively, these fragments might play a regulatory role. For example, fragments from fibronectin and aggrecan have been reported to correlate with joint diseases (Homandberg et al., 1997a; Homandberg et al., 1997b; Struglics et al., 2009). Interestingly, these two proteins were also found in this study (Table I). It is not clear whether they form a protein complex together with lubricin or just happened to be co-purified with lubricin.

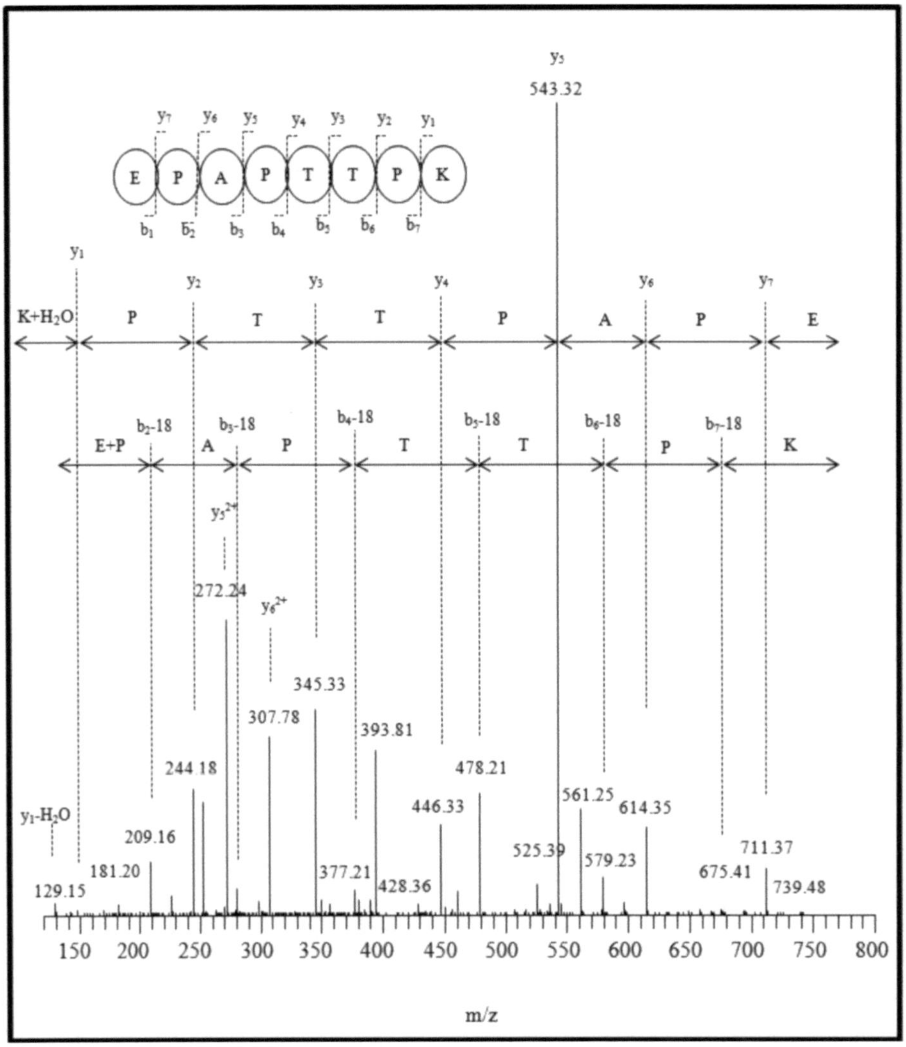

Fig. 8. MS[2] spectrum of the peptide derived after desialylated and *O*-glycanase treated lubricin sample searched against UniProt and NCBI human protein database using GPM software. The *m/z* 420.73 is the $[M+H]^{2+}$ precursor ion. The assigned ID number for the peptide in the GPM database is 3740. This peptide sequence is in the mucin domain of lubricin and is repeated 18 times in lubricin.

Besides two flanking protein domains, in the middle of lubricin there is a mucin-like domain. To our knowledge, this is the first report of a protein sequence within this domain (Fig. 7 and 8). It should be noted that among 59 imperfect repeat units, 18 have a perfect repeating unit of EPAPTTPK (Fig. 7 and 8). *O*-glycanase treatment greatly increased the recovery. As discussed above, proteolytic cleavage sites on lubricin are probably located within the mucin-like domain, and here we show that the mucin domain of lubricin is indeed accessible to proteolytic enzymes. This is probably due to a dispersed *O*-glycosylation in contrast to continuous *O*-glycosylation as the heavily bottle-brush-like *O*-glycosylation on traditional mucins, which will hinder the access to the cleavage site. Being able to sequence mucin-like domain in lubricin will facilitate the mapping of authentic proteolytic cleavage sites on lubricin *in situ* and to investigate the effect of cytokine regulated proteases on synovial lubricin during joint diseases.

3. Conclusion

In summary, using glycoproteomics we fully characterized the major glycoprotein in SF as lubricin. With knowledge of *O*-glycosylation and proteomic properties of lubricin, it allowed us to identify RA or OA-specific glyco-epitopes and fragments, enabling us to better understand how the glycosylation of lubricin is influenced by inflammation of the joint.

4. Acknowledgment

This work was supported by the Swedish Research Council (621-2010-5322), EU Marie Curie Program (PIRG-GA-2007-205302) and Reumatikerförbundet (R-85481). The mass spectrometers were obtained by grants from the Swedish Research Council (342-2004-4434) and from Knut and Alice Wallenberg's foundation (KAW2007.0118).

5. References

Arnett, F. C., Edworthy, S. M., Bloch, D. A., McShane, D. J., Fries, J. F., Cooper, N. S., Healey, L. A., Kaplan, S. R., Liang, M. H., Luthra, H. S., Medsger, T. A., Mitchell, D. M., Neustadt, D. H., Pinals, R. S., Schaller, J. G., Sharp, J. T., Wilder, R. L. & Hunder, G. G. (1988). The American Rheumatism Association 1987 revised criteria for the classification of rheumatoid arthritis. *Arthritis Rheum*, Vol.31, No.3, (Mar 1988), pp. 315-24, ISSN 0004-3591

Bao, J. P., Chen, W. P. & Wu, L. D. (2011). Lubricin: a novel potential biotherapeutic approaches for the treatment of osteoarthritis. *Mol Biol Rep*, Vol.38, No.5, (Jan 2011), pp. 2879-85, ISSN 0301-4851

Bayless, K. J., Meininger, G. A., Scholtz, J. M. & Davis, G. E. (1998). Osteopontin is a ligand for the alpha4beta1 integrin. *J Cell Sci*, Vol.111, No.9, (May 1998), pp. 1165-74, ISSN 0021-9533

Brockhausen, I. & Anastassiades, T. P. (2008). Inflammation and arthritis: perspectives of the glycobiologist. *Expert Rev Clin Immunol*, Vol.4, No.2, (Mar 2008), pp. 173-91, ISSN 1744-8409

Burkhardt, H., Rehkopf, E., Kasten, M., Rauls, S. & Heimann, P. (1988). Interaction of polymorphonuclear leukocytes with cartilage in vitro. Catabolic effects of serine proteases and oxygen radicals. *Scand J Rheumatol*, Vol.17, No.3, (Jan 1988), pp. 183-95, ISSN 0300-9742

De Clerck, L. S., De Gendt, C. M., Bridts, C. H., Van Osselaer, N. & Stevens, W. J. (1995). Expression of neutrophil activation markers and neutrophil adhesion to chondrocytes in rheumatoid arthritis patients: relationship with disease activity. *Res Immunol*, Vol.146, No.2, (Feb 1995), pp. 81-7, ISSN 0923-2494

Elsaid, K. A., Jay, G. D. & Chichester, C. O. (2007). Reduced expression and proteolytic susceptibility of lubricin/superficial zone protein may explain early elevation in the coefficient of friction in the joints of rats with antigen-induced arthritis. *Arthritis Rheum*, Vol.56, No.1, (Jan 2007), pp. 108-16, ISSN 0004-3591

Elsaid, K. A., Jay, G. D., Warman, M. L., Rhee, D. K. & Chichester, C. O. (2005). Association of articular cartilage degradation and loss of boundary-lubricating ability of synovial fluid following injury and inflammatory arthritis. *Arthritis Rheum*, Vol.52, No.6, (Jun 2005), pp. 1746-55, ISSN 0004-3591

Estrella, R. P., Whitelock, J. M., Packer, N. H. & Karlsson, N. G. (2010). The glycosylation of human synovial lubricin: implications for its role in inflammation. *Biochem J*, Vol.429, No.2, (Jul 2010), pp. 359-67, ISSN 1470-8728

Fernandez, G. C., Ilarregui, J. M., Rubel, C. J., Toscano, M. A., Gomez, S. A., Beigier Bompadre, M., Isturiz, M. A., Rabinovich, G. A. & Palermo, M. S. (2005). Galectin-3 and soluble fibrinogen act in concert to modulate neutrophil activation and survival: involvement of alternative MAPK pathways. *Glycobiology*, Vol.15, No.5, (May 2005), pp. 519-27, ISSN 0959-6658

Flannery, C. R., Hughes, C. E., Schumacher, B. L., Tudor, D., Aydelotte, M. B., Kuettner, K. E. & Caterson, B. (1999). Articular cartilage superficial zone protein (SZP) is homologous to megakaryocyte stimulating factor precursor and Is a multifunctional proteoglycan with potential growth-promoting, cytoprotective, and lubricating properties in cartilage metabolism. *Biochem Biophys Res Commun*, Vol.254, No.3, (Jan 1999), pp. 535-41, ISSN 0006-291X

Flannery, C. R., Zollner, R., Corcoran, C., Jones, A. R., Root, A., Rivera-Bermudez, M. A., Blanchet, T., Gleghorn, J. P., Bonassar, L. J., Bendele, A. M., Morris, E. A. & Glasson, S. S. (2009). Prevention of cartilage degeneration in a rat model of osteoarthritis by intraarticular treatment with recombinant lubricin. *Arthritis Rheum*, Vol.60, No.3, (Mar 2009), pp. 840-7, ISSN 0004-3591

Flato, B., Lien, G., Smerdel, A., Vinje, O., Dale, K., Johnston, V., Sorskaar, D., Moum, T., Ploski, R. & Forre, O. (2003). Prognostic factors in juvenile rheumatoid arthritis: a case-control study revealing early predictors and outcome after 14.9 years. *J Rheumatol*, Vol.30, No.2, (Feb 2003), pp. 386-93, ISSN 0315-162X

Gobezie, R., Kho, A., Krastins, B., Sarracino, D. A., Thornhill, T. S., Chase, M., Millett, P. J. & Lee, D. M. (2007). High abundance synovial fluid proteome: distinct profiles in health and osteoarthritis. *Arthritis Res Ther*, Vol.9, No.2, (Apr 2007), pp. R36, ISSN 1478-6362

Goldring, M. B. & Goldring, S. R. (2007). Osteoarthritis. *J Cell Physiol*, Vol.213, No.3, (Dec 2007), pp. 626-34, ISSN 1097-4652

Hasegawa, M., Hirata, H., Sudo, A., Kato, K., Kawase, D., Kinoshita, N., Yoshida, T. & Uchida, A. (2004). Tenascin-C concentration in synovial fluid correlates with radiographic progression of knee osteoarthritis. *J Rheumatol*, Vol.31, No.10, (Oct 2004), pp. 2021-6, ISSN 0315-162X

Hasegawa, M., Nakoshi, Y., Iino, T., Sudo, A., Segawa, T., Maeda, M., Yoshida, T. & Uchida, A. (2009). Thrombin-cleaved osteopontin in synovial fluid of subjects with rheumatoid arthritis. *J Rheumatol*, Vol.36, No.2, (Feb 2009), pp. 240-5, ISSN 0315-162X

Hayes, C. A., Karlsson, N. G., Struwe, W. B., Lisacek, F., Rudd, P. M., Packer, N. H. & Campbell, M. P. (2011). UniCarb-DB: a database resource for glycomic discovery. *Bioinformatics*, Vol.27, No.9, (May 2011), pp. 1343-4, ISSN 1367-4811

Homandberg, G. A., Davis, G., Maniglia, C. & Shrikhande, A. (1997a). Cartilage chondrolysis by fibronectin fragments causes cleavage of aggrecan at the same site as found in osteoarthritic cartilage. *Osteoarthritis Cartilage*, Vol.5, No.6, (Nov 1997a), pp. 450-3, ISSN 1063-4584

Homandberg, G. A., Hui, F., Wen, C., Purple, C., Bewsey, K., Koepp, H., Huch, K. & Harris, A. (1997b). Fibronectin-fragment-induced cartilage chondrolysis is associated with release of catabolic cytokines. *Biochem J*, Vol.321, No.3, (Feb 1997b), pp. 751-7, ISSN 0264-6021

Hrkal, Z., Kuzelova, K., Muller-Eberhard, U. & Stern, R. (1996). Hyaluronan-binding properties of human serum hemopexin. *FEBS Lett*, Vol.383, No.1-2, (Mar 1996), pp. 72-4, ISSN 0014-5793

Humbria, A., Diaz-Gonzalez, F., Campanero, M. R., Arroyo, A. G., Laffon, A., Gonzalez-Amaro, R. & Sanchez-Madrid, F. (1994). Expression of L-selectin, CD43, and CD44 in synovial fluid neutrophils from patients with inflammatory joint diseases. Evidence for a soluble form of L-selectin in synovial fluid. *Arthritis Rheum*, Vol.37, No.3, (Mar 1994), pp. 342-8, ISSN 0004-3591

Ikegawa, S., Sano, M., Koshizuka, Y. & Nakamura, Y. (2000). Isolation, characterization and mapping of the mouse and human PRG4 (proteoglycan 4) genes. *Cytogenet Cell Genet*, Vol.90, No.3-4, (Aug 2000), pp. 291-7, ISSN 0301-0171

Issa, S., Moran, A. P., Ustinov, S. N., Lin, J. H., Ligtenberg, A. J. & Karlsson, N. G. (2010). O-linked oligosaccharides from salivary agglutinin: Helicobacter pylori binding sialyl-Lewis x and Lewis b are terminating moieties on hyperfucosylated oligo-N-acetyllactosamine. *Glycobiology*, Vol.20, No.8, (Aug 2010), pp. 1046-57, ISSN 1460-2423

Jasin, H. E. & Taurog, J. D. (1991). Mechanisms of disruption of the articular cartilage surface in inflammation. Neutrophil elastase increases availability of collagen type II epitopes for binding with antibody on the surface of articular cartilage. *J Clin Invest*, Vol.87, No.5, (May 1991), pp. 1531-6, ISSN 0021-9738

Jay, G. D. (1992). Characterization of a bovine synovial fluid lubricating factor. I. Chemical, surface activity and lubricating properties. *Connect Tissue Res*, Vol.28, No.1-2, (Jan 1992), pp. 71-88, ISSN 0300-8207

Jay, G. D., Harris, D. A. & Cha, C. J. (2001). Boundary lubrication by lubricin is mediated by O-linked beta(1-3)Gal-GalNAc oligosaccharides. *Glycoconj J*, Vol.18, No.10, (Oct 2001), pp. 807-15, ISSN 0282-0080

Jones, A. R. C., Hughes, C. E., Wainwright, S. D., Flannery, C. R., Little, C. B. & Caterson, B. (2003). Degradation of PRG4/SZP by matrix proteases [abstract]. *Trans Orthop Res Soc*, Vol.28, (Feb 2003), pp. 133, ISSN 0065-9533

Kamphorst, J. J., van der Heijden, R., DeGroot, J., Lafeber, F. P., Reijmers, T. H., van El, B., Tjaden, U. R., van der Greef, J. & Hankemeier, T. (2007). Profiling of endogenous peptides in human synovial fluid by NanoLC-MS: method validation and peptide identification. *J Proteome Res*, Vol.6, No.11, (Nov 2007), pp. 4388-96, ISSN 1535-3893

Kantor, A. B., Wang, W., Lin, H., Govindarajan, H., Anderle, M., Perrone, A. & Becker, C. (2004). Biomarker discovery by comprehensive phenotyping for autoimmune diseases. *Clin Immunol*, Vol.111, No.2, (May 2004), pp. 186-95, ISSN 1521-6616

Kuhn, E., Wu, J., Karl, J., Liao, H., Zolg, W. & Guild, B. (2004). Quantification of C-reactive protein in the serum of patients with rheumatoid arthritis using multiple reaction monitoring mass spectrometry and 13C-labeled peptide standards. *Proteomics*, Vol.4, No.4, (Apr 2004), pp. 1175-86, ISSN 1615-9853

Kuster, B., Wheeler, S. F., Hunter, A. P., Dwek, R. A. & Harvey, D. J. (1997). Sequencing of *N*-linked oligosaccharides directly from protein gels: in-gel deglycosylation followed by matrix-assisted laser desorption/ionization mass spectrometry and normal-phase high-performance liquid chromatography. *Anal Biochem*, Vol.250, No.1, (Jul 1997), pp. 82-101, ISSN 0003-2697

Liao, H., Wu, J., Kuhn, E., Chin, W., Chang, B., Jones, M. D., O'Neil, S., Clauser, K. R., Karl, J., Hasler, F., Roubenoff, R., Zolg, W. & Guild, B. C. (2004). Use of mass spectrometry to identify protein biomarkers of disease severity in the synovial fluid and serum of patients with rheumatoid arthritis. *Arthritis Rheum*, Vol.50, No.12, (Dec 2004), pp. 3792-803, ISSN 0004-3591

Marcelino, J., Carpten, J. D., Suwairi, W. M., Gutierrez, O. M., Schwartz, S., Robbins, C., Sood, R., Makalowska, I., Baxevanis, A., Johnstone, B., Laxer, R. M., Zemel, L., Kim, C. A., Herd, J. K., Ihle, J., Williams, C., Johnson, M., Raman, V., Alonso, L. G., Brunoni, D., Gerstein, A., Papadopoulos, N., Bahabri, S. A., Trent, J. M. & Warman, M. L. (1999). CACP, encoding a secreted proteoglycan, is mutated in camptodactyly-arthropathy-coxa vara-pericarditis syndrome. *Nat Genet*, Vol.23, No.3, (Nov 1999), pp. 319-22, ISSN 1061-4036

Nagase, H. & Woessner, J. F., Jr. (1999). Matrix metalloproteinases. *J Biol Chem*, Vol.274, No.31, (Jul 1999), pp. 21491-4, ISSN 0021-9258

O'Regan, A. & Berman, J. S. (2000). Osteopontin: a key cytokine in cell-mediated and granulomatous inflammation. *Int J Exp Pathol*, Vol.81, No.6, (Dec 2000), pp. 373-90, ISSN 0959-9673

Ohshima, S., Kuchen, S., Seemayer, C. A., Kyburz, D., Hirt, A., Klinzing, S., Michel, B. A., Gay, R. E., Liu, F. T., Gay, S. & Neidhart, M. (2003). Galectin 3 and its binding protein in rheumatoid arthritis. *Arthritis Rheum*, Vol.48, No.10, (Oct 2003), pp. 2788-95, ISSN 0004-3591

Oldberg, A., Franzen, A. & Heinegard, D. (1986). Cloning and sequence analysis of rat bone sialoprotein (osteopontin) cDNA reveals an Arg-Gly-Asp cell-binding sequence. *Proc Natl Acad Sci U S A*, Vol.83, No.23, (Dec 1986), pp. 8819-23, ISSN 0027-8424

Rees, S. G., Davies, J. R., Tudor, D., Flannery, C. R., Hughes, C. E., Dent, C. M. & Caterson, B. (2002). Immunolocalisation and expression of proteoglycan 4 (cartilage superficial zone proteoglycan) in tendon. *Matrix Biol*, Vol.21, No.7, (Nov 2002), pp. 593-602, ISSN 0945-053X

Rhee, D. K., Marcelino, J., Al-Mayouf, S., Schelling, D. K., Bartels, C. F., Cui, Y., Laxer, R., Goldbach-Mansky, R. & Warman, M. L. (2005a). Consequences of disease-causing mutations on lubricin protein synthesis, secretion, and post-translational processing. *J Biol Chem*, Vol.280, No.35, (Sep 2005a), pp. 31325-32, ISSN 0021-9258

Rhee, D. K., Marcelino, J., Baker, M., Gong, Y., Smits, P., Lefebvre, V., Jay, G. D., Stewart, M., Wang, H., Warman, M. L. & Carpten, J. D. (2005b). The secreted glycoprotein lubricin protects cartilage surfaces and inhibits synovial cell overgrowth. *J Clin Invest*, Vol.115, No.3, (Mar 2005b), pp. 622-31, ISSN 0021-9738

Ruiz-Romero, C. & Blanco, F. J. (2010). Proteomics role in the search for improved diagnosis, prognosis and treatment of osteoarthritis. *Osteoarthritis Cartilage*, Vol.18, No.4, (Apr 2010), pp. 500-9, ISSN 1522-9653

Schmid, T., Homandberg, G., Madsen, L., Su, J. & Kuettner, K. (2002). Superficial zone protein (SZP) binds to macromolecules in the lamina splendens of arthicular cartilage [abstract]. *Trans Orthop Res Soc*, Vol.27, (Feb 2002), pp. 359, ISSN 0065-9533

Schmid, T., Lindley, K., Su, J., Soloveychik, V., Block, J., Kuettner, K. & Schumacher, B. (2001). Superficial zone protein (SZP) is an abundant glycoprotein in human synovial fluid and serum. *Trans Orthop Res Soc*, Vol.26, 2001), pp. 82,

Schmidt, T. A., Gastelum, N. S., Han, E. H., Nugent-Derfus, G. E., Schumacher, B. L. & Sah, R. L. (2008). Differential regulation of proteoglycan 4 metabolism in cartilage by IL-1alpha, IGF-I, and TGF-beta1. *Osteoarthritis Cartilage*, Vol.16, No.1, (Jan 2008), pp. 90-7, ISSN 1063-4584

Schmidt, T. A., Plaas, A. H. & Sandy, J. D. (2009). Disulfide-bonded multimers of proteoglycan 4 PRG4 are present in normal synovial fluids. *Biochim Biophys Acta*, Vol.1790, No.5, (May 2009), pp. 375-84, ISSN 0006-3002

Schulz, B. L., Packer, N. H. & Karlsson, N. G. (2002). Small-scale analysis of O-linked oligosaccharides from glycoproteins and mucins separated by gel electrophoresis. *Anal Chem*, Vol.74, No.23, (Dec 2002), pp. 6088-97, ISSN 0003-2700

Schumacher, B. L., Block, J. A., Schmid, T. M., Aydelotte, M. B. & Kuettner, K. E. (1994). A novel proteoglycan synthesized and secreted by chondrocytes of the superficial zone of articular cartilage. *Arch Biochem Biophys*, Vol.311, No.1, (May 1994), pp. 144-52, ISSN 0003-9861

Schumacher, B. L., Hughes, C. E., Kuettner, K. E., Caterson, B. & Aydelotte, M. B. (1999). Immunodetection and partial cDNA sequence of the proteoglycan, superficial zone protein, synthesized by cells lining synovial joints. *J Orthop Res*, Vol.17, No.1, (Jan 1999), pp. 110-20, ISSN 0736-0266

Schumacher, B. L., Schmidt, T. A., Voegtline, M. S., Chen, A. C. & Sah, R. L. (2005). Proteoglycan 4 (PRG4) synthesis and immunolocalization in bovine meniscus. *J Orthop Res*, Vol.23, No.3, (May 2005), pp. 562-8, ISSN 0736-0266

Sinz, A., Bantscheff, M., Mikkat, S., Ringel, B., Drynda, S., Kekow, J., Thiesen, H. J. & Glocker, M. O. (2002). Mass spectrometric proteome analyses of synovial fluids and plasmas from patients suffering from rheumatoid arthritis and comparison to reactive arthritis or osteoarthritis. *Electrophoresis*, Vol.23, No.19, (Sep 2002), pp. 3445-56, ISSN 0173-0835

Struglics, A., Larsson, S., Hansson, M. & Lohmander, L. S. (2009). Western blot quantification of aggrecan fragments in human synovial fluid indicates differences in fragment patterns between joint diseases. *Osteoarthritis Cartilage*, Vol.17, No.4, (Apr 2009), pp. 497-506, ISSN 1522-9653

Sun, Y., Berger, E. J., Zhao, C., Jay, G. D., An, K. N. & Amadio, P. C. (2006). Expression and mapping of lubricin in canine flexor tendon. *J Orthop Res*, Vol.24, No.9, (Sep 2006), pp. 1861-8, ISSN 0736-0266

Swann, D. A., Silver, F. H., Slayter, H. S., Stafford, W. & Shore, E. (1985). The molecular structure and lubricating activity of lubricin isolated from bovine and human synovial fluids. *Biochem J*, Vol.225, No.1, (Jan 1985), pp. 195-201, ISSN 0264-6021

Swann, D. A., Slayter, H. S. & Silver, F. H. (1981). The molecular structure of lubricating glycoprotein-I, the boundary lubricant for articular cartilage. *J Biol Chem*, Vol.256, No.11, (Jun 1981), pp. 5921-5, ISSN 0021-9258

Teeple, E., Elsaid, K. A., Jay, G. D., Zhang, L., Badger, G. J., Akelman, M., Bliss, T. F. & Fleming, B. C. (2011). Effects of supplemental intra-articular lubricin and hyaluronic acid on the progression of posttraumatic arthritis in the anterior cruciate ligament-deficient rat knee. *Am J Sports Med*, Vol.39, No.1, (Jan 2011), pp. 164-72, ISSN 1552-3365

Tilleman, K., Van Beneden, K., Dhondt, A., Hoffman, I., De Keyser, F., Veys, E., Elewaut, D. & Deforce, D. (2005). Chronically inflamed synovium from spondyloarthropathy and rheumatoid arthritis investigated by protein expression profiling followed by tandem mass spectrometry. *Proteomics*, Vol.5, No.8, (May 2005), pp. 2247-57, ISSN 1615-9853

Ungethuem, U., Haeupl, T., Witt, H., Koczan, D., Krenn, V., Huber, H., von Helversen, T. M., Drungowski, M., Seyfert, C., Zacher, J., Pruss, A., Neidel, J., Lehrach, H., Thiesen, H. J., Ruiz, P. & Blass, S. (2010). Molecular signatures and new candidates to target the pathogenesis of rheumatoid arthritis. *Physiol Genomics*, Vol.42A, No.4, (Nov 2010), pp. 267-82, ISSN 1531-2267

Yamamoto, N., Nakashima, T., Torikai, M., Naruse, T., Morimoto, J., Kon, S., Sakai, F. & Uede, T. (2007). Successful treatment of collagen-induced arthritis in non-human primates by chimeric anti-osteopontin antibody. *Int Immunopharmacol*, Vol.7, No.11, (Nov 2007), pp. 1460-70, ISSN 1567-5769

Yokosaki, Y., Matsuura, N., Sasaki, T., Murakami, I., Schneider, H., Higashiyama, S., Saitoh, Y., Yamakido, M., Taooka, Y. & Sheppard, D. (1999). The integrin alpha(9)beta(1) binds to a novel recognition sequence (SVVYGLR) in the thrombin-cleaved amino-terminal fragment of osteopontin. *J Biol Chem*, Vol.274, No.51, (Dec 1999), pp. 36328-34, ISSN 0021-9258

Young, A. A., McLennan, S., Smith, M. M., Smith, S. M., Cake, M. A., Read, R. A., Melrose, J., Sonnabend, D. H., Flannery, C. R. & Little, C. B. (2006). Proteoglycan 4 downregulation in a sheep meniscectomy model of early osteoarthritis. *Arthritis Res Ther*, Vol.8, No.2, (Jan 2006), pp. R41, ISSN 1478-6362

Zhang, C. C., Rogalski, J. C., Evans, D. M., Klockenbusch, C., Beavis, R. C. & Kast, J. (2011). In silico protein interaction analysis using the global proteome machine database. *J Proteome Res*, Vol.10, No.2, (Feb 2011), pp. 656-68, ISSN 1535-3907

9

Profiling Inflammatory Genes and Signaling Pathways in Rheumatoid Synoviocytes for RA Light Therapy

Yasuko Shibata and Yoshimitsu Abiko
Department of Biochemistry and Molecular Biology
Nihon University School of Dentistry at Matsudo
Japan

1. Introduction

Rheumatoid arthritis (RA) is an autoimmune joint disease characterized by inflammation and destruction of the articular surfaces and bone. During joint movement, synovial tissues contribute to mechanical load bearing by changing their shape. These elastic synovial membranes are an early target of rheumatic inflammation, and together with chondrocytes, become a primary source of inflammatory factors (e.g., cytokines) that enter the synovial fluid (Dayer, 2004, Firestein, 2007). The pathophysiological steps leading to RA include inflammation, proliferation of synovial cells, and attachment to and invasion of adjacent cartilage and bone by fibroblast-like cells derived from rheumatoid synoviocytes (RA-FLSs) (Firestein, 1996, Pap et al., 2000, Tolboom et al., 2005, Bartok & Firestein, 2010).

In the healthy synovium, one to three layers of synoviocytes, the macrophage-like type A and the more abundant fibroblast-like type B (also referred to as synovial fibroblasts), form the synovial lining layer separating the synovial sublining layer of loose connective tissue from the joint cavity (Iwanaga et al., 2000). The joint damage observed in RA is mainly mediated by macrophage/macrophage-like cell-derived cytokines, such as interleukin (IL)-1, IL-6 and tumor necrosis factor (TNF)-α, which induce neutral protease production by FLSs and articular chondrocytes (Houssiau et al., 1988, Feldmann & Maini, 1999, Dayer, 2002). Although IL-1 and TNF-α share many biological activities that are relevant in RA, early studies of experimental arthritis models have demonstrated that IL-1 plays a predominant role in cartilage destruction via inflammatory processes that include the activation of matrix metalloproteinases (MMPs) (Borghaei et al., 1998) and the inhibition of the synthesis of extracellular matrix (ECM) molecules (Mauviel et al., 1988). In particular, IL-1β is readily detected, long after the onset of RA, at high levels in the synovial fluid of RA patients. IL-1β can significantly alter the expression of a variety of genes, including inflammatory mediators such as cytokines and MMPs (Sun & Yokota, 2002, Suzuki et al., 2010). In addition, IL-1 stimulates bone resorption by activating osteoclasts (Goldring, 2003). That said, there is little comprehensive information available on the effects of IL-1β on fibroblast-like synoviocytes (FLSs).

RA-FLSs not only mediate tissue destruction, but also are considered to play a major role in initiating and driving RA in concert with inflammatory cells (Huber, 2006, Bartok &

Firestein, 2010). However, the original roles of single RA-FLS, and their relationship with macrophage-like type B cells in the rheumatoid synovium are poorly understood, although many case reports of RA patients, and many experimental reports using the synovium tisuues/cells from RA patients have been published. The utilization of cells such as the MH7A human RA-FLSs (Cell Bank, Riken Bioresource Center, Ibaraki, Japan), which are established cells isolated from the knee joint of an RA patient that retain the morphological and functional characteristics of primary synovial cells should provide guidance to clarify the mechanisms of onset of RA and to the development of useful treatments for RA. The MH7A cells are an immortalized RA-FLS line that stains positively for IL-1R, intercellular adhesion molecule-1 (ICAM-1), CD16, CD40, CD80, and CD95 and has been used extensively to investigate the molecular mechanisms underlying RA (Miyazawa et al., 1998). It has been shown, for example, that IL-1β enhances the production of IL-6, IL-8, and MMPs in MH7A cells (Shibata et al., 2005, Han et al., 2006) in a manner similar to that seen in the parental FLSs, although the immortalized cells grow more rapidly than the parental cells. These results clearly indicate the usefulness of MH7A cells for investigating the regulation of rheumatoid FLSs and the IL-1 signal transduction pathway to develop a future RA therapy.

In what is becoming known as the "post-genomic era", many new technologies and methodologies are being developed to take advantage of the recent progress in genomic research. Among these, gene expression profiling has become an invaluable tool in functional genomics. DNA microarrays, cDNA subtraction, and the serial analysis of gene expression have all emerged as leading transcript profiling technologies for the global analysis of biological systems. One of the high throughput technologies, high-density oligonucleotide genechip microarrays, makes it possible to simultaneously measure the relative abundance of numerous mRNAs within a cell. To better understand the direct IL-1β-induced changes in gene expression that might promote inflammatory responses in MH7A cells, in the present study we used an Affymetrix HG-8500 Focus array GeneChip to analyze the patterns of gene expression, and then used the Ingenuity Pathway Analysis (IPA) software program to investigate the signaling pathways leading to the IL-1β-induced gene expression. In addition, we used a biotin label-based antibody array to measure the levels of 507 human target proteins, including cytokines, chemokines, growth factors, angiogenic factors, proteases, and soluble receptors, among others, in the cell culture supernatants. We analyzed the expression profiles of both the genes and proteins to identify the key molecules involved in articular rheumatism, which could be related to the induction of inflammation and pannus formation in the synovial tissues of RA patients. In addition, we propose the possibility of a new therapy using linear polarized infrared light, that induces the suppression of inflammation and pain for RA patients with no apparent side-effects.

2. Microarray analysis

MH7A human RA-FLSs (Riken Bioresource Center, Ibaraki) were maintained in RPMI 1640 medium supplemented with 10% fetal calf serum (FCS) and penicillin-streptomycin at 37°C under a 5% CO_2 atmosphere. Total RNA from the MH7A cells was treated according to the manufacturer's protocol, and then hybridized to a Human Genome Focus Array HG-8500 GeneChip (Affymetrix Inc.).

Our aims were to identify potential mediators of RA inflammation and joint destruction induced by the inflammatory cytokine IL-1β, and to investigate the mechanisms responsible for their stimulation. Of the 8,746 genes on the Focus array HG-8500 GeneChip, 4,909 from untreated cells and 5,073 from IL-1β-treated cells were classified as marginally expressed or present. After the cut-offs for induction (≥2.0-fold) and suppression (≤0.5-fold) by IL-1β were applied, 120 genes (74 upregulated and 46 downregulated genes) were identified as being affected by IL-1β. When we then classified the IL-1β-inducible gene expression in MH7A cells with respect to six functionalities based on BiologicalProcess words, we found that IL-1β conspicuously increased the expression of inflammation and apoptosis/proliferation-related genes, although the largest group of genes affected by IL-1β was signaling-related (Fig. 1).

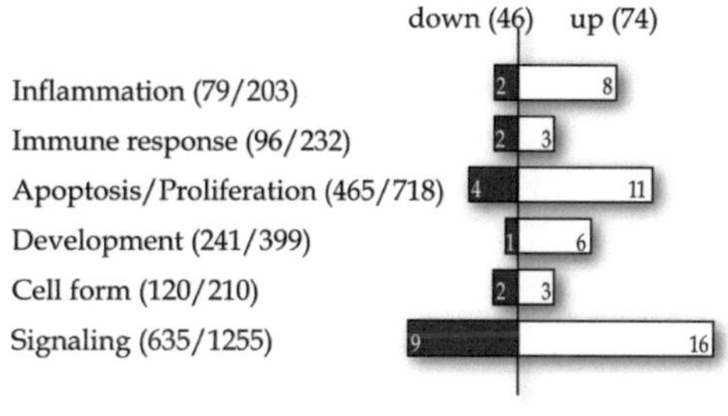

The genes that were upregulated (n=74) or down-regulated (n=46) by IL-1β were classified into 6 groups based on the GO-BiologicalProcess terms listed in the GeneSpring 6.2 software program.

Fig. 1. Classification of genes whose expression in MH7A cells was affected by IL-1β.

We used IPA to gain a better understanding of how differentially expressed genes were integrated into specific regulatory and signaling networks. A data set containing gene identifiers adhering to the 2-fold (120 genes) change used in microarray experiments was uploaded into the IPA software application. Each gene identifier was mapped to its corresponding gene object and then overlaid onto a global molecular network developed from information contained in the Ingenuity Pathways Knowledge Base. The networks of these genes were then algorithmically generated based on their connectivity, after which a functional analysis of the networks identified the biological functions that were the most significant.

2.1 IL-1β-induced inflammatory signaling pathways

We attempted to visualize the IL-1β-induced genes within the canonical IPA pathway, which involves IL-1β, IL-6, and TNF-α signaling (Fig. 2A, canonical pathway name: IL-6 signaling). Four IL-1β-inducible genes (>2.0-fold), IL-1β, IL-6, IL-8, and IκB, were situated within this atlas. As shown in Fig. 2A, activation of NF-κB signaling is also important for the secretion of IL-8, IL-1β and IL-6. We previously used an ELISA to show that TNF-α was not expressed in MH7A cells, regardless of whether they were exposed to IL-1β (0.1 unit/ml) (Shibata et al., 2005). Likewise, the results we obtained using the GeneChip microarray indicated no expression of TNF-α in MH7A cells under our experimental conditions. IL-1β did induce its own expression, which may be important for its accumulation during the inflammation in RA. Furthermore, high levels of NF-IL6 (CEBPB) expression were consistently observed.

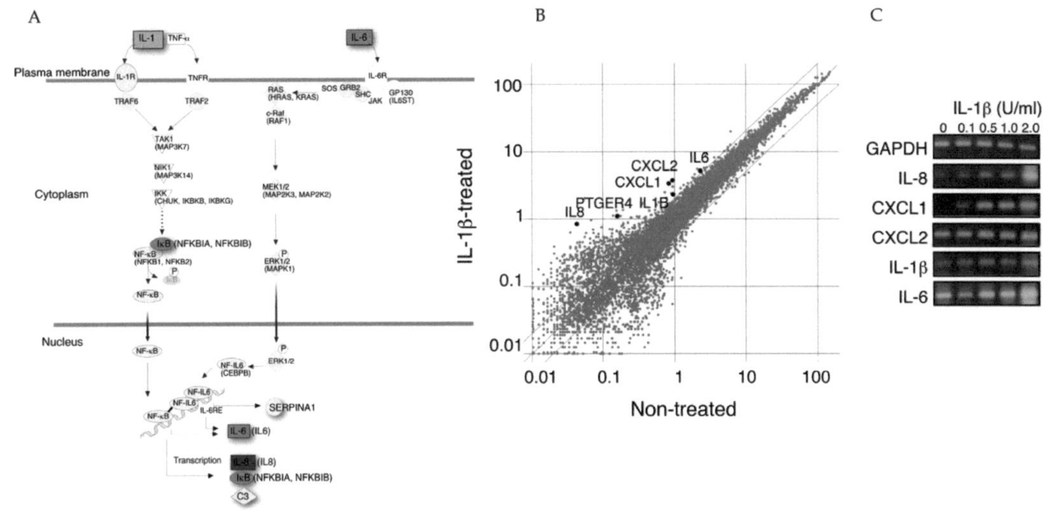

A. The IL-1β and IL-6 signaling pathways as determined by IPA analysis. Grayed symbols indicate genes that were upregulated by IL-1β; white symbols indicate genes whose expression was not increased by IL-1β. **B.** A scatter plot of 8,793 genes. Genes whose expression ratio was changed by >2-fold by IL-1β are positioned outside the lines. **C.** Dose-dependent effects of IL-1β on the gene expression. MH7A cells were examined after treatment with fresh medium containing the indicated concentration of IL-1β, and the cells were incubated for an additional 2 hr.

Fig. 2. The IL-1β and IL-6 signaling pathways and the results of the RT-PCR analysis

Based on the structural analysis, the chemokine superfamily can be divided into two groups: the C-X-C and the C-C subfamilies (Baggiolini et al., 1994). IL-8 belongs to the first group and acts mainly on neutrophils (Hebert & Baker, 1993). Our microarray experiments showed that IL-8 transcription was the most dramatically upregulated (20.8 fold) in MH7A cells exposed to IL-1β. It is also noteworthy that the expression of other chemokines, including CXCL-1 (4.1-fold), -2 (4.0-fold) and -3 (2.7-fold), three potent stimulators of neutrophil activation and tissue infiltration was also enhanced. Leukocyte recruitment from the microvasculature to sites of inflammation is a sequential process that includes rolling, activation, firm adhesion, and finally, transmigration through the vessel wall (King & Hammer, 2001). Although macrophages, neutrophils, and endothelial cells are all thought to be primary sources of IL-8, which is known to be elevated at inflammatory sites such as the synovial fluid of RA patients, fibroblast-like and macrophage-like cells of the synovial membrane, together with the infiltrating leucocytes, are the major source of these mediators in the rheumatoid synovial pannus (Rathanaswami et al., 1993). In the GeneChip microarray experiment, an IL-1β concentration close to the levels seen clinically was used to stimulate the MH7A cells. The gene expression of IL-8, Gro-α (CXCL1), Gro-β (CXCL2), IL-1β, and IL-6 in scatter plots is shown in Fig. 2B. According to a RT-PCR analysis, the levels of IL-8, CXCL1, CXCL2, IL-1β, and IL-6 mRNA in MH7A cells were all found to be dose-dependently increased by IL-1β (Fig. 2C). Therefore, IL-8 appears to play a major role in the initiation and maintenance of inflammatory responses.

Within the 5′-flanking region of the human IL-8 promoter are a number of motifs with the potential to bind various transcription factors in a cell and stimulus-dependent manner. In particular, the transcription factors NF-κB and NF-IL-6 are both involved in stimulus-induced IL-8 expression (Matsusaka et al., 1993). We would therefore anticipate that these transcription factors would play an important role in the increased expression of IL-8 mRNA elicited by IL-1β, but no increases in the expression for NFKB1 (NF-κB), RELA (RelA), or CEBPB (NF-IL-6) were seen in the microarray experiment. On the other hand, in resting cells, NF-κB is trapped in the cytoplasm through its interaction with its inhibitor, IkB, and a crucial step in the activation of NF-κB is the stimulus-induced phosphorylation of IκB by IκB kinases (IKKs). To study the extent to which IKKs modulate IL-1β induced IL-8 production, MH7A cells were pretreated with Bay11-7085, an inhibitor of IκB phosphorylation, for 1 hr before stimulation with IL-1β (Shibata et al., 2009a). As shown in Fig. 3, Bay11-7085 completely blocked the release of IL-8 from IL-1β-stimulated MH7A cells.

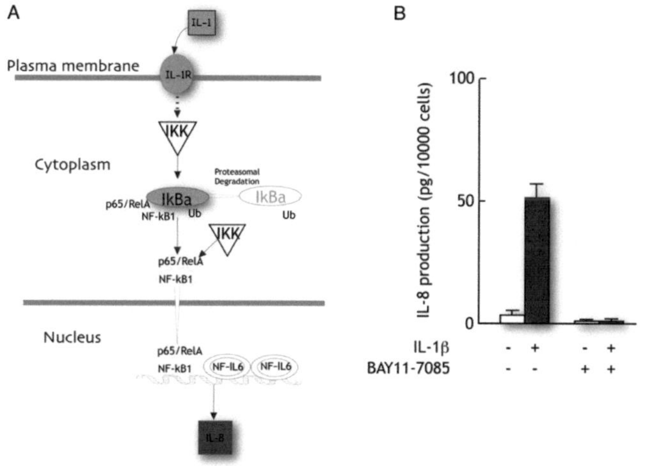

A. The IL-1β-induced signal transduction pathways leading to the production of IL-8. Gray symbols indicate genes that were up-regulated by IL-1β. White symbols indicate genes whose expression was increased less than 2.0-fold by IL-1β. **B.** The effects of Bay11-7085 on the production of IL-8. MH7A cells were first incubated with the IKKα/β inhibitor Bay11-7085 for 1 hr, and then with IL-1β for 2 hr. The levels of IL-8 in medium conditioned by the cells were measured using an ELISA. [This figure is modified from (Shibata et al., 2009a)]

Fig. 3. The effect of Bay11-7085 on the production of IL-8

2.2 Arithmetic IL-8 production through the PGE_2 receptor synthesis

PGE_2, a product of the cyclooxygenation of arachidonic acid, is a potent mediator of the immune response and inflammation, and contributes to the pathogenesis of RA (Robinson et al., 1975, Trebino et al., 2003). PGE_2 also displays a complex regulatory function affecting IL-8 gene expression, which is dependent on the concentration of PGE_2 and on the specific cell type involved. At physiological and pathological concentrations of up to 100 μM, PGE_2 is capable of upregulating endogenous IL-8 expression in human colonic epithelial cells (Yu & Chadee, 1998). However, there have been many reports that PGE_2 has no effect on neutrophil-derived IL-8 induced by LPS (Wertheim et al., 1993); that it down-regulates IL-8 in response to LPS in human alveolar macrophages and blood monocytes (Standiford et al., 1992); and suppresses the production of chemokines, including IL-8, in human macrophages

(Takayama et al., 2002). Furthermore, PGE_2 alone had little detectable effect on IL-8, although a small enhancement of the mRNA and protein levels of IL-6 has been observed in human synovial fibroblasts (Agro et al., 1996). In RA research, while PGE_2 alone has limited effects on synovial cell production of IL-8, its effects are significant in the context of IL-1α stimulation; endogenous PGE_2 may alter the cytokines secreted by mesenchymally-derived cells.

A variety of transcription factors, including NF-κB, NF-IL6, activator protein-1 and octamer-1, have been shown to regulate IL-8 gene transcription (Matsusaka et al., 1993). Caristi *et al* (Caristi et al., 2005) have shown that, in human T cells, PGE_2 induces IL-8 synthesis through an NF-κB-independent pathway via its EP1- and EP4-type receptors (PGE2EP1 and PGE2EP4, respectively). We have demonstrated that PGE_2 at physiological, as well as pathological, concentrations induced IL-8 production thorough the increased expression of PGE2EP4 receptors in synovial fibroblasts of RA *in vitro* (Shibata et al., 2009b). The present results were of particular interest, since the effect of PGE_2 on IL-8 production was found in the IL-1β-pretreated MH7A cells. We demonstrated that the newly expressed-PGE_2 receptors are involved in this process.

These findings show the complexity with which PGE_2 regulates IL-8 synthesis by inhibiting or enhancing its production depending on the cell types and environmental conditions. Therefore, we proposed that, in IL-1β-stimulated synovial fibroblasts in RA patients, PGE_2 induces IL-8 mRNA transcription by the activation of different signal transduction pathways from the conventional IL-1β-stimulated pathways, including PGE_2 receptor EP4-triggered pathways. IL-1β enhanced the gene expression of IL8 and PTGER4 (Shibata et al., 2009b), subsequently IL-8 production was enhanced by IL-1β and PGE_2 from environmental neutrophils/macrophages in the synovial tissues. These results may therefore highlight a new important role for PGE_2 in regulating IL-8 production by the synovial fibroblasts of RA patients, confirming the pro-inflammatory activity of this prostaglandin.

2.3 Apoptotic signaling

Inflammation of the synovial membrane results in the development of aggressive granulation tissue, called "pannus". Pannus tissue is composed mainly of inflammatory cells such as macrophages and FLSs. By a microarray analysis, the apoptosis/proliferation-related molecules included those involved in processes associated with negative/positive regulation of cell proliferation, apoptosis/anti-apoptosis, cell death, cell proliferation and regulation of the cell cycle, and a large number of these genes were influenced by IL-1β (Fig. 1). Interestingly, whereas the expression of the gene encoding the apoptosis inhibitor cIAP (BIRC3) was enhanced (4.8-fold), the expression of those encoding the cell death inducing molecule FOSL2 (FOS-like antigen 2, 0.4-fold)) and the cell proliferation-related molecule EDNRA (endothelin receptor type A, 0.2-fold) were both suppressed. We attempted to apply the IL-1β-inducible genes to a typical pathway atlas involving apoptotic signaling (Fig. 4A). The expression of BIRC3, which encodes the anti-apoptotic protein cIAP, implies that IL-1β signaling leads to inhibition of apoptotic signaling, as expression of cIAP should exert an inhibitory effect on caspase 3 activity (Rothe et al., 1995, Budihardjo et al., 1999). To confirm the increased cIAP production in MH7A cells, we found that levels of the BIRC3 transcript were substantially increased in the IL-1β-induced MH7A cells (Fig. 4B).

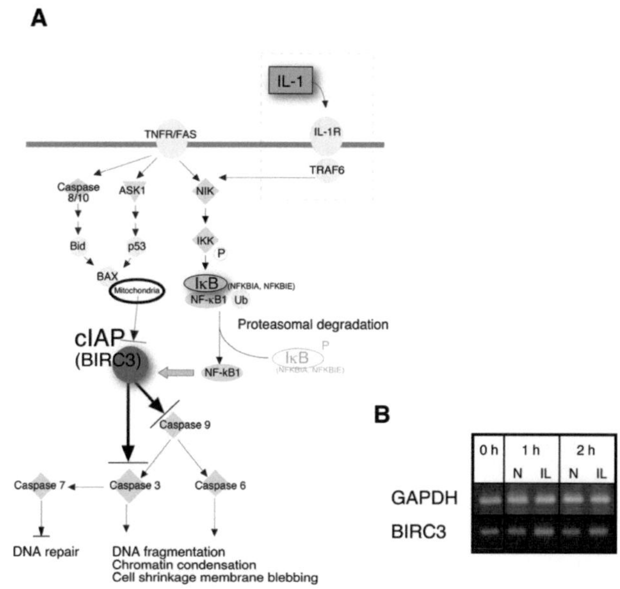

A. The gray symbols indicate the IL-1β-inducible genes (>2.0-fold) in the apoptosis signaling pathway.
B. The time-dependent effects of IL-1β on the gene expression of cIAP (BIRC3), which negatively regulates apoptotic signaling, were examined using MH7A cells.

Fig. 4. An atlas of an apoptosis signaling pathway

It has been suggested that RA is driven by a network of closely connected interdependent pathogenic mechanisms involving innate and adaptive immunity that ultimately lead to synovial inflammation and aggressive synovial overproliferation during the terminal destructive phase (Firestein, 2003). Furthermore, in a chronically inflamed microenvironment, these destructive changes are driven by invasive synovial hyperplasia and neovascularization (pannus formation) at the interface between the synovium and intra-articular space. During the process of synovial pannus formation, FLSs actively contribute to the inflamed and destructive local microenvironment by secreting a variety of inflammatory mediators, which lead to tissue degradation. In response to IL-1 and TNF-α, FLSs also secrete angiogenic growth factors, such as vascular endothelial growth factor (VEGF) (Nagashima et al., 1999) and basic fibroblast growth factor (bFGF), which are essential for the pathophysiological neovascularization in RA joints. In addition, we have identified that BIRC3 is upregulated, making it a candidate mediator of FLS overproliferation in RA. BIRC3 encodes cIAP, which is a key negative regulator of apoptotic signaling in FLSs. The resulting inhibition of FLS apoptosis in the inflamed area would be expected to contribute to the formation of the pannus in the RA joint.

3. Protein chip analysis

3.1 ECM degradation

A RayBio biotin label-based human antibody array I (RayBiotech, Inc.) was used to measure the expression levels of 507 proteins in culture medium conditioned by MH7A cells. Table 1 presents the results of the biotin label-based antibody array analysis of secreted proteins that categorized interleukins, and molecules involved in ECM metabolism. IL-12 p70 and IL-8 were both abundantly expressed in the IL-1β-induced MH7A cells (57.8- and 12.6-fold increases, respectively). IL-12 is a heterodimer expressed in RA synovial tissue (Morita et al., 1998); dendritic cells and macrophages produce IL-12 within minutes of activation, and it plays a central role in the development of Th1 responses (Hunter, 2005). The biological functions of these cells are not yet fully understood, but they are known to play a role in the differentiation and proliferation of T cells of the Th1 phenotype. Th1 responses in turn are deemed to be of particular importance in inflammatory arthritis, including RA. This induction of IL-12p70 by IL-1β in MH7A cells may be the first *in vitro* evidence of IL-12 expression in RA. This is noteworthy, because Connell & McInnes (Connell & McInnes, 2006) suggested in their review that IL-12 likely contributes to the pathology of inflammatory joint disease. If this is the case, it may represent a potentially useful therapeutic target.

Fold	Protein Name	Non-treated		IL-1b-treated	
		Normalized	Raw (n=3)	Normalized	Raw (n=3)
ILs					
57.8	IL-12 p70	0.01	*nd*	0.58	3384 ± 104
12.6	IL-8	0.01	*nd*	0.13	737 ± 104
2.6	IL-16	0.01	49 ± 99	0.03	162 ± 54
MMPs					
3.7	MMP-10	0.01	*nd*	0.04	219 ± 44
2.3	MMP-11 (Stromelysin-3)	0.01	*nd*	0.02	134 ± 26
TIMPs					
0.3	TIMP-1	0.72	3270 ± 1051	0.24	1395 ± 129
0.4	TIMP-3	0.28	1296 ± 65	0.11	643 ± 296

RayBio biotin label-based human antibody array I (RayBiotech, Inc.) was used to measure the expression levels of 507 proteins in culture medium conditioned by MH7A cells. The cell were cultured for 16 h and then treated with IL-1β (0.1 U/ml) for 3 h. The cultured medium from five wells was then combined and dialyzed against PBS (pH 8.0), and an internal control protein was added to the 400 μl of dialyzed sample medium. The procedure used for biotin labeling, blocking and incubation of the antibody array, as well as fluorescence detection were carried out according to the operating manual from RayBiotech. The images were captured using an Axon GenePix laser scanner. Biotinylation of the internal control protein yielded a positive control signals that was used to identify the orientation of the results and help normalize them for comparison of those from the untreated and IL-1β-treated MH7A cell arrays. Values below 0.01 were set to 0.001.

Table 1. IL-1β-induced protein.

On the other hand, the levels of two MMP family enzymes, MMP-10, and MMP-11 were upregulated by IL-1β, while the levels of TIMP-1 and -3 were downregulated. As the overall MMP activity reflects a balance between the amount of MMPs and TIMPs present, the reduction in TIMP-1 and TIMP-3 levels seen in MH7A cells would be expected to shift the balance in favor of increased MMP activity. Taken together, these data suggest that IL-1β elicits a series of responses in the synovial fluid, leading to the pathology seen in RA, including enhanced expression of inflammatory cytokines and enzymes, and a reduction in the ability to protect against the destruction of the tissue ECM.

4. Medical treatments for RA

Several disease-modifying anti-rheumatic drugs (DMARDs) have been used to control the progression of RA. While the majority of these drugs act as immunomodulatory agents, some also act by inhibiting cytokines and endothelial cell proliferation (Cozzolino et al., 1993, Volin et al., 1999). Newly developed biological response modifiers (biologics) offer even more hope, having a greater potential to suppress disease activity, and improve the quality of life of RA patients.

4.1 Disease-modifying anti-rheumatic drugs, TNF-α blockers, and other agents

Guidelines advocate treatment with DMARDs as soon as RA is diagnosed to control symptoms and delay disease progression (Smolen & Steiner, 2003, O'Dell, 2004, Saag et al., 2008). DMARDs slow the progression of the joint damage that leads to loss of function, whereas drugs such as nonsteroidal antiinflammatory drugs and corticosteroids only control the symptoms (Kirwan & Power, 2007). On the other hand, targeted inhibition of TNF-α is an effective therapy widely used against RA and other rheumatic diseases. The advent of TNF blockers has led to substantial improvement in the management of active RA refractory to conventional DMARDs. While on a patient-population level, the efficacy of the TNF blockers infliximab, etanercept, and adalimumab seems comparable, on an individual level, there are no clear-cut methods for assessing whether there will be a response to anti-TNF therapy, let alone which agent would yield the best outcome. The updated consensus statement on biological agents for the treatment of rheumatic diseases states that the optimal treatment for anti-TNF refractory RA remains to be determined. However, most importantly, it is not yet possible to identify prior to therapy which patients will fail to respond or who are at increased risk for adverse drug reactions (Mendonça et al., 2011). Given the important role that TNF-α antagonists play in managing rheumatoid arthritis and the concern for safety during long-term therapy, such factors need to be determined as soon as possible.

Glucocorticoids have potent immunosuppressive effects and have been widely used in the management of chronic inflammatory diseases such as severe RA. A number of studies have focused on the cellular and molecular mechanisms underlying the anti-inflammatory effects of glucocorticoids such as dexamethasone (Dex). Glucocorticoids exert their effects via intracellular receptors that act as potent transcriptional activators of genes that possess glucocorticoid responsive elements. By regulating gene expression, glucocorticoids suppress the production of pro-inflammatory proteins, such as cytokines, chemokines and some enzymatic mediators. However, the therapeutic management of long-term pathological conditions with steroids is often linked to unwanted side effects involving the cardiovascular system (Suissa et al., 2006).

4.2 Proposal of RA therapy using linear polarized infrared light

It is unclear whether early treatment with biologics should continue to be recommended, given their potential to slow disease progression and extend productivity on the one hand, while causing unwanted side effects and risks due to drug-associated health care utilization on the other. Therefore, we examined the potential of photodynamic therapy using a linear polarized infrared light (LPIL). Laser therapy is a new arthroscopic technique to treat inflammation of the synovial membrane. Following gallium-aluminum-arsenide (Ga-Al-As) laser treatment, histological examination of the irradiated synovial membranes showed flattening of the epithelial cells, decreased villous proliferation, narrower vascular lumens and less infiltration by inflammatory cells than was seen in non-irradiated synovia. An alternative approach makes use of a linear polarized infrared light (LPIL) instrument (Super Lizer™, Tokyo Iken Co., Ltd), which has been used clinically with good effects in several patients with inflammatory disease. LPIL can be applied during physical therapy to relieve pain, and several studies have shown that such irradiation also relieves temporomandibular joint pain (Yokoyama & Oku, 1999), improves the structure of stored human erythrocytes (Yokoyama & Sugiyama, 2003), and improves the flexibility of shoulder and ankle joints (Demura et al., 2002). A fuller understanding of the anti-inflammatory mechanism of LPIL in rheumatoid synoviocytes could serve as the basis for improved treatment of RA patients in the future.

We treated MH7A cells IL-1β (0.1 U/ml) and/or Dex (1 μM) or LPIL (3.8 J/cm^2). Microarray experiments were then carried out using the Affymetrix Focus Array HG-8500 GeneChip. As shown in Fig. 5A, the transcription of numerous genes was up- or down-regulated to a greater degree in cells treated with Dex than in those treated with LPIL. Likewise, the effects of LPIL irradiation on the transcription levels of many genes were smaller than those of IL-1β. In total, 120 (IL-1β), 561 (Dex), 877 (Dex/IL-1β), 88 (LPIL) and 90 (LPIL/IL-1β) genes were up- or downregulated by the different treatments (Fig. 5B).

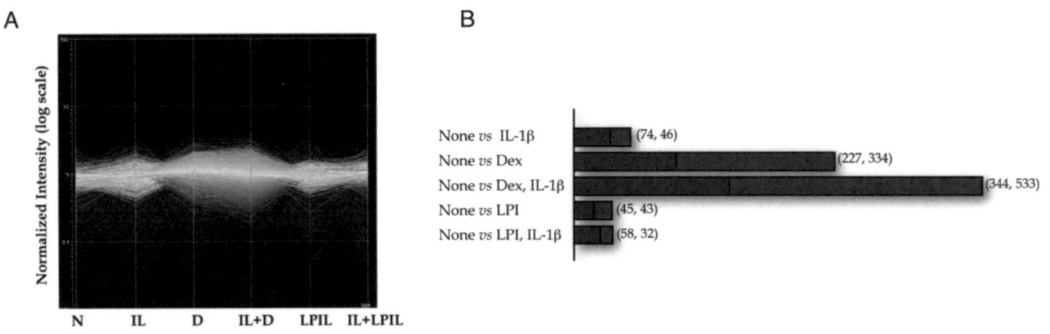

The global gene expression in MH7A cells. The normalized gene expression is shown. MH7A cells were treated with Dex or LPIL in the presence or absence of IL-1β before the extraction of their RNA. N, untreated cells; IL, IL-1β-treated cells; D, Dex-treated cells. **B.** The numbers of up- and down-regulated genes. Genes whose expression was increased or decreased by over two-fold are indicated. [This figure is modified from (Shibata et al., 2009b)]

Fig. 5. Microarray data analysis.

We focused on the genes that were up-regulated by at least 2.0-fold in cells treated with IL-1β and then suppressed by the anti-inflammatory treatments. IL-8 transcripts showed the largest increase (20.8 fold), and LPIL and Dex each suppressed this gene expression. Others genes, including CXCL1, 2, 3, IL6, and IL1B, which respectively encode Gro-α, Gro-β, Gro-γ, IL-6 and IL-1β, were also suppressed by LPIL to the same extent as by Dex (Table 2). Thus, although for the most part LPIL irradiation did not alter the transcription levels to the same degree as Dex did, IL-1β inducible genes, such as the CXCL type chemokines, IL6 and IL1B, were clearly suppressed by LPIL irradiation. To evaluate the

Gene	Title Affy	IL-1β/None			IL-1β+Dex /None	IL-1β+LPIL /None
		Fold	Normalized intensity	Raw Data	Fold	Fold
IL8	interleukin 8, CXCL8	20.2	0.86/0.04	(P/A)	5.6	7.6
CXCL1	chemokine (C-X-C motif) ligand 1, GRO1	4.1	3.36/0.82	(P/P)	3.2	1.8
CXCL2	chemokine (C-X-C motif) ligand 2, GRO2	4.0	3.78/0.94	(P/P)	2.4	3.1
CXCL3	chemokine (C-X-C motif) ligand 3, GRO3	2.7	0.85/0.32	(M/A)	3.2	2.1
IL6	Interleukin 6	2.7	5.51/2.07	(P/P)	1.0	2.2
IL1B	Interleukin 1, beta	2.5	2.33/0.92	(P/M)	1.4	1.5

Table 2. Inhibitory effects of anti-inflammatory treatments on IL-1β-induced gene expression

inhibitory effects of LPIL irradiation on IL-1β inducible inflammation, we next used an ELISA to monitor IL-1β induced IL-8 synthesis and secretion from MH7A cells. We found that IL-1β strongly induced IL-8 production, and that the effect was similarly suppressed by Dex or LPIL (Fig. 6). We compared the effects of one-time LPIL irradiation and Dex administration on the production of IL-8. Even one period of exposure to LPIL irradiation diminished the IL-1β-induced production of IL-8 to the same extent as administration of 1 μM Dex to the cells. Furthermore, using end-point PCR and real-time PCR, we determined that there were corresponding decreases in the expression of IL-8 mRNA (Fig. 6). It is also noteworthy that the inhibitory effects on IL-8 transcription increased with increasing optical pulse energy.

The genes whose products are involved in NF-κB signaling (e.g., NFKB1, RelA, and C/EBP-β) were not induced by IL-1β stimulation as determined by the microarray analysis. On the other hand, increasing evidence has highlighted the importance of NF-κB modification in the regulation of its transcriptional activity. For instance, it appears that NF-κB activity can be modulated by phosphorylation of the RelA subunit. Recent evidence indicates that the phosphorylation of the RelA subunit on S276 and S536 is physiologically induced by various proinflammatory stimuli. Zhong *et al.* (2002) found that LPS stimulates protein kinase A-dependent phosphorylation of RelA on S276 and subsequently recruits the transcription coactivator CREB binding protein (CBP)/p300 to stimulate NF-κB-mediated transcription. Furthermore, it appears that S536 of endogenous cytoplasmic RelA is phosphorylated in response to a wide variety of NF-κB stimuli and is then rapidly dephosphorylated in the nucleus (Sakurai et al., 1999, Sakurai, 2003, Yang et al., 2003, Mattioli et al., 2004).

Because transduction of the IL-1β signal is tightly regulated in MH7A cells via a network involving NF-κB, we tried to measure the levels of NF-κB phosphorylation. As shown in Fig. 7, the total levels of NF-κB-bound RelA were nearly the same in all of the treated MH7A cells (right panel). Phosphorylation of the RelA subunit on both S276 and S536 was significantly increased by IL-1β stimulation, and was decreased in the presence of Bay11-

7085 (left and center panels). Interestingly, LPIL irradiation suppressed the phosphorylation of both S276 to the same degree as Dex in IL-1β-stimulated MH7A cells.
The extent to which the risk of side-effects may be driven by drugs that decrease immune surveillance (notably, DMARDs including TNF-α blockers, and glucocorticoid agents), is not completely clear. This issue has gained interest in light of reports of serious infections in patients receiving newer RA therapies.

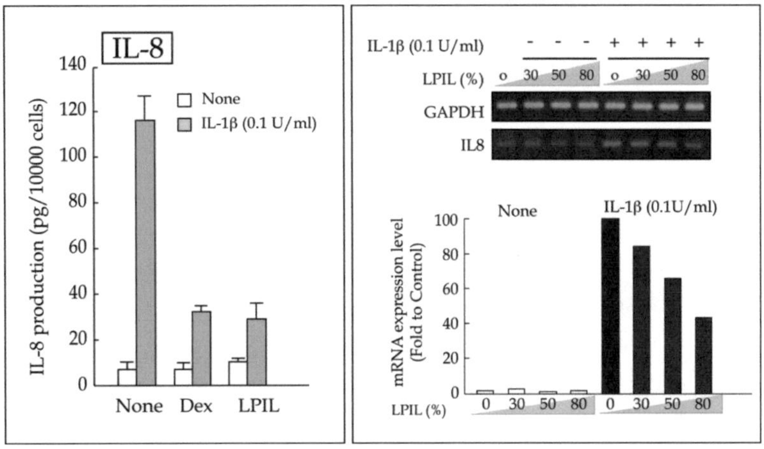

The inhibitory effects of LPIL or Dex on the production of IL-8 in MH7A cells. An end-point PCR analysis shows that LPIL irradiation inhibits IL8, but not GAPDH, gene expression. The power level of the irradiation was changed by adjusting the power dial on the Super Lizer™ to 30%, 50%, or 80%. The duration of the irradiation was the same for all wells. A real-time PCR analysis shows the dose-dependent inhibitory effects of LPIL on IL-8 gene expression. [This figure is modified from (Shibata et al., 2009a)]

Fig. 6. The transcriptional regulation of IL-8 by LPIL and Dex in IL-1β-stimulated MH7A cells.

5. Conclusion

To study the pathophysiological mechanisms involved in chronic inflammatory disorders such as RA, *in vitro* culture systems using IL-1β-activated FLSs from RA patients have become useful models of the first step in RA-induced joint deterioration. Our findings demonstrate the utility of profiling the gene expression in IL-1β stimulated-MH7A cells, with the supposition that it is representative of the early disease stage of RA. By employing GeneChips and IPA, we were able to show that autocrine induction of IL-1β gene expression may underlie the strong expression of several inflammatory cytokines, including IL-8, IL-1β and IL-6, and suggest that continuous IL-1β production has an exacerbating effect on RA. In addition, we have identified upregulation of the BIRC3 gene as a candidate mediator of the FLS overproliferation in RA. BIRC3 encodes cIAP, which is a key negative regulator of apoptotic signaling in FLSs. The resulting inhibition of FLS apoptosis in the inflamed area would be expected to contribute to the formation of the pannus in the RA joint. It is our expectation that further studies of the comprehensive information provided by the GeneChip/IPA analysis and antibody array systems will provide a means to ease the suffering caused by RA.

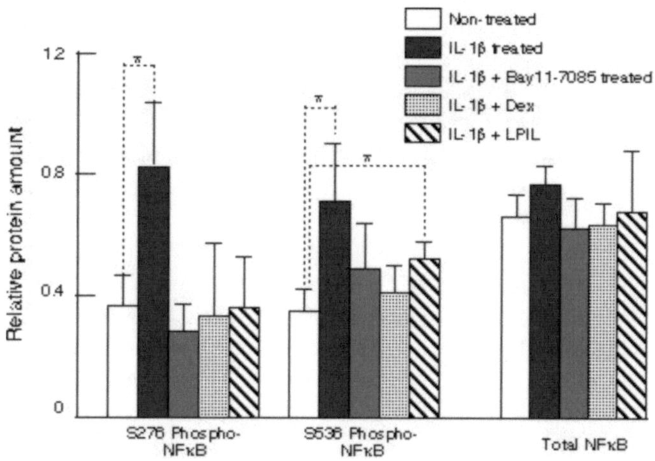

MH7A cells were cultured for 16 h in 96 well plates and then used to assess the phosphorylation of the NF-kB RelA subunit. Cells were irradiated with LPIL for 680 s immediately after stimulation with IL-1b for 2 h, or Dex was added to cells at the same time as IL-1b. Some cells were pretreated with Bay11-7085 for 1 h before addition of the IL-1b. After stimulation with IL-1b, the culture medium was removed, the cells were fixed by microwaving, and the levels of phosphorylation of the NF-kB RelA subunit on S276 and S536 were measured using a Cellular Activating of Signaling ELISA CASE™ kit. The results are expressed as the means ± SD (n=6); *P < 0.005 vs. untreated. [This figure is modified from (Shibata et al., 2009a)]

Fig. 7. The effects of Bay11-7085, LPIL or Dex on the phosphorylation of S536 and S276 of the NF-kB RelA subunit

IL-8, originally called monocyte-derived neutrophil chemotactic factor, is a potent chemokine, causing recruitment and infiltration of neutrophils and T cells into local inflammatory sites. The infiltration of neutrophils contributes to inflammation and has been implicated in various diseases. The transcription factors NF-κB, AP-1, and NF-IL-6 are all involved in the stimulus-induced expression of IL-8. Subsequent IPA revealed that NF-κB signaling was likely important for the synthesis and release of the IL-8 protein. We then found that IL-1β-induced IL-8 release from MH7A cells requires the activation of the canonical NF-κB pathway and kinases catalyzing its phosphorylation. Furthermore, treatments with Dex or LPIL suppressed the phosphorylation of S276 of the RelA subunit, which would in turn inhibit the translocation of NF-κB into the nucleus, where it could interact with the promoter region of the IL8 gene.

6. Acknowledgements

We gratefully acknowledge the assistance of Mrs Asayo Imaoka with the microarray technology. This research was supported in part by "Academic Frontier" Project for Private Universities: matching fund subsidy from Ministry of Education, Culture, Sports, Science and Technology in 2007-2011, the Grants-in-Aid for Scientific Research (Kakenhi: 21390497, 22592078).

7. References

Agro, A., Langdon, C., Smith, F. & Richards, C. D. (1996). Prostaglandin E_2 enhances interleukin 8 (IL-8) and IL-6 but inhibits GMCSF production by IL-1 stimulated human synovial fibroblasts in vitro. *J Rheumatol*, Vol. 23, No. 5, pp. (862-868), issn 0315-162X.

Baggiolini, M., Dewald, B. & Moser, B. (1994). Interleukin-8 and related chemotactic cytokines - CXC and CC chemokines, In: *Adv Immunol, Vol 55*, pp. 97-179).

Bartok, B. & Firestein, G. S. (2010). Fibroblast-like synoviocytes: key effector cells in rheumatoid arthritis. *Immunol Rev*, Vol. 233, No. 1, pp. (233-255), issn 1600-065X (Electronic), 0105-2896 (Linking).

Borghaei, R. C., Rawlings, P. L. & Mochan, E. (1998). Interleukin-4 suppression of interleukin-1-induced transcription of collagenase (MMP-1) and stromelysin 1 (MMP-3) in human synovial fibroblasts. *Arthritis Rheum*, Vol. 41, No. 8, pp. (1398-1406), issn 0004-3591.

Budihardjo, I., Oliver, H., Lutter, M., Luo, X. & Wang, X. D. (1999). Biochemical pathways of caspase activation during apoptosis. *Annu Rev Cell Dev Biol*, Vol. 15, No., pp. (269-290), issn 1081-0706.

Caristi, S., Piraino, G., Cucinotta, M., Valenti, A., Loddo, S. & Teti, D. (2005). Prostaglandin E_2 induces interleukin-8 gene transcription by activating C/EBP homologous protein in human T lymphocytes. *J Biol Chem*, Vol. 280, No. 15, pp. (14433-14442), issn 0021-9258.

Connell, L. & McInnes, I. B. (2006). New cytokine targets in inflammatory rheumatic diseases. *Best Pract Res Clin Rheumatol*, Vol. 20, No. 5, pp. (865-878), issn 1521-6942.

Cozzolino, F., Torcia, M., Lucibello, M., Morbidelli, L., Ziche, M., Platt, J., Fabiani, S., Brett, J. & Stern, D. (1993). Interferon-alpha and interleukin 2 synergistically enhance basic fibroblast growth factor synthesis and induce release, promoting endothelial cell growth. *J Clin Invest*, Vol. 91, No. 6, pp. (2504-2512), issn 0021-9738 (Print), 0021-9738 (Linking).

Dayer, J. M. (2002). The saga of the discovery of IL-1 and TNF and their specific inhibitors in the pathogenesis and treatment of rheumatoid arthritis. *Joint Bone Spine*, Vol. 69, No. 2, pp. (123-132), issn 1297-319X.

Dayer, J. M. (2004). The process of identifying and understanding cytokines: from basic studies to treating rheumatic diseases. *Best Pract Res Clin Rheumatol*, Vol. 18, No. 1, pp. (31-45), issn 1521-6942.

Demura, S., Yamaji, S. & Ikemoto, Y. (2002). Effect of linear polarized near-infrared light irradiation on flexibility of shoulder and ankle joints. *J Sports Med Phys Fitness*, Vol. 42, No. 4, pp. (438-445), issn 0022-4707 (Print), 0022-4707 (Linking).

Feldmann, M. & Maini, R. N. (1999). The role of cytokines in the pathogenesis of rheumatoid arthritis. *Rheumatology*, Vol. 38, No., pp. (3-7), issn 1462-0324.

Firestein, G. S. (1996). Invasive fibroblast-like synoviocytes in rheumatoid arthritis. Passive responders or transformed aggressors? *Arthritis Rheum*, Vol. 39, No. 11, pp. (1781-1790), issn 0004-3591.

Firestein, G. S. (2003). Evolving concepts of rheumatoid arthritis. *Nature*, Vol. 423, No. 6937, pp. (356-361), issn 0028-0836.

Firestein, G. S. (2007). Biomedicine: Every joint has a silver lining. *Science*, Vol. 315, No. 5814, pp. (952-953), issn 0036-8075, 1095-9203.

Goldring, S. R. (2003). Pathogenesis of bone and cartilage destruction in rheumatoid arthritis. *Rheumatology*, Vol. 42, No., pp. (11-16), issn 1462-0324.

Han, S. K., Jeon, S. J., Miyazawa, K., Yi, S. Y. & Yoo, Y. S. (2006). Enhancement of anti-inflammatory tendency by SB203580, p38alpha specific inhibitor, in human fibroblast-like synoviocyte cell line, MH7A. *Rheumatol Int,* Vol. 26, No. 11, pp. (972-978), issn 0172-8172 (Print), 0172-8172 (Linking).

Hebert, C. A. & Baker, J. B. (1993). Interleukin-8 - a review. *Cancer Invest,* Vol. 11, No. 6, pp. (743-750), issn 0735-7907.

Houssiau, F. A., Devogelaer, J. P., Van Damme, J., de Deuxchaisnes, C. N. & Van Snick, J. (1988). Interleukin-6 in synovial fluid and serum of patients with rheumatoid arthritis and other inflammatory arthritides. *Arthritis Rheum,* Vol. 31, No. 6, pp. (784-788), issn 0004-3591 (Print), 0004-3591 (Linking).

Huber, L. C. (2006). Synovial fibroblasts: key players in rheumatoid arthritis. *Rheumatology,* Vol. 45, No. 6, pp. (669-675), issn 1462-0324, 1462-0332.

Hunter, C. A. (2005). New IL-12-family members: IL-23 and IL-27, cytokines with divergent functions. *Nat Rev Immunol,* Vol. 5, No. 7, pp. (521-531), issn 1474-1733.

Iwanaga, T., Shikichi, M., Kitamura, H., Yanase, H. & Nozawa-Inoue, K. (2000). Morphology and functional roles of synoviocytes in the joint. *Arch Histol Cytol,* Vol. 63, No. 1, pp. (17-31), issn 0914-9465 (Print), 0914-9465 (Linking).

Kirwan, J., & Power L. (2007). Glucocorticoids: action and new therapeutic insights in rheumatoid arthritis. Curr Opin Rheumatol, Vol. 19, No. 3, pp. (233-237).

King, M. R. & Hammer, D. A. (2001). Multiparticle adhesive dynamics: Hydrodynamic recruitment of rolling leukocytes. *Proc Natl Acad Sci USA,* Vol. 98, No. 26, pp. (14919-14924), issn 0027-8424.

Matsusaka, T., Fujikawa, K., Nishio, Y., Mukaida, N., Matsushima, K., Kishimoto, T. & Akira, S. (1993). Transcription factors NF-IL6 and NF-kappa B synergistically activate transcription of the inflammatory cytokines, interleukin 6 and interleukin 8. *Proc Natl Acad Sci USA,* Vol. 90, No. 21, pp. (10193-10197), issn 0027-8424 (Print), 0027-8424 (Linking).

Mattioli, I., Sebald, A., Bucher, C., Charles, R. P., Nakano, H., Doi, T., Kracht, M. & Schmitz, M. L. (2004). Transient and selective NF-kappa B p65 serine 536 phosphorylation induced by T cell costimulation is mediated by I kappa B kinase beta and controls the kinetics of p65 nuclear import. *J Immunol,* Vol. 172, No. 10, pp. (6336-6344), issn 0022-1767 (Print), 0022-1767 (Linking).

Mauviel, A., Teyton, L., Bhatnagar, R., Penfornis, H., Laurent, M., Hartmann, D., Bonaventure, J., Loyau, G., Saklatvala, J. & Pujol, J. P. (1988). Interleukin-1 alpha modulates collagen gene expression in cultured synovial cells. *Biochem J,* Vol. 252, No. 1, pp. (247-255), issn 0264-6021 (Print), 0264-6021 (Linking).

Mendonça, J. A., Marques-Neto, J. F., Samara, A. M. & Appenzeller, S. (2011). Increased levels of rheumatoid factors after TNF inhibitor in rheumatoid arthritis. *Rheumatol Int,* Vol., No.), issn 0172-8172, 1437-160X.

Miyazawa, K., Mori, A. & Okudaira, H. (1998). Establishment and characterization of a novel human rheumatoid fibroblast-like synoviocyte line, MH7A, immortalized with SV40 T antigen. *J Biochem,* Vol. 124, No. 6, pp. (1153-1162), issn 0021-924X (Print), 0021-924X (Linking).

Morita, Y., Yamamura, M., Nishida, K., Harada, S., Okamoto, H., Inoue, H., Ohmoto, Y., Modlin, R. L. & Makino, H. (1998). Expression of interleukin-12 in synovial tissue from patients with rheumatoid arthritis. *Arthritis Rheum,* Vol. 41, No. 2, pp. (306-314), issn 0004-3591.

Nagashima, M., Yoshino, S., Aono, H., Takai, M. & Sasano, M. (1999). Inhibitory effects of anti-rheumatic drugs on vascular endothelial growth factor in cultured rheumatoid synovial cells. *Clin Exp Immunol,* Vol. 116, No. 2, pp. (360-365), issn 0009-9104.

O'Dell, J. R. (2004). Therapeutic strategies for rheumatoid arthritis. *N Engl J Med,* Vol. 350, No. 25, pp. (2591-2602), issn 1533-4406 (Electronic), 0028-4793 (Linking).

Pap, T., Muller-Ladner, U., Gay, R. E. & Gay, S. (2000). Fibroblast biology. Role of synovial fibroblasts in the pathogenesis of rheumatoid arthritis. *Arthritis Res,* Vol. 2, No. 5, pp. (361-367), issn 1465-9913.

Rathanaswami, P., Hachicha, M., Sadick, M., Schall, T. J. & McColl, S. R. (1993). Expression of the cytokine RANTES in human rheumatoid synovial fibroblasts. Differential regulation of RANTES and interleukin-8 genes by inflammatory cytokines. *J Biol Chem,* Vol. 268, No. 8, pp. (5834-5839), issn 0021-9258 (Print), 0021-9258 (Linking).

Robinson, D. R., Tashjian, A. H. & Levine, L. (1975). Prostaglandin-stimulated bone-resorption by rheumatoid synovial: possible mechanism for bone destruction in rheumatoid-arthritis. *J Clin Invest,* Vol. 56, No. 5, pp. (1181-1188), issn 0021-9738.

Rothe, M., Pan, M. G., Henzel, W. J., Ayres, T. M. & Goeddel, D. V. (1995). The TNFR2-TRAF signaling complex contains two novel proteins related to baculoviral inhibitor of apoptosis proteins. *Cell,* Vol. 83, No. 7, pp. (1243-1252), issn 0092-8674 (Print), 0092-8674 (Linking).

Saag, K. G., Teng, G. G., Patkar, N. M., Anuntiyo, J., Finney, C., Curtis, J. R., Paulus, H. E., Mudano, A., Pisu, M., Elkins-Melton, M., Outman, R., Allison, J. J., Almazor, M. S., Bridges, S. L., Chatham, W. W., Hochberg, M., Maclean, C., Mikuls, T., Moreland, L. W., O'Dell, J., Turkiewicz, A. M. & Furst, D. E. (2008). American College of Rheumatology 2008 recommendations for the use of nonbiologic and biologic disease-modifying antirheumatic drugs in rheumatoid arthritis. *Arthritis Rheum,* Vol. 59, No. 6, pp. (762-784), issn 00043591, 15290131.

Sakurai, H., Chiba, H., Miyoshi, H., Sugita, T. & Toriumi, W. (1999). IkappaB kinases phosphorylate NF-kappaB p65 subunit on serine 536 in the transactivation domain. *J Biol Chem,* Vol. 274, No. 43, pp. (30353-30356), issn 0021-9258 (Print), 0021-9258 (Linking).

Sakurai, H. (2003). Tumor Necrosis Factor- -induced IKK Phosphorylation of NF- B p65 on Serine 536 Is Mediated through the TRAF2, TRAF5, and TAK1 Signaling Pathway. *J Biol Chem,* Vol. 278, No. 38, pp. (36916-36923), issn 0021-9258, 1083-351X.

Shibata, Y., Ogura, N., Yamashiro, K., Takashiba, S., Kondoh, T., Miyazawa, K., Matsui, M. & Abiko, Y. (2005). Anti-inflammatory effect of linear polarized infrared irradiation on interleukin-1 beta-induced chemokine production in MH7A rheumatoid synovial cells. *Lasers Med Sci,* Vol. 20, No. 3-4, pp. (109-113), issn 0268-8921.

Shibata, Y., Araki, H., Oshitani, T., Imaoka, A., Matsui, M., Miyazawa, K. & Abiko, Y. (2009a). Effects of linear polarized infrared light irradiation on the transcriptional regulation of IL-8 expression in IL-1 beta-stimulated human rheumatoid synoviocytes involves phosphorylation of the NF-kappa B RelA subunit. *J Photochem Photobiol B-Biol,* Vol. 94, No. 3, pp. (164-170), issn 1011-1344.

Shibata, Y., Kasai, H., Shimada, M., Koitabashi, T., Arai, T., Sai, R., Terao, H., Horikiri, M., Negishi, H., Miyazawa, K. & Abiko, Y. (2009b). IL-1 beta stimulates IL-8 production, including prostaglandin E_2 receptor EP4-triggered pathways, in synoviocyte MH7A cells. *Mol Med Rep*, Vol. 2, No. 3, pp. (359-363), issn 1791-2997.

Smolen, J. S. & Steiner, G. (2003). Therapeutic strategies for rheumatoid arthritis. *Nat Rev Drug Discov*, Vol. 2, No. 6, pp. (473-488), issn 14741776, 14741784.

Standiford, T. J., Kunkel, S. L., Rolfe, M. W., Evanoff, H. L., Allen, R. M. & Strieter, R. M. (1992). Regulation of human alveolar macrophage-derived and blood monocyte-derived interleukin-8 by prostaglandin-E2 and dexamethasone. *Am J Respir Cell Mol Biol*, Vol. 6, No. 1, pp. (75-81), issn 1044-1549.

Suissa, S., Bernatsky, S. & Hudson, M. (2006). Antirheumatic drug use and the risk of acute myocardial infarction. *Arthritis Rheum*, Vol. 55, No. 4, pp. (531-536), issn 0004-3591 (Print), 0004-3591 (Linking).

Sun, H. B. & Yokota, H. (2002). Reduction of cytokine-induced expression and activity of MMP-1 and MMP-13 by mechanical strain in MH7A rheumatoid synovial cells. *Matrix Biol*, Vol. 21, No. 3, pp. (263-270), issn 0945-053X.

Suzuki, M., Hashizume, M., Yoshida, H., Shiina, M. & Mihara, M. (2010). IL-6 and IL-1 synergistically enhanced the production of MMPs from synovial cells by up-regulating IL-6 production and IL-1 receptor I expression. *Cytokine*, Vol. 51, No. 2, pp. (178-183), issn 10434666.

Takayama, K., Garcia-Cardena, G., Sukhova, G. K., Comander, J., Gimbrone, M. A. & Libby, P. (2002). Prostaglandin E_2 suppresses chemokine production in human macrophages through the EP4 receptor. *J Biol Chem*, Vol. 277, No. 46, pp. (44147-44154), issn 0021-9258.

Tolboom, T. C. A., van der Helm-Van Mil, A. H. M., Nelissen, R. G. H. H., Breedveld, F. C., Toes, R. E. M. & Huizinga, T. W. J. (2005). Invasiveness of fibroblast-like synoviocytes is an individual patient characteristic associated with the rate of joint destruction in patients with rheumatoid arthritis. *Arthritis Rheum*, Vol. 52, No. 7, pp. (1999-2002), issn 0004-3591, 1529-0131.

Trebino, C. E., Stock, J. L., Gibbons, C. P., Naiman, B. M., Wachtmann, T. S., Umland, J. P., Pandher, K., Lapointe, J. M., Saha, S., Roach, M. L., Carter, D., Thomas, N. A., Durtschi, B. A., McNeish, J. D., Hambor, J. E., Jakobsson, P. J., Carty, T. J., Perez, J. R. & Audoly, L. P. (2003). Impaired inflammatory and pain responses in mice lacking an inducible prostaglandin E synthase. *Proc Natl Acad Sci USA*, Vol. 100, No. 15, pp. (9044-9049), issn 0027-8424.

Volin, M. V., Harlow, L. A., Woods, J. M., Campbell, P. L., Amin, M. A., Tokuhira, M. & Koch, A. E. (1999). Treatment with sulfasalazine or sulfapyridine, but not 5-aminosalicyclic acid, inhibits basic fibroblast growth factor-induced endothelial cell chemotaxis. *Arthritis Rheum*, Vol. 42, No. 9, pp. (1927-1935), issn 0004-3591 (Print), 0004-3591 (Linking).

Wertheim, W. A., Kunkel, S. L., Standiford, T. J., Burdick, M. D., Becker, F. S., Wilke, C. A., Gilbert, A. R. & Strieter, R. M. (1993). Regulation of neutrophil-derived Il-8. The role of prostaglandin E_2, dexamethasone, and Il-4. *J Immunol*, Vol. 151, No. 4, pp. (2166-2175), issn 0022-1767.

Yang, F., Tang, E., Guan, K. & Wang, C. Y. (2003). IKK beta plays an essential role in the phosphorylation of RelA/p65 on serine 536 induced by lipopolysaccharide. *J Immunol*, Vol. 170, No. 11, pp. (5630-5635), issn 0022-1767 (Print), 0022-1767 (Linking).

Yokoyama, K. & Oku, T. (1999). Rheumatoid arthritis-affected temporomandibular joint pain analgesia by linear polarized near infrared irradiation. *Can J Anaesth,* Vol. 46, No. 7, pp. (683-687), issn 0832-610X (Print), 0832-610X (Linking).

Yokoyama, K. & Sugiyama, K. (2003). Influence of linearly polarized near-infrared irradiation on deformability of human stored erythrocytes. *J Clin Laser Med Surg,* Vol. 21, No. 1, pp. (19-22), issn 1044-5471 (Print), 1044-5471 (Linking).

Yu, Y. & Chadee, K. (1998). Prostaglandin E_2 stimulates IL-8 gene expression in human colonic epithelial cells by a posttranscriptional mechanism. *J Immunol,* Vol. 161, No. 7, pp. (3746-3752), issn 0022-1767.

Zhong, H., May, M. J., Jimi, E. & Ghosh, S. (2002). The phosphorylation status of nuclear NF-kappa B determines its association with CBP/p300 or HDAC-1. *Mol Cell,* Vol. 9, No. 3, pp. (625-636), issn 1097-2765 (Print), 1097-2765 (Linking).

10

The Role of miRNA in Rheumatoid Arthritis

Seiji Kawano and Yuji Nakamachi
Kobe University
Japan

1. Introduction

MicroRNAs (miRNAs) are a well-established class of small (~22 nucleotides) endogenous non-coding RNAs that influence the stability and translation of messenger RNA (mRNA) (van Rooij et al., 2007). Hundreds of miRNA have been identified in numerous animal species. The miRNA genes are transcribed by RNA polymerase II as primary miRNA (pri-miRNA). The RNase III enzyme Drosha then processes the nuclear pri-miRNA, to precursor miRNA (pre-miRNA), which is exported from the nucleus with the help of exportin. Maturation of the pre-miRNA into miRNA is then mediated by the cytoplasmic enzyme Dicer, after which the single-stranded mature miRNA is loaded into the RNA-induced silencing complex (RISC). Once loaded, the miRNA guides this complex to the 3'-untranslated region (3'-UTR) of target mRNA (Figure 1). The socalled 'seed region' (nucleotides 2–8) of miRNA is most important for target recognition and silencing. miRNA usually binds with imperfect complementarity to its target, which is called the 'seed sequence'. Association of miRNA with its target mRNA silences expression via at least three mechanisms: inhibition of translation, inhibition of the initiation of translation and destabilization of target mRNA.

Recent advances have shown that miRNA expression during development is highly tissue-specific, which suggests that miRNA may be involved in specifying and maintaining tissue identity. Recent studies have shown that a single miRNA can generate a huge impact to the whole profile of protein expression (Selbach et al., 2008; Baek et al., 2008). For most interactions, microRNAs act as 'rheostats' to make fine-scale adjustments to protein output (Baek et al., 2008). Several miRNAs have been shown to regulate the 3'-UTR of mRNA that encode transcription factors, and a circuit that sequentially involves miRNA and transcription factors in a mutual negative feedback loop has been described (Tsang et al., 2008). The role of miRNA on protein expression, therefore, is not one-directional: from miRNA to protein. If we consider, however, a simple setting of miRNA and its direct target mRNA, the miRNA upregulated in a particular cell type from patients with specific disease possibly put the cell in short of a group of proteins which are necessary to maintain the physiological homoeostasis by targeting the translation of those proteins. In contrast, the miRNA downregulated in a particular cell type from patients with specific disease might allow the cell to increase translation of a group of proteins that are suppressed at low levels in normal conditions.

In 2009, the direct involvement of single nucleotide polymorphisms of a miRNA in human hereditary disease was reported for the first time (Mencia et al., 2009). They found that two different single nucleotide polymorphisms of miR-96 are related the hearing loss found in two families. Their report was the start of a new era, in which the involvement of genetic

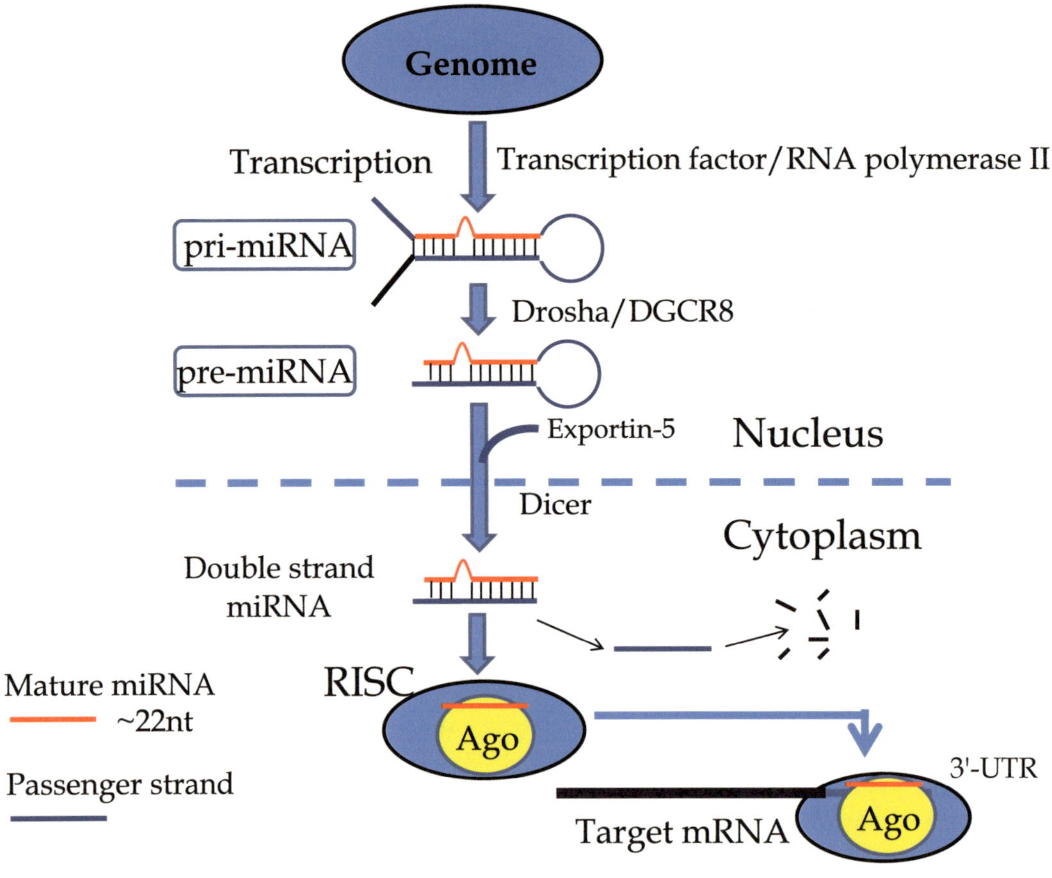

Fig. 1. Biogenesis of miRNA

changes of non-coding RNAs in hereditary diseases and possibly multifactorial disorders such as autoimmune diseases should be considered. As we discuss in this review, our understanding of RA pathogenesis has been enriched by recent miRNA studies, it is now obvious that miRNAs play important roles in the critical aspects of RA pathogenesis such as joint destruction, inflammation, proliferation of synoviocytes, and chemotaxis of inflammatory cells. We summarize the recent advances of RA studies focusing on miRNAs, and provide the current understanding of the role of miRNAs in RA pathogenesis.

2. Immunity and miRNA

More than 100 miRNAs are expressed by cells of the immune system, and they have the potential to broadly influence the molecular pathways that control the development and function of innate and adaptive immune responses (O'Connell et al., 2010). miRNA levels are dynamically regulated during lineage differentiation of haematopoietic stem cells and also during the course of the immune response, including innate immunity and acquired immunity. Animal experiments of the ablating-specific miRNA genes have shown that miRNA expression in haematopoietic cells is critical for mounting an appropriate immune response. In innate immunity, miRNAs have unique effects on granulocytes, monocytes/

macrophages, dendritic cells and natural killer cells. In particular, miR-146, miR-155, miR-147, miR-21 and miR-9 have been reported to regulate the macrophage activation via a Toll-like receptor pathway or cytokine production. miRNAs are also involved in acquired immunity by modulating the differentiation and function of T and B cells. miR-17-92 cluster targeting BIM and PTEN and miR-181a targeting DUSP5, DUSP6, SHP2 and PTPN22 are important for T-cell development in the thymus. For T-cell function, miR-142, miR-146, miR-150, miR-155, and others have been reported to regulate the development of functional T cells such as Th1, Th2, Th17, and Treg.
Recently, mutant mice with a targeted deletion of miR-146a (Boldin et al., 2011) have been created. *Baldin et al* have found that miR-146a is expressed predominantly in immune tissues, and its expression can be induced in immune cells upon cell maturation and/or activation. Lack of miR-146a expression results in hyperresponsiveness of macrophages to bacterial Lipopolysaccharide (LPS) and leads to an exaggerated inflammatory response in endotoxin-challenged mice. In contrast, overexpression of miR-146a in monocytes has the opposite effect. Interestingly, miR-146a–null mice developed a spontaneous autoimmune disorder, characterized by splenomegaly, lymphadenopathy, and multiorgan inflammation, resulting in premature death. Using a combination of gain and loss of function approaches, they confirmed TRAF6 and IRAK1 genes as miR-146a targets, whose derepression in miR-146a-null mice might account for some of the observed immune phenotypes. In addition, they found that miR-146a seems to play a role in the control of immune cell proliferation; aging miR-146a–null mice display an excessive production of myeloid cells and develop frank tumors in their secondary lymphoid organs, suggesting that miR-146a can function as a tumor suppressor in the context of the immune system. Their results showed that miR-146a as an important negative regulator of inflammation, myeloid cell proliferation, and cancer.

2.1 miRNA and Rheumatoid Arthritis

Rheumatoid arthritis (RA) is a chronic disease of unknown cause that presents a characteristic inflammatory features, including synoviocyte hyperplasia, which results in pannus formation and joint destruction. The local production of cytokines and chemokines accounts for many of the pathological and clinical manifestations of RA. In culture, RA fibroblast like synoviocytes (FLS) proliferate and secrete a variety of cytokines/ chemokines/angiogenic factors, including fibroblast growth factor, granulocyte-macrophage colony stimulating factor, interleukin 6 (IL-6), IL-8, monocyte chemoattractant protein 1 (MCP-1) and macrophage inflammatory proteins 1α, and they present various adhesion molecules on their surfaces. Since the first report by *Stanczyk et al* in 2008, several reports have described the altered miRNAs in the joint and/or peripheral blood leucocytes of patients with RA, including miR-155, miR-146 and others (Table 1) (Stanczyk, et al., 2008; Nakasa, et al., 2008; Pauley, et al., 2008; Murata, et al., 2010; Li, et al., 2010; Fulci, et al., 2010; Nakamachi, et al., 2009. Niimoto, et al., 2010).

2.1.1 Overexpressed miRNAs in RA

Stanczyk et al reported that constitutive expression of miR-155 and miR-146a was higher in RA synovial fibroblasts (RASF) than in those from patients with osteoarthritis (OA), and expression of miR-155 was induced by tumour necrosis factor α (TNF-α), IL-1β, LPS, polyinosinic/polycytidylic acid. Enforced expression of miR-155 in RASF was found to repress the levels of matrix metalloproteinase 3 (MMP-3) and reduce the induction of MMP-3 and MMP-1 by Toll-like receptor ligands and cytokines. Moreover, RA synovial fluid monocytes displayed higher levels of miR-155 than peripheral blood monocytes. *Nakasa et al* reported that miR-146 is expressed in RA synovial tissue and its expression is induced by stimulation with TNF-α and IL-1β. They also showed by in situ hybridisation that CD68-positive macrophages and CD3 T cells strongly express miR-146 (Nakasa et al., 2008). *Pauley et al* reported that peripheral blood mononuclear cells (PBMCs) from patients with RA exhibit significantly increased expression levels of miR-16, miR-132, miR-155 and miR-146a compared with healthy and disease control individuals (Pauley et al., 2008). Furthermore, they demonstrated that high levels of miR-16 and miR-146a expression correlated with active disease. Although miR-146a expression is increased in patients with RA, levels of the two established miR-146a targets, TNF receptor-associated factor 6 (TRAF-6) and IL-1 receptor-associated kinase 1(IRAK-1), in patients with RA are similar to those in control individuals. Recently, *Murata et al* reported that synovial fluid concentrations of miR-16, miR-146a miR-155 and miR-223 in patients with RA were significantly higher than those in patients with OA. In addition, plasma miRNAs or ratio of synovial fluid miRNAs to plasma miRNAs, including miR-16 and miR-146a, significantly correlated with tender joint counts and 28-joint Disease Activity Score (DAS-28) (Murata et al., 2010).

Upregulated miRNA	Downregulated miRNA	tissue	Ref.
miR-146, miR-155		SF	Stanczyk et al, 2008
miR-146		ST	Nakasa et al, 2008
miR-16, miR-132, miR-146a, miR-155		PBMC	Pauley et al, 2008
miR-16, miR-146a, miR-155, miR-223		JF	Murata et al, 2010
miR-146a	miR-363, miR-498	CD4T	Li et al, 2010
miR-223		CD4T	Fulci et al, 2010
Let-7a, miR-26, miR-146a/b, miR-150, miR-155		IL-17+CD4 T	Niimoto et al, 2010
miR-133a, miR-146a, miR-142-3p, miR-142-5p, miR-223	miR-124a	SF	Nakamachi et al, 2009

SF: Synival fibroblast, ST: Synovial tissue, PBMC: Peripheral blood mononuclear cell, JF: Joint fluid, CD4T: peripheral blood CD4+T cells.

Table 1. miRNA expression in Rheumatoid Arthritis

These studies showed that miR-146 is strongly expressed in synovial fibroblasts and mononuclear cells from patients with RA. *Li et al* reported that the level of miR-146a expression was positively correlated with levels of TNF-α, and in vitro studies showed that TNF-α upregulated miR-146a expression in T cells (Li et al., 2010). They also reported that miR-146a overexpression was found to suppress Jurkat T-cell apoptosis. Interestingly,

transcriptome analysis of miR-146a overexpression in T cells identified Fas associated factor 1 as a miR-146a-regulated gene, which was critically involved in modulating T-cell apoptosis. *Niimoto et al* reported that six miRNAs, let-7a, miR-26, miR-146a/b, miR-150, and miR-155 were significantly upregulated in the IL-17 producing CD4+ T cells from RA patient (Niimoto et al, 2010). miR-146a was intensely expressed in RA synovium in comparison to OA. miR-146a expressed intensely in the synovium with hyperplasia and high expression of IL-17 from the patients with high disease activity. Double staining revealed that miR-146a was expressed in IL-17 expressing cells. These results indicated that miR-146a was associated with IL-17 expression in the PBMC and synovium in RA patients. Recently, *Nasaka et al* reported that the number of TRAP-positive multinucleated cells in human PBMCs was significantly reduced by miR-146a in a dose-dependent manner when isolated PBMCs from healthy volunteers were transfected with double-stranded miR-146a and cultured in the presence of M-CSF and either TNF-α or RANKL (Nasaka et al., 2011). The expression of c-Jun, NF-ATc1, PU.1, and TRAP in PBMCs was significantly down-regulated by miR-146a. Their results suggest that miR-146a might suppress the osteoclastgenesis form human monocytes. Thus, our knowledge about the roles of miR-146a has been expanding to various cell types including not only synoviocytes, monocytes, lymphocytes but also differentiated functional cells such as Th17 cells and osteoclasts.
Taken together, several miRNAs have been repeatedlydescribed as upregulated in RA studies. Among those, the most redundant miRNA has been miR-146 and miR-155. Interestingly, miR-146 is downregulated in PBMCs from patients with systemic lupus erythematosus (SLE) (Tsang et al., 2009). This contrast is attractive in illustrating a difference in the cytokine profiles of RA and SLE, with type I interferon playing a dominant role in SLE, whereas TNF-α, IL-1 and IL-6 are the principal cytokines in RA (Chan et al., 2009).

2.1.2 Manipulation of overexpressed miRNAs in arthritis models

Several groups have been focused on particular miRNAs upregulated in human RA tissues. They downregulated those upregulated miRNAs in human RA by targeting miRNA expression in mouse models of inflammatory arthritis and examined if the suppression of those miRNAs could regulate the arthritis development. *Nasaka et al* reported that administration of miR-146a prevented joint destruction in mice with collagen-induced arthritis (CIA) when double-stranded miR-146a or nonspecific double-stranded RNA was administered twice by intravenous injection, although it did not completely ameliorate inflammation (Nasaka et al., 2011). Their results indicate that expression of miR-146a inhibits osteoclastogenesis and that administration of double-stranded miR-146a prevents joint destruction in arthritic mice. *Blüml et al* examined the role of miRNA in the pathogenesis of autoimmune arthritis, using CIA and K/BxN serum-transfer arthritis in wild-type (WT) and miR-155-null mice (Blüml et al, 2011). They found that the miR-155-null mice did not develop CIA. Deficiency in miR-155 prevented the generation of pathogenic autoreactive B and T cells, since anti-collagen antibodies and the expression levels of antigen-specific T cells were strongly reduced in miR-155-null mice. Moreover, Th17 polarization of miR-155-null mouse T cells was impaired, as shown by a significant decrease in the levels of IL-17 and IL-22. In the K/BxN serum-transfer arthritis model, which only depends on innate effector mechanisms, miR-155-null mice showed significantly reduced local bone destruction, attributed to reduced generation of osteoclasts, although the severity of joint inflammation was similar to that in WT mice. They concluded that miR-155 is essentially involved in the adaptive and innate immune reactions leading to autoimmune arthritis. These two reports implicate that the manipulation of overexpressed miRNAs in PBMCs or synoviocytes such as miR-146a and miR-155, may provide a novel target for the treatment of patients with RA.

2.1.3 Suppressed miRNA in RA

There have been two reports regarding the suppressed miRNAs in RA. *Li et al* reported that miR-146a expression was significantly upregulated while miR-363 and miR-498 were downregulated in CD4+ T cells of RA patients (Li et al., 2010). However, their analyses were focused on miR-146a but not on miR-363 and miR-498. We compared synovial fibroblast derived from patients with RA (RASF) with those from patients with OA (OASF) for their expression of a panel of 156 miRNAs with quantitative stem-loop RT-RCR (Nakamachi et al., 2009). We found that the miR-124a level significantly decreased in RASF. Five other miRNAs (miR-146a, miR-223, miR-142-3p, miR-142-5p and miR-133a) were, on the other hand, expressed more strongly in RA than in OA. In published reports, the expression of miR-124a has been restricted to the brain and nerve tissues of animals and insects (Kloosterman et al., 2006). In those tissues, miR-124a contributes to the differentiation of neural progenitors into mature neurons through degradation of non-neuronal transcripts. In addition to neural tissue development, miR-124a also appears to be involved in carcinogenesis (Agirre et al., 2009).

To investigate the function of miR-124a in RA, we started with the transfection of precursor miR-124a (pre-miR-124a) into RASF and it significantly suppressed their proliferation and arrested the cell cycle at the G1 phase. Interestingly, transfection with pre-miR-124a suppressed proliferation of RASF, but did not induce cell death. These results suggest that the low expression of miR-124a in RASF might protect them from cell-cycle arrest, thereby promoting cell proliferation. For comparison, we transfected pre-miR-146a, pre-miR-223, premiR-142-3p and pre-miR-133a, all of which were elevated in RASF, into OASF, but transfection of these pre-miRNAs did not promote the proliferation of OASF.

A computer search with miRanda 3.0 database (http://microrna.sanger.ac.uk/) to find possible target mRNAs for miR-124a binding in the 3′-UTR, identified a putative consensus site in cyclin-dependent kinase 2 (CDK-2) mRNA. The induction of precursor miR-124a (pre-miR-124a) in RA synoviocytes significantly suppressed the production of the CDK-2 proteins. A luciferase reporter assay demonstrated that miR-124a specifically suppressed the reporter activity driven by the 3′-UTR of CDK-2 mRNA but not reporters driven by the mutant of 3′-UTR of CDK-2 mRNA. We also found that CDK-6 protein, another CDK that regulates the G1-S phase, was suppressed by miR-124a. These results suggest that miR-124a has a key role in regulating the proliferation of RASF. Based on these results, we assumed that the suppressed expression of miR-124a resulted in high expression of a group of proteins, especiallycell-cycle-related proteins. We next measured the levels of cytokines/chemokines in culture medium conditioned with RASF after overexpression of miR-124a, and we detected changes in the levels of three of them: MCP-1, angiogenin and vascular endothelial growth factor (VEGF). While VEGF levels were increased compared with those in medium conditioned with control cells, MCP-1 and angiogenin levels were significantly decreased in the presence of miR-124a overexpression. We also transfected precursors of miR-133a, miR-142-3p, miR-146a and miR-223 into OASF and analysed the culture media for cytokines/chemokines.

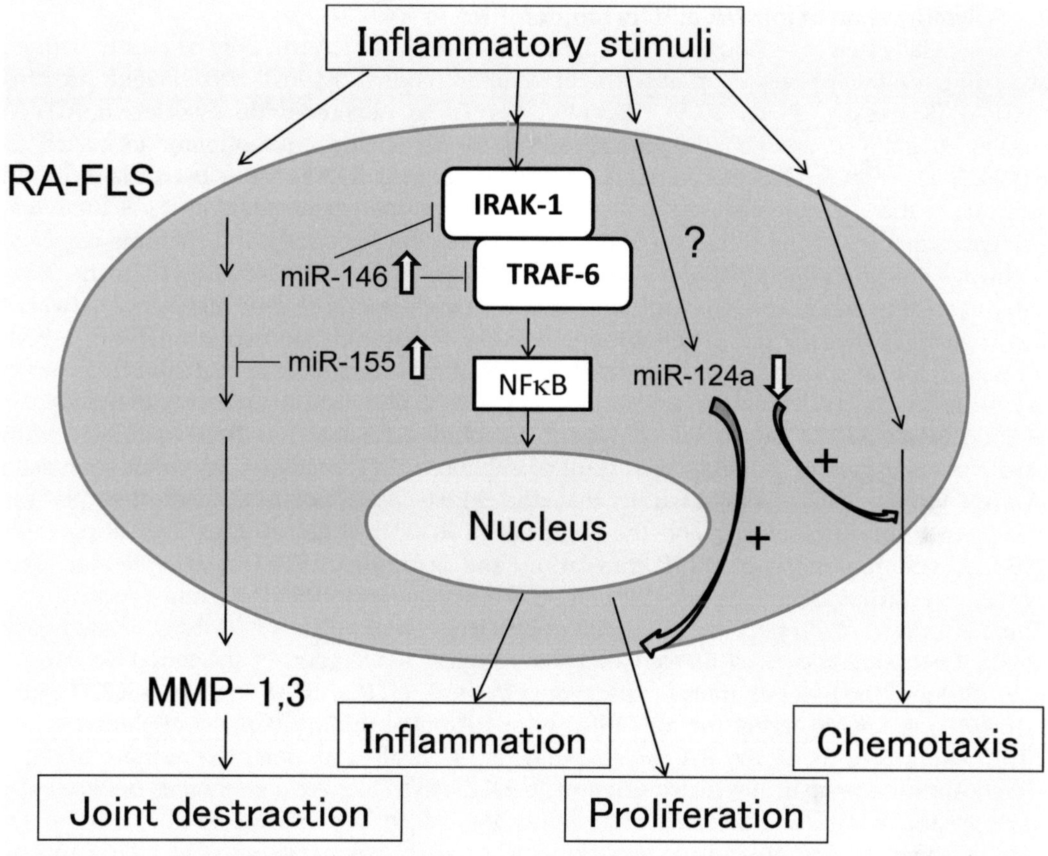

Fig. 2. The role of miRNAs in RASF

In contrast to the findings with pre-miR-124a, the overexpression of these pre-miRNAs did not stimulate any cytokine/chemokine secretion from OASF. We then used the miRanda 3.0 database to search for the 3′-UTR sequences of the mRNA encoding MCP-1, angiogenin and VEGF, and found that only MCP-1 mRNA contained a seed sequence for miR-124a. Subsequent luciferase assays showed that miR-124a specifically suppressed the luciferase activity driven by the 3′-UTR of MCP-1 mRNA. To elucidate the question what kind of stimulants depress the expression of miR-124a, we treated RASF and OASF with TNF-α, IL-1β, IL-6, IL-12, IL-17, IL-18, interferon α or lipopolysaccharide. However, none of these mediators elicited a change in miR-124a level. Possibly this unresponsiveness is the result of the silencing by hypermethylation of miR-124a loci, since the loci in cancer cell lines have been reported to be hypermethylated (Lujambio et al., 2007). Demethylation treatment with 5-aza-2′-cytidine (5-azaC) did not suppress the proliferation of RASF, and methylation-sensitive PCR revealed that the CpG islands of miR-124a loci in RASF were not methylated (Nakamachi Y, unpublished data, 2009). The hypomethylated status of miR-124a loci reflects the suggestion of *Karouzakis et al* that genes are frequently hypomethylated in RA (Karouzakis et al., 2009). At present, the search for factors or epigenetic events that can induce the suppression of miR-124a in RA pathogenesis is underway.

2.2 Polymorphism of miRNA and its target mRNA in RA

RA is clinically heterogeneous, but two disease subgroups of RA can now be clearly defined according to the presence or absence of auto-antibodies against citrullinated proteins (ACPA) (Klareskog et al., 2009). Recently, thanks to genome-wide association (GWA) studies to analyze the genetic predisposition to RA, many susceptibility loci such as PTPN22, TRAF1-C5, OLIG3-TNFAIP3, CD40, CCL21 and STAT4 have been identified in addition to the well established HLA-DRB1 shared epitope alleles (Stahl et al., 2010). Now, evidence emerges of the existence of different genetic backgrounds and immune-response pathways contributing to the development of RA in ACPA-positive and ACPA-negative subgroups of patients. The interruption of miRNAs in the arena of gene regulatory networks has triggered interest from geneticists for looking at naturally occurring miRSNP, a SNP located at or near a miRNA binding site in 3′-UTR of the target gene or in a miRNA (Ryan et al., 2010). *Martin et al* demonstrated that the +1166 A/C polymorphism occurs in the 3′-UTR of the human AT1R(angiotensin II type 1 receptor) gene that has been associated with cardiovascular disease, possibly as a result of enhanced AT1R activity, for unknown reason (Martin et al., 2007). They assume that the +1166 A/C polymorphism disrupts the basepairing complementarity and the ability of miR-155 to interact, thus alleviating miR-155-mediated repression of AT1R translation, and leading to AT1R over-expression, and possibly to cardiovascular disease. Several other examples of miRSNP are now reported.

There is an only one report analyzing the polymorphism of miRNA and its associated gene in RA. *Chatzikyriakidou et al* investigated the potential association of the miR-146a variant rs2910164 and the two polymorphisms located in the 3′-UTR of IRAK-1 gene (rs3027898 and rs1059703), a known target for miR-146a, with RA susceptibility (Chatzikyriakidou et al., 2010). Using cohorts of 136 RA patients and of 147 healthy donors, the authors found a significant difference in the distribution of IRAK-1 rs3027898 A>C genotypes between RA patients and controls. The same association was recently reported by the authors for psoriasic arthritis and ankylosing spondylitis (PsA) (Chatzikyriakidou et al., 2009) and by others for atherothrombotic cerebral infraction (Yamada et al., 2008). However, no difference was observed in the distribution of IRAK-1 rs1059703 and miR-146a rs2910164 variants between RA and control individuals. Thus, no miRSNP has yet been found functionally associated with RA. Therefore, it would be of real interest to assess whether the observed polymorphism has potential consequences on IRAK-1 expression levels and to link a mutation in the 3′-UTR of IRAK-1 with putative binding site for other miRNAs than miR-146a. Another track would be to search for 3'-UTR motif(s) located in the vicinity of the miRNA target sequence, which may be coupled to regulation by miRNA, as it is suggested by a recent publication (Jacobsen et al., 2010).

Finally, although five groups have published since 2008 that miR-146a is over-expressed in RA tissues; it is not a RA-specific miRNA, as it has been found deregulated in many other human disorders. There is thus much room for studies identifying at RA-specific miRNAs and investigating the impact of miRSNPs on RA in particular and on human pathologies in general for the next decade.

2.3 Epigenetics of miRNA in RA

Another important and emerging field of study for autoimmune diseases, including RA, is represented by epigenetics. The three main mechanisms of epigenetic control (DNA methylation, histone modifications, and miRNA regulation) interact in the development of the RA-synovial fibroblast phenotype (Karouzakis et al., 2009a). RA synoviocytes show epigenetic abnormalities, mainly represented by DNA hypomethylation and histone hyperacetylation, thus leading to synovial proliferation (Brooks et al., 2010). In RA synovial cells overexpression of histone deacetylase has been demonstrated at the transcriptional level, and the use of histone deacetylase small-interfering RNA has revealed that this enzyme plays an important role in the synoviocyte proliferation and apoptosis (Horiuchi et al., 2009). Another study showed that synoviocyte hyperacetylation was associated with an increase of histone acetyl transferases, without variation of the histone deacetylases (Huber et al., 2007). DNA hypomethylation is another epigenetic modification that can occur in RA, leading to the up-regulation of genes coding for growth factors, receptors, adhesion molecules, and other components responsible for the inflammatory milieu and active phenotype of RASFs (Karouzakis et al., 2009b).

PCR–based screening of 260 individual miRNAs which were differentially expressed miRNAs in RASF versus OASF revealed that expression of miR-203 was higher in RASF than in OASF or fibroblasts from healthy donors (Stanczyk et al., 2011). Levels of miR-203 did not change upon stimulation with IL-1β, TNF-α, or LPS; however, DNA demethylation with 5-azaC increased the expression of miR-203. Enforced expression of miR-203 led to significantly increased levels of MMP-1 and IL-6. Induction of IL-6 by miR-203 overexpression was inhibited by blocking of the NF-κB pathway. Basal expression levels of IL-6 correlated with basal expression levels of miR-203. These results showed that the production of miR-223 exerts its role as a pro-inflammatory miRNA in response to the signal via NFκB pathway and its level is influenced by methylation/ demethylation status. These observations show that epigenetic control is deficient in RA joint cells, suggesting that broader analysis is required to better understand the role of these mechanisms in the pathogenesis of RA, the identification of epigenetic biomarkers, and the development of specific therapies targeting key molecules of the epigenetic process.

3. Biomarkers for RA

A biomarker is a physical sign or cellular, biochemical, molecular or genetic alteration by which a normal or abnormal biologic process can be recognized or monitored, or both, and that might have diagnostic or prognostic utility (Illei et al., 2004). Biomarkers have several potential applications in rheumatic diseases. Genetic markers can predict or quantify the risk or the severity of diseases in populations or individuals. Classical examples include the increased risk of ankylosing spondylitis in carriers of the HLA-B27 allele (Thomas and Brown, 2010), and the association between the 'shared epitope' and RA (de Vries et al., 2005). An increasing number of genetic polymorphisms have been identified as risk factors for autoimmune diseases in general (Gregersen and Olsson, 2009; Mackay, 2009) as well as for specific diseases (Scofield, 2009). Autoantibodies are frequently used to establish or confirm a diagnosis. Some, such as anti-cyclic citrullinated peptide (CCP) antibodies in RA, are fairly specific for a particular disease, whereas others, such as antinuclear antibodies and anti-Ro (SS-A) antibody are present, albeit at different frequencies and levels, in a number of conditions (Schulte-Pelkum et al., 2009).

Once a diagnosis is established, some biomarkers provide prognostic information regarding disease progression and severity. For example, the combination of anti-CCP antibody positivity and the presence of the shared epitope defines a subset of patients with a severe form of RA (Kaltenhauser et al., 2007; Sanmarti et al., 2007), whereas the presence of specific autoantibodies define distinct subsets of inflammatory myopathies (Gunawardena et al.,

2009). Other biomarkers are used to monitor the degree of immunologic activity or inflammation. Measures of levels of complement activation and of anti-double stranded DNA autoantibodies are commonly used to monitor disease activity in lupus nephritis, and nonspecific markers of inflammation, such as the erythrocyte sedimentation rate or CRP levels, are measured in many diseases. Some of the biggest challenges, especially in the late stages of most chronic rheumatic diseases, include distinguishing between ongoing inflammation and irreversible organ damage, and assessing the impact of comorbidities or the adverse effects of treatments. Probably most needed are biomarkers that predict response to a particular therapy. Such markers could be used to optimize the risk to benefit ratio of a treatment in individual patients. If a strong correlation between a biomarker and a change in clinical activity can be established, a biomarker could act as a surrogate marker of a clinically important end point. Monitoring that surrogate end point could permit the use of targeted preemptive therapy if the measurement predicts relapse, or could be used as a guide to discontinue therapy if it denotes remission.

3.1 Detection of miRNAs in body fluids

Since 2008, several studies have evidenced the possibility of detecting miRNAs in body fluids including serum, plasma, urine, saliva, tears, amniotic and placental fluids, thus opening up major opportunities for a novel type of diagnostic molecules (Chen et al., 2008; Gilad et al., 2008; Mitchell et al., 2008). Since RA is a systemic chronic inflammatory disorder for which peripheral blood gene expression signature has been reported and molecular biomarkers are of great interest, identification of miRNA-based signatures is indeed a major issue. Most of the studies supporting the clinical utility of miRNAs as biomarkers in body fluids or diseased tissues have been conducted in cancer. High concentrations of cell-free miRNAs originating from the primary tumour have been found in the plasma of cancer patients, and several lines of evidence indicate that circulating miRNAs represent a promising source of cancer biomarkers (White et al., 2010). Indeed, correlations between miRNA expression levels and the development of malignancies, disease severity and aggressiveness, metastatic potential, therapeutic response and survival are reported in various cancer types. Interestingly, tumour-associated miRNomes appear highly tissue-specific.

The detection of miRNAs in serum was quite unexpected as RNA molecules are unstable in the circulation. Studies (Chen et al., 2008; Mitchell et al., 2008; Mraz et al., 2009) showed that miRNAs exhibit high stability in the serum and plasma as they circulate within membrane vesicles such as exosomes or microparticles which protect them from endogenous RNase activity (Hunter et al., 2008). These microvesicles are resistant to drastic conditions and express tissue-specific markers. Although it is easily accessible and of great interest for new biomarker discovery, very few studies report the optimisation of extraction and detection of miRNAs in plasma or serum (Gilad et al., 2008; Mitchell et al., 2008). Several technical challenges in miRNA extraction, detection and quantification in serum or plasma are still underinvestigated. Moreover, all the miRNAs detected in total blood samples are not found in serum or plasma, and/or the low concentration of most of the miRNAs in serum or plasma precludes their detection, thus limiting the panel of miRNAs for solid profiling. Indeed, it is currently estimated that 20 miRNAs are needed for solid definition of biomarker signatures. For all these reasons, and mainly technical reasons, whole blood profiling is to be definitively the main focus in future studies on biomarker discovery, as opposed to plasma- or serum-based signatures. Although it seems to be very close, many more studies are needed before the use of miRNAs can fulfil criteria for their use as reliable tools in diagnostic and prognostic settings.

3.2 miRNAs as biomarkers for RA management

Although the potential value of miRNAs as molecular biomarkers for diagnosis, prognosis, and prediction of therapeutic response is widely documented in cancer, it is still largely unexplored in RA. The identification of abnormal miRNA expression in the circulation or inflamed joints of RA patients is still in its beginning. Until now there has been only one publication in which the concentrations of 5 miRNAs in RA patients' body fluids were measured, bringing the first proof for the use of miRNA biomarker potential in RA (Murata et al., 2010). In the report, synovial fluid miRNAs were present and as stable as plasma miRNAs for storage at -20°C and freeze-thawing from -20°C to 4°C. In RA and OA, synovial fluid concentrations of miR-16, miR-132, miR-146a, and miR-223 were significantly lower than their plasma concentrations, and there were no correlation between plasma and synovial fluid miRNAs. Interestingly, synovial tissues, fibroblast-like synoviocytes, and mononuclear cells secreted miRNAs in distinct patterns. The expression patterns of miRNAs in synovial fluid of OA were similar to miRNAs produced by synovial tissues. Plasma miR-132 of healthy controls (HC) was significantly higher than that of RA or OA. Synovial fluid concentrations of miR-16, miR-146a miR-155 and miR-223 of RA were significantly higher than those of OA. Plasma miRNAs or ratio of synovial fluid miRNAs to plasma miRNAs, including miR-16 and miR-146a, significantly correlated with tender joint counts and DAS-28. Therefore, plasma miRNAs had distinct patterns from synovial fluid miRNAs, which appeared to originate from synovial tissue. Plasma miR-132 well differentiated HC from patients with RA or OA, while synovial fluid miRNAs differentiated RA and OA. Furthermore, plasma miRNAs correlated with the disease activities of RA. Thus, synovial fluid and plasma miRNAs have potential as diagnostic biomarkers for RA and OA and as a tool for the analysis of their pathogenesis. However, this study shows that only miR-132 plasma concentrations were significantly lower in RA than in HC, but certainly not useful as diagnostic biomarkers since miR-132 plasma concentrations were not correlated with DAS28 and not disease-specific, since miR-132 plasma concentrations were also significantly lower in OA than in HC. Further investigations are required to find more suitable miRNAs for utilizing as biomarkers for diagnosis, predicting drug efficacy in order to plan optimal management of RA patients.

4. Conclusion

Our understanding of RA pathogenesis has been enriched by recent miRNA studies. We modified the schematic diagram described by *Furer et al* (Furer et al., 2010) to explain the mechanism of miRNA in RASF in Figure 2. It is obvious that miRNAs have important roles in the critical aspects of RA pathogenesis such as joint destruction, inflammation, proliferation of synoviocytes, and chemotaxis of inflammatory cells. Taking the involvement of miRNAs in leucocyte functions into account, miRNA has become one of necessary tools to address many unanswered questions as well as to envision the whole story of RA pathogenesis. It has been proposed that a gene transfer system which provides a direct delivery of nucleic acid into an affected joint may be useful for RNA therapy (Adriaansen et al., 2006). Therefore, developing a method for direct and selective transfer of specific

miRNA or inhibitor of miRNA into lymphocyte, synovial fibroblast, or DC may be a possible candidate for future treatment of RA rather than a systemic administration of miRNA which may cause off-target or harmful effects to different tissues and cell types.
In the meantime, miR-124a is unique in that it is downregulated in RASF and directly associated with cell-cycle regulation. When you consider the proliferative nature of RASF, miR-124a may have a good candidacy for a novel drug for RA treatment. Therefore, developing a drug delivery system for direct and selective transfer of miR-124a into RASF, such as intra-articular injection, is an attractive idea, since systemic administration of miR-124a may possibly cause 'off-target effects' or harmful side effects on different tissues and cell types. Besides the miRNAs described in this article, it is expected that new biomarkers and therapeutic tools will be developed in the near future based on the research generated from miRNAs.

5. Acknowledgment

This work was supported in part by a Grant-in-aid for Scientific Research (18591109, 23591436) from the Japan Society for the Promotion of Science.

6. References

Agirre, X.; Vilas-Zornoza, A.; Jiménez-Velasco, A.; Martin-Subero, J. I.; Cordeu, L.; Gárate, L.; San José-Eneriz, E.; Abizanda, G.; Rodríguez-Otero, P.; Fortes, P.; Rifón, J.; Bandrés, E.; Calasanz, M.J.; Martín, V.; Heiniger, A.; Torres, A.; Siebert, R.; Román-Gomez, J., & Prósper F. (2009). Epigenetic silencing of the tumor suppressor microRNA Hsa-miR-124a regulates CDK6 expression and confers a poor prognosis in acute lymphoblastic leukemia. *Cancer Res*, Vol. 69, No. 10, (May 2009), pp. 4443-53. ISSN 0008-5472.

Baek, D.; Villén, J.; Shin, C.; Camargo, F.D.; Gygi, S.P., & Bartel, D.P. (2008). The impact of microRNAs on protein output. *Nature,* Vol. 455, Issue 7209, (July 2008): pp. 64–71. ISSN 0028-0836.

Blüml, S. Bonelli, M.; Niederreiter, B.; Puchner, A.; Mayr, G.; Hayer, S.; Koenders, M.I. ; van den Berg, W.B.; Smolen, J., & Redlich K. Essential role of microRNA-155 in the pathogenesis of autoimmune arthritis in mice. (2011). *Arthritis Rheum,* Vol. 63, No. 5, (May 2011), pp. 1281–8. ISSN 0004-3591.

Boldin, M.; Konstantin, P.; Taganov, D.; Rao, D.S.; Yang, L.; Zhao, J.L.; Kalwani, M.; Garcia-Flores, Y.; Luong, M.; Devrekanli, A.; Xu, J.; Sun, G.; Tay, J.; Linsley, P.S., & Baltimore, D. (2011) miR-146a is a significant brake on autoimmunity, myeloproliferation, and cancer in mice. *J Exp Med,* Vol. 208, No. 6, pp. 1189-1201. ISSN 0022-1007.

Brooks, W.H.; Le Dantec, C.; Pers, J.O.; Youinou, P., & Renaudineau, Y. (2010). Epigenetics and autoimmunity. *J Autoimmun,* Vol.34, J207–J219. ISSN 0896-8411.

Chan, E.K.; Satoh, M., & Pauley, K.M. (2009). Contrast in aberrant microRNA expression in systemic lupus erythematosus and rheumatoid arthritis: is microRNA-146 all we need? *Arthritis Rheum,* Vol. 60, No.4, (October 2009), pp. 912–5. ISSN 0004-3591.

Chatzikyriakidou, A.; Voulgari, P.V.; Georgiou, I., & Drosos, A.A. (2010a). A polymorphism in the 3'-UTR of interleukin-1 receptor-associated kinase (IRAK1), a target gene of miR-146a, is associated with rheumatoid arthritis susceptibility. *Joint Bone Spine*, Vol. 77, No.5, (October, 2010), pp. 411-3. ISSN 1297-319X.

Chatzikyriakidou, A.; Voulgari, P.V.; Georgiou, I., & Drosos, A.A. (2010b). The role of microRNA-146a (miR-146a) and its target IL-1R-associated kinase (IRAK1) in psoriatic arthritis susceptibility. *Scand J Immunol*, Vol. 71 No. 5, (May 2010), pp. 382-5. ISSN 0300-9475.

Ma, L.; Cai, X.; Yin, Y.; Wang, K.;Guo, J.; Zhang, Y.; Chen, J.; Guo, X.; Li,Q.; Li, X.; Wang, W.; Zhang,Y.; Wang, J.; Jiang, X.; Xiang, Y.; Xu, C.; Zheng, P.; Zhang, J.; Li, R.; Zhang, H.; Shang, X.; Gong, T.; Ning, G.; Wang, J.; Zen, K., Zhang, J., & Zhang, C.Y. (2008). Characterization of microRNAs in serum: a novel class of biomarkers for diagnosis of cancer and other diseases. *Cell Res*. Vol. 18, No. 10, (October 2008), pp. 997–1006. ISSN:1001-0602.

de Vries, R. R.; Huizinga, T. W., & Toes, R. E. (2005). Redefining the HLA and RA association: to be or not to be anti-CCP positive. *J Autoimmun*, 25 (Suppl.), pp. 21–5. ISSN 0896-8411.

Furer, V.; Greenberg, J.D.; Attur, M.; Abramson, S.B., & Pillinger, M.H. (2010). The role of microRNA in rheumatoid arthritis and other autoimmune diseases. *Clin Immunol*,Vol.36, No.1, (July 2010), pp. 1–15. ISSN 1521-6616.

Fulci, V.; Scappucci, G.; Sebastiani, G.D.; Giannitti, C.; Franceschini, D.; Meloni, F.; Colombo, T.; Citarella, F.; Barnaba, V.; Minisola, G.; Galeazzi, M., & Macino, G. (2010). miR-223 is overexpressed in T-Lymphocytes of patients affected by rheumatoid arthritis. *Hum Immunol*, Vol. 71, No. 2, (Februally 2010), pp. 206–11. ISSN 0198-8859.

Gilad, S.; Meiri, E.; Yogev, Y.; Benjamin, S.; Lebanony, D.; Yerushalmi, N.; Benjamin, H., Kushnir,M.; Cholakh,H.; Melamed,N.; Bentwich, Z.; Hod, M.; Goren,Y., & Chajut,A. (2008). Serum microRNAs are promising novel biomarkers. *PLoS ONE*, Vol. 3, No. 9, (September 2008), e3148. ISSN 1932-6203.

Gregersen, P. K. & Olsson, L. M. (2009). Recent advances in the genetics of autoimmune disease. *Annu Rev Immunol*, Vol. 27, pp. 363–391. ISSN 0732-0582.

Gunawardena, H.; Betteridge, Z. E., & McHugh, N. J. (2009). Myositis-specific autoantibodies: their clinical and pathogenic significance in disease expression. *Rheumatology (Oxford)*, Vol. 48, No. 6, (June 2009), pp. 607-12. ISSN 1462-0324.

Horiuchi, M.; Morinobu, A.; Chin, T.; Sakai, Y.; Kurosaka, M., & Kumagai, S (2009) Expression and function of histone deacetylases in rheumatoid arthritis synovial fibroblasts. *J Rheumatol*, Vol. 36, pp. 1580–89. ISSN 0315-162X.

Huber, L.C.; Brock, M.; Hemmatazad, H.; Giger, O.T.; Moritz, F.; Trenkmann, M.; Distler, J.H.; Gay, R.E.; Kolling, C.; Moch, H.; Michel, B.A.; Gay, S.; Distler, O., & Jüngel, A. (2007). Histone deacetylase/acetylase activity in total synovial tissue derived from rheumatoid arthritis and osteoarthritis patients. *Arthritis Rheum*, Vol. 56, No. 4, (April 2007), pp. 1087–93. ISSN 0004-3591.

Hunter, M.P.; Ismail, N.; Zhang, X.; Aguda, B.D.; Lee, E.J.; Yu, L.; Xiao, T.; Schafer, J.; Lee, M.L.; Schmittgen, T.D.; Nana-Sinkam, S.P.; Jarjoura, D., & Marsh, C.B. (2008). Detection of microRNA expression in human peripheral blood microvesicles. *PLoS ONE*, Vol. 3, No. 11, (November 2008), e3694. ISSN 1932-6203.

Illei, G. G.; Tackey, E.; Lapteva, L., & Lipsky, P. E. (2004). Biomarkers in systemic lupus erythematosus. I. General overview of biomarkers and their applicability. *Arthritis Rheum*, Vol. 50, No. 6, (June 2004), pp. 1709–20. ISSN 0004-3591.

Jacobsen, A.; Wen, J.; Marks, D., & Krogh, A. (2010). Signatures of RNA binding proteins globally coupled to effective microRNA target sites. *Genome Res,* Vol. 21, No. 7, (July2010), pp. 1010-19. ISSN 1088-9051.

Kaltenhauser, S.; Pierer, M.; Arnold, S.; Kamprad, M.; Baerwald, C.; Häntzschel, H., & Wagner, U. (2007). Antibodies against cyclic citrullinated peptide are associated with the DRB1 shared epitope and predict joint erosion in rheumatoid arthritis. *Rheumatology (Oxford),* Vol. 46, No. 1, (January 2007), pp 100–4. ISSN 1462-0324.

Karouzakis, E.; Gay, R.E.; Gay, S., & Neidhart, M. (2009a). Epigenetic control in rheumatoid arthritis synovial fibroblasts. *Nat Rev Rheumatol,* Vol. 5, pp. 266–72. ISSN 1759-4790.

Karouzakis, E.; Gay R.E.; Michel, B.A.; Gay, S., & Neidhart, M. (2009b). DNA hypomethylation in rheumatoid arthritis synovial fibroblasts. *Arthritis Rheum,* 2009, Vol. 60, No. 12, (December 2009), pp. 3613– 22. ISSN 0004-3591.

Klareskog, L.; Catrina, A.I., & Paget, S. Rheumatoid arthritis. *Lancet,* Vol. 373, No.9664, (February 2009), pp. 659–72. ISSN 0099-5355.

Kloosterman, W.P., & Plasterk, R.H. (2006). The diverse functions of microRNAs in animal development and disease. *Dev Cell,* Vol. 11, No. 4, (October 2006), pp. 441–50. ISSN 1534-5807.

Li, J.; Wan, Y.; Guo, Q.; Zou, L.; Zhang, J.; Fang, Y.; Zhang, J.; Zhang, J.; Fu, X.; Liu, H.; Lu, L., & Wu, Y. *(2010).* Altered microRNA expression profile with miR-146a upregulation in CD4+ T cells from patients with rheumatoid arthritis. *Arthritis Res Ther,* Vol.12, No.3, (May 2010), R81. ISSN 1478-6354.

Lujambio, A., & Esteller, M. (2007). CpG island hypermethylation of tumor suppressor microRNAs in human cancer. *Cell Cycle,* Vol. 6, No. 12, (June 2007), pp. 1455–9. ISSN 1538-4101.

Mackay, I. R. Clustering and commonalities among autoimmune diseases. (2009). *J Autoimmun,* Vol. 33, No. 3-4, (November-December 2009), pp. 170–7. ISSN 0896-8411.

Martin, M.M.; Buckenberger, J.A.; Jiang, J.; Malana, G.E.; Nuovo, G.J.; Chotani, M.; Feldman, D.S.; Schmittgen, T.D., & Elton, T.S. (2007). The human angiotensin II type 1 receptor +1166 A/C polymorphism attenuates microRNA-155 binding. *J Biol Chem,* Vol. 282, No. 33, (August 2007), pp. 24262–9. ISSN 1067-8816.

Mencía, A.; Modamio-Høybjør, S.; Redshaw, N.; Morín, M.; Mayo-Merino, F.; Olavarrieta, L.; Aguirre, L.A.; del Castillo, I.; Steel, K.P.; Dalmay, T.; Moreno, F., & Moreno-Pelayo, M.A. (2009). Mutations in the seed region of human miR-96 are responsible for nonsyndromic progressive hearing loss. *Nat Genet,* Vol. 41, No. 5, (April 2009), pp. 609–13. ISSN 1061-4036.

Mitchell, P.S.; Parkin, R.K.; Kroh, E.M.; Fritz, B.R.; Wyman, S.K.; Pogosova-Agadjanyan, E.L.; Peterson, A.; Noteboom, J.; O'Briant, K.C.; Allen, A.; Lin, D.W.; Urban, N; Drescher, C.W.; Knudsen, B.S.; Stirewalt, D.L.; Gentleman, R,; Vessella, R.L.; Nelson, P.S.; Martin, D.B., & Tewari, M. (2008). Circulating microRNAs as stable blood-based markers for cancer detection. *Proc Natl Acad Sci. U S A,* Vol. 105, No. 30, (July 2008), pp. 10513–8. ISSN 0027-8424.

Mraz, M.; Malinova, K.; Mayer, J., & Pospisilova, S. (2009). MicroRNA isolation and stability in stored RNA samples. *Biochem Biophys Res Commun,* Vol. 390, No.1, (December 2009), pp. 1–4. ISSN 0006-291X.

Murata, K.; Yoshitomi, H.; Tanida, S.; Ishikawa, M.; Nishitani, K.; Ito, H., & Nakamura, T. *(2010)*. Plasma and synovial fluid microRNAs as potential biomarkers of rheumatoid arthritis and osteoarthritis. *Arthritis Res Ther,* Vol. 12, No. 3, (May 2010), R86. ISSN 1478-6354.

Nakamachi, Y.; Kawano, S.; Takenokuchi, M.; Nishimura, K.; Sakai, Y.; Chin, T.; Saura, R.; Kurosaka, M., & Kumagai, S. (2009). MicroRNA-124a is a key regulator of proliferation and monocyte chemoattractant protein 1 secretion in fibroblast-like synoviocytes from patients with rheumatoid arthritis. *Arthritis Rheum,* Vol. 60, No. 5, (May 2009), pp. 1294–304, ISSN 0004-3591.

Nakasa, T.; Miyaki, S.; Okubo, A.; Hashimoto, M.; Nishida, K.; Ochi, M., & Asahara, H. Expression of microRNA-146 in rheumatoid arthritis synovial tissue. *Arthritis Rheum,* Vol. 58, No. 5, (May 2008), pp. 1284–92. ISSN 0004-3591

Nakasa, T.; Shibuya, H.; Nagata, Y.; Niimoto, T., & Ochi, M. The inhibitory effect of microRNA-146a expre ssion on bone destruction in collagen-induced arthritis. (2011). *Arthritis Rheum,* Vol. 63, No. 6, (Jun 2011), pp. 1582-90. ISSN 0004-3591.

Niimoto, T.; Nakasa, T.; Ishikawa, M.; Okuhara, A.; Izumi, B.; Deie, M.; Suzuki, O.; Adachi, N., & Ochi, M. MicroRNA-146a expresses in interleukin-17 producing T cells in rheumatoid arthritis patients. *BMC Musculoskelet Disord,* Vol. 11, (September 2010), 209.

Nishimura, K.; Sugiyama, D.; Kogata, Y.; Tsuji, G.; Nakazawa, T.; Kawano, S.; Saigo, K.; Morinobu, A.; Koshiba, M.; Kuntz, K.M.; Kamae, I., & Kumagai, S. (2007). Meta-analysis: diagnostic accuracy of anti-cyclic citrullinated peptide antibody and rheumatoid factor for rheumatoid arthritis. *Ann Intern Med,* Vol. 146, No. 11, (June 2007), pp. 797–808. ISSN 0003-4819.

O'Connell R.M.; Rao, D.S.; Chaudhuri A.A., & Baltimore, D. (2010).Physiological and pathological roles for microRNAs in the immune system. *Nat Rev Immunol,* Vol. 10, No. 2, (February 2010), pp. 111–22. ISSN 1474-1733.

Pauley, K.M.; Satoh, M.; Chan, A.L.; Bubb, M.R.; Reeves, W.H., & Chan, E.K. (2008), Upregulated miR-146a expression in peripheral blood mononuclear cells from rheumatoid arthritis patients. *Arthritis Res Ther,* Vol. 10, No. 4, (August 2008), R101. ISSN 1478-6354.

Sanmarti, R.; Gómez-Centeno, A.; Ercilla, G.; Larrosa, M.; Viñas, O.; Vazquez, I.; Gómez-Puerta, J.A.; Gratacós, J.; Salvador, G., & Cañete, J.D. (2007). Prognostic factors of radiographic progression in early rheumatoid arthritis: a two year prospective study after a structured therapeutic strategy using DMARDs and very low doses of glucocorticoids. *Clin Rheumatol,* Vol. 26, No. 7, (July 2007), pp. 1111–8. ISSN 0770-3198.

Schulte-Pelkum, J.; Fritzler, M., & Mahler, M. (2009). Latest update on the Ro/SS-A autoantibodysystem. *Autoimmun Rev,* Vol. 8, pp. 632–637. ISSN 1568-9972.

Scofield, R. H. (2009). Genetics of systemic lupus erythematosus and Sjogren's syndrome. *Curr Opin Rheumatol,* Vol. 21, pp. 448-53. ISSN 1040-8711.

Selbach, M.; Schwanhäusser, B.; Thierfelder, N. Fang, Z.; Khanin, R., & Rajewsky N. (2008).Widespread changes in protein synthesis induced by microRNAs. *Nature,* Vol. 455, Issue 7209, (September 2008), pp. 58–63, ISSN 0028-0836.

Stahl, E.A.; Raychaudhuri, S.; Remmers, E.F.; Xie, G.; Eyre, S.; Thomson, B.P.; Li Y.; Kurreeman, F.A.; Zhernakova, A.; Hinks, A.; Guiducci, C.; Chen, R.; Alfredsson, L.;

Amos, C.I.; Ardlie, K.G.; BIRAC Consortium; Barton, A.; Bowes, J.; Brouwer, E.; Burtt, N.P.; Catanese, J.J.; Coblyn, J.; Coenen, M.J.; Costenbader, K.H.; Criswell, L.A.; Crusius, J.B.; Cui, J.; de Bakker, P.I.; De Jager, P.L.; Ding, B.; Emery, P.; Flynn, E.; Harrison, P.; Hocking, L.J.; Huizinga, T.W.; Kastner, D.L.; Ke, X.; Lee, A.T.; Liu, X.; Martin, P.; Morgan, A.W.; Padyukov, L.; Posthumus, M.D.; Radstake, T.R.; Reid, D.M.; Seielstad, M.; Seldin, F.; Shadick, N.A.; Steer, S.; Tak, P.P.; Thomson, W.; van der Helm-van Mil, A.H.; van der Horst-Bruinsma, I.E.; van der Schoot, C.E.; van Riel, P.L.; Weinblatt, M.E.; Wilson, A.G.; Wolbink, G.J.; Wordsworth, B.P.; YEAR Consortium; Wijmenga, C.; Karlson, E.W.; Toes, R.E.; de Vries, N.; Begovich, A.B.; Worthington, J.; Siminovitch, K.A.; Gregersen, P.K.; Klareskog, L., & Plenge, R.M. (2010). Genome-wide association study meta-analysis identifies seven new rheumatoid arthritis risk loci. *Nat Genet*, Vol. 42, pp. 508–14. ISSN 1061-4036.

Stanczyk, J.; Pedrioli, D.M.; Brentano, F.; Sanchez-Pernaute, O.; Kolling, C.; Gay, R.E.; Detmar, M.; Gay, S., & Kyburz, D. (2008). Altered expression of MicroRNA in synovial fibroblasts and synovial tissue in rheumatoid arthritis. *Arthritis Rheum,* Vol. 58, No. 4, (April 2008), pp. 1001–9. ISSN 0004-3591.

Stanczyk, J.; Ospelt, C.; Karouzakis, E.; Filer, A.; Raza, K.; Kolling, C.; Gay, R.; Buckley, C.D.; Tak, P.P.; Gay, S., & Kyburz D. (2011). Altered Expression of microRNA-203 in Rheumatoid Arthritis Synovial Fibroblasts and Its Role in Fibroblast Activation. *Arthritis Rheum,* Vol. 63, No. 2, (February 2011), pp. 373–81. ISSN 0004-3591.

Tang, Y.; Luo, X.; Cui, H.; Ni, X.; Yuan, M.; Guo, Y.; Huang, X.; Zhou, H.; de Vries, N.; Tak, PP.; Chen, S., & Shen, N. (2009). MicroRNA-146a contributes to abnormal activation of the type I interferon pathway in human lupus by targeting the key signaling proteins. *Arthritis Rheum,* Vol. 60, No. 4 (April 2009), pp. 1065–75. ISSN 0004-3591.

Thomas, G. P. & Brown, M. A. (2010). Genetics and genomics of ankylosing spondylitis. *Immunol Rev,* Vol. 233, No. 1, (January 2010), pp. 162–180. ISSN 0105-2896.

Tsang, J.; Zhu, J., & van Oudenaarden, A. (2007) MicroRNA-mediated feedback and feedforward loops are recurrent network motifs in mammals. *Mol Cell,* Vol. 26, No. 5, (Jun 2008), pp. 753–67. ISSN 1097-2765.

van Rooij, E. & Olson, E.N. (2007). MicroRNAs: powerful new regulators of heart disease and provocative therapeutic targets. *J Clin Invest,* Vol. 117, Issue 9, (September 2007), pp.2369–76., ISSN 0021-9738.

White, M.A.; Fatoohi, E.; Metias, M.; Jung, K.; Stephan, C., & Yousef G.M. (2011). Metastamirs: a stepping stone towards improved cancer management. *Nature Reviews Clinical Oncology,* Vol. 8, No. 2, (February 2011), pp. 75-84. ISSN 1759-4774.

Yamada, Y.; Metoki, N.; Yoshida, H.; Satoh, K.; Kato, K.; Hibino, T.; Yokoi, K.; Watanabe, S.; Ichihara, S.; Aoyagi, Y.; Yasunaga, A.; Park, H.; Tanaka, M., & Nozawa, Y. (2008). Genetic factors for ischemic and hemorrhagic stroke in Japanese individuals. *Stroke,* Vol. 39, No. 8 (August 2008), pp. 2211–8. ISSN 0039-2499

Part 2

Consequences and Co-Morbidities

11

Rheumatoid Arthritis: A Historical and Biopsychosocial Perspective

Yulia Zyrianova
University College Dublin
Ireland

1. Introduction

Rheumatoid arthritis (RA) is a relatively common, disabling, autoimmune disease that is characterized by progressive joint disorder, significant pain and functional disability. Its prevalence is estimated at 0.5 - 1.0 percent of adults worldwide (Kvein, 2004), and the disease continues to cause significant morbidity and premature mortality.

Symmetric highly inflammatory polyarthritis of peripheral joints is the hallmark of the disease. The condition is also systemic in that it often affects many extra-articular tissues throughout the body, including skin, blood vessels, heart, lungs, and muscles. The gradual involvement of multiple joints into pathophysiological process eventually results in articular destruction, ensuing instability, deformity and collateral pain. As the pathology progresses, chronic pain and functional disability dominates one's life and lessens everyday enjoyment and comforts.

Physical in nature, the disease also exacts an emotional toll that often leads to unfortunate psychiatric sequelae. It is not at all surprising that in addition to joint deformity, disability, dolour, and excess mortality, on average one in five patients with rheumatoid arthritis will experience depression.

Many new insights into epidemiology, pathogenesis, outcomes measurement, and pharmacologic treatment of rheumatoid arthritis have occurred in recent years. Applications of historical analyses to the development of a cogent etiologic theory of rheumatoid arthritis have been limited to date (Entezami et al, 2011). In this chapter, the author presents the major points of evidence and conclusions that have been drawn from historical, clinical and research material in the study of rheumatic diseases.

2. Historical conceptualisation

2.1 Nosology in evolution

Although the appearance of rheumatoid arthritis was noted in radiological examination of skeletal remains of Tennessee Indians from as early as 4500 BC, we do not find documented evidence until much later. It is said that realisation of how "taxing" arthritis can be, made Roman Emperor Diocletian free his citizens with the disorder from paying taxes. The term *'rheumatism'* dates back to 1630, and is derived from the Greek *'rheumatos'* that means 'flowing'. It signified an evil humour or mucus that was thought to flow from the brain to the joints, causing inflammation, pain and deformities. Short (Short, 1974) traced the first adequate description of what was probably rheumatoid arthritis to Thomas Sydenham (1624-1689) and emphasised that medical literature before Sydenham's time may have confused gout and other forms of polyarthritis as manifestations of the same disease.

Analysis of the hands in the Flemish paintings and works attributed to Peter Paul Rubens seems to show hand lesions resembling those of rheumatoid arthritis. To illustrate this, on the reproduction here, swelling of three metacarpophalangeal joints are clearly visible on the right hand of Erasmus of Rotterdam painted by the Flemish Quinten Metsys in 1529, (FIG.1). Disiderius Erasmus (1467-1536), the Dutch renaissance scholar is often quoted for his famous aphorism "prevention is better than cure" and is recognised as the Prince of Humanists for his progressive writings of the time. This painting is testimony to the high cultural climate of the time, and evidence of the links between two great humanist thinkers, Erasmus of Rotterdam and Sir Thomas More, both of whom contributed to the publication of Utopia.

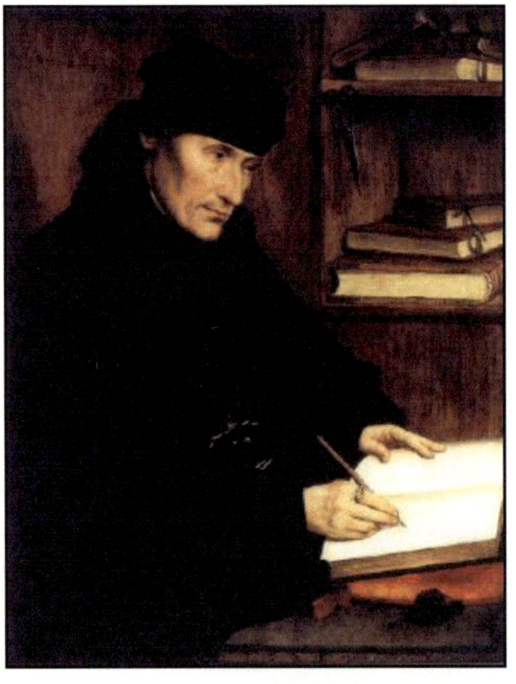

Fig. 1. **Quinten Metsys, Portrait of Erasmus of Rotterdam, 1517.** *Oil on panel, 59 x 46.5 cm.* Reproduced with permission from National Gallery of Antique Art, Rome.

While none of the deformities or swellings is indisputable examples of rheumatoid arthritis, they do at least suggest that the painters must have been confronted with rheumatoid-like lesions in their models. It is established that Rubens was well qualified to accurately depict arthritic deformities, as he had a personal familiarity with arthritis. Although history is uncertain as to who suffered from the disease, Rubens or his long-term co-author, it is easy to imagine artists' working surroundings at the time: ancient damp art studios, oils, powders and drying canvases everywhere - a portrayal of an "ideal" environment for triggering a rheumatic flare-up and causing inflammation.

These observations suggest that rheumatoid arthritis is not a modern disease and was present several centuries before its description as a separate entity by Augustine-Jacob Landré Beauvais' in 1800 (Dequeker J. 1977; Appelboom T. et al, 1981; Dequeker J, Rico H. 1992). A generation later, in 1859, Sir Alfred Garrod, a physician from Ipswich who later was appointed Professor of Materia Medica and Therapeutics and of Medicine, coined the name 'rheumatoid arthritis'. In his renowned treatise with illustrations (Garrod, 1859), he considered the main differential diagnosis, including rheumatic gout of Fuller, chronic rheumatism of Heberden, scorbutic rheumatism and rheumalgia, and rejected them all in favour of 'rheumatoid arthritis' the name he chose for the disease. He divided it into two types: generalised and localised and identified three forms: acute, chronic and irregular. The name has remained ever since.

2.2 Diagnostically diverse group of disorders

Rheumatoid arthritis belongs to a diverse group of musculoskeletal disorders ("arthritis"): there are more than 200 types of these diseases that also encompass osteoarthritis, Still's disease, ankylosing spondylitis, and Reiter's syndrome. Some sources also name Felty's syndrome and Sjogren's syndrome as related disorders (Wilson et al, 1991). Some of these are very serious diseases that can be difficult to diagnose and treat. For instance, hemochromatosis (build up of iron in the body) was misdiagnosed as rheumatoid arthritis in the past (Espinosa-Morales et al, 1998).

Skeletal evidence of primary ankle (kaki) **osteoarthritis** has been discovered in dinosaurs! In 1715 William Musgrave published the second edition of his most important medical work '*De arthritide symptomatica*' which concerned arthritis and its effects (Cameron, 2004). A common feature in all osteoarthritis is a loss of cartilage in association with bone features such as osteophytes and subchondral bone sclerosis. Large epidemiologic studies of osteoarthritis performed over a period of 30 years (Peyron, 1986) have confirmed that osteoarthritis is a ubiquitous condition, that it is linked to age, that it is more frequent and more widespread in women older than 45 years of age, and that the mechanical overuse of the joints is probably instrumental in the occurrence and the location of certain cases of osteoarthritis. Epidemiologic evidence points to the existence of an entity of "generalised osteoarthritis" composed of three or more locations with involvement of the interphalangeals. Heredity, in cases associated with distal interphalangeal osteoarthritis, and inflammation, in cases with proximal interphalangeal osteoarthritis, are the factors found to be most closely correlated to generalised osteoarthritis. Surveys of several series of osteoarthritis of the hip have pointed to the existence of several clinicoradiologic subsets that could have different clinical correlates and various pathophysiological mechanisms. Interestingly, according to a Boston University study (Hunter *et al*, 2004), ever since their invention five thousand years ago, chopsticks have been a source of osteoarthritis. This epidemiologic study investigated the relationship of chopsticks use to hand arthropathy. The results suggest that chopsticks use is associated with an increased prevalence of osteoarthritis in the interphalangeal joint of the thumb, and in the second and third interphalangeal and metacarpophalangeal joints.

In 1897 Sir George Frederick Still published a paper entitled 'On a form of chronic joint disease in children', that was the subject of his MD thesis, where he described several types of juvenile rheumatoid arthritis (FIG.2) and introduced an previously unrecognizable disease, known, as it is today, as **Still's disease** or systemic-onset juvenile rheumatoid

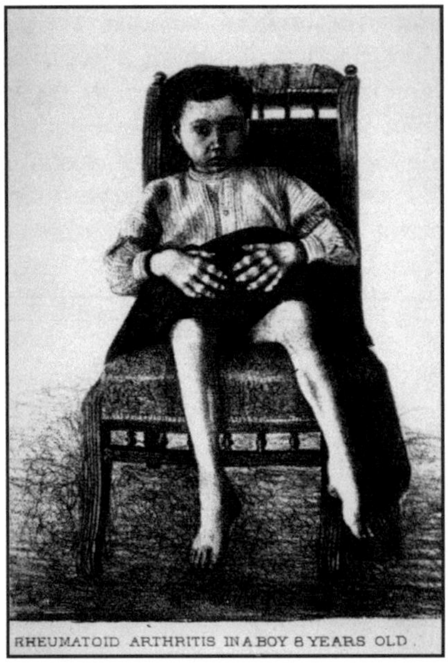

Fig. 2. Rheumatoid arthritis in an 8 yr old boy. From a slide collection of images from Still's *'On a form of chronic joint disease in children'* reproduced with permission from Professor Patricia Woo.

arthritis. He defined the condition as a 'chronic progressive enlargement of joints, associated with general enlargement of glands and enlargement of spleen' with the onset 'almost always before the second dentition' (Still, 1897). Still concluded that this condition differed from rheumatoid arthritis in adults in the enlargement of glands and spleen and in the absence of bony change.

Since then adult onset Still's disease (AOSD) has been described as an acute febrile illness in young adults. It usually affects multiple organs, but is a diagnosis of exclusion. The aetiology of AOSD is unknown; however, a number of infectious triggers have been suggested, including viruses and bacterial pathogens including Mycoplasma pneumoniae. Clinical features include a high fever, arthralgia and arthritis, phayngitis, typical rash (evanescent salmon-coloured, macular or maculopapular eruption), lymphadenopathy, and serositis. Chronic arthritis and constitutional symptoms are common. The triad of fever, rash, and arthralgia are often absent during the first month of the illness. A quotidian (daily, spiking) or "double-quotidian" fever curve is a hallmark of the disease. The usual joints affected are wrists, knees, and ankles in descending order. Several diagnostic criteria sets for AOSD have been proposed. Two of these sets of criteria are shown in the TABLE 1.1. 1987 and 1992 Criteria for the Classification of Adult Onset of Still's Disease.

It is interesting that a recent case series identified patients with **ankylosing spondylitis** who also meet the criteria of adult onset Still's disease (Akkoc et al, 2008). The ankylosing spondylitis existed since ancient times, as verified by the skeletal remains of a 5000-year-old Egyptian mummy with evidence of 'bamboo spine' (Calin, 1985). It is a chronic, painful, degenerative, inflammatory arthritis primarily affecting the spine and sacroiliac joints; the ossification of joints and entheses primarily of the axial skeleton are known as 'bamboo spine'. It was recognised as distinct from arthritis by Galen as early as the second century

Diagnostic Criteria I	Diagnostic Criteria II
Requires ALL of the following: • Fever > 39 degrees • Arthralgia or arthritis • Rheumatoid factor < 1:80 • ANA < 1:100 **In addition to ANY TWO of the following:** • WBC count > 15,000 • Stills rash • Pleuritis or Pericarditis • Hepatomegaly, Splenomegaly, or Lymphadenopathy	**Presence of 5 or more criteria**, of which at least 2 are Major - yields 96% sensitivity; 92% specificity **Major Criteria** • Fever > 39 degrees > 1 week • Arthralgia/arthritis > 2 weeks • Typical rash • WBC > 10 K with 80% PMN's **Minor Criteria** • Sore throat • Lymphadenopathy • Increased LFT's • RF and ANA negative
According to: Cush JJ, Medsger TA, Jr, Christy WC, et al. Adult-onset Still's disease: Clinical course and outcome. Arthritis Rheum 30:186, 1987.	According to: Yamaguchi M, Ohta A, Tsunematsu T, et al. Preliminary criteria for classification of adult Still's disease. J Rheumatol 19:424, 1992.

Table 1.1 Diagnostic Criteria

(Dieppe, 1988), and the anatomist and surgeon Realdo Colombo characterised the condition in 1559 (Benoist, 1995). However, it was not until 1892, when Russian neurologist Vladimir Michailovich Bekhterev published a series of papers, that the syndrome was fully described (Bechterev, 1892). Later, Adolf Strümpel of Germany (1897) and Pierre Marie of France (1898) also gave adequate descriptions which permitted an accurate diagnosis of ankylosing spondylitis prior to severe spinal deformity. For this reason, ankylosing spondylitis is also known as Bekhterev's Disease or Marie-Strümpel Disease. Bekhterev advocated physiotherapy and the benefits of hypnosis for the patients with rheumatic spondylitis, the latter treatment method he studied under the direction of Professor Jean-Martin Charcot in Salpetriere (Kannabikh, 1925).

Reiter's syndrome was named after Hans Reiter (Reiter, 1916), who reported a case of a soldier with the triad of urethritis, arthritis and conjunctivitis, following an episode of bloody diarrhea. However, the history of this constellation of signs actually predates his description. Urethritis, arthritis and conjunctivitis have subsequently remained as the essential components of this syndrome, but some feel that the eye involvement is so often minimal or insignificant that it need not necessarily be present to make the diagnosis (Gaston & Lillicrap, 2003). Although Reiter's syndrome and psoriatic arthritis are ordinarily two rather discrete entities, there is a significant zone of diagnostic overlap in patients with cutaneous lesions. Both diseases may coexist in the same patient, or Reiter's syndrome seemingly may evolve into psoriatic arthritis. Reiter's syndrome in recent medical literature is simply referred to as reactive arthritis which may or may not be accompanied by extraintestinal manifestations. Salmonella has been the most frequently studied bacteria associated with reactive arthritis. Overall, studies have found rates of Salmonella-associated reactive arthritis to vary between 6 and 30% (Hill Gaston, & Lillicrap, 2003). The term Reiter's syndrome has fallen into disfavour, owning to its author's reputation as a high-ranking Nazi official who was responsible for medical experiments in concentration camps (Panush, et al., 2003; Petersel & Sigal, 2005).

Felty's syndrome is an uncommon extra-articular manifestation of rheumatoid arthritis. First described in 1924, Felty syndrome is a potentially serious condition that is associated with seropositive rheumatoid arthritis. Felty syndrome is characterized by the triad of rheumatoid arthritis, splenomegaly, and granulocytopenia. Although many patients are asymptomatic, some develop serious and life-threatening infections secondary to granulocytopenia. It is more prevalent among women around 60 with a long history of severe articular disease, positive rheumatoid factor, and who carry the HLA-DR4 allele (Ghavami *et al*, 2005).

In 1933, Swedish physician Henrik Sjögren observed a large number of his female patients were experiencing dry eyes and mouths along with their arthritis symptoms. The condition became known as **Sjögren's syndrome**. Primary Sjögren's syndrome is defined when only the ocular (ketratoconjunctivities sicca) and oral (xerostomia) components are present, while the secondary form refers to the association with a connective tissue disorder, especially rheumatoid arthritis, or other illness such as AIDS, hepatitis C infection, or biliary cirrhosis. In recent years, Sjögren's syndrome has also been reported to be associated with chronic graft-versus-host disease after allogeneic bone marrow transplantation. Sjögren's syndrome is a common, but often overlooked disorder. Patients with severe disease run a forty-times risk of developing lymphoma usually of the B cell type (Parke and Buchanan, 1998).

2.2.1 Formation of rheumatology as a speciality

The important work of the time by Boyle, Richardson and Doll on 'The Scientific Method' (Boyle, 1954; Doll, 1954) illustrate the beginning of a change in the practice of physical medicine in UK. The evolution of rheumatology as a subspecialty of General Medicine in England since the 1960s was happening alongside the progressive developments in clinical science, and in academic provision across the country. This initiative aimed at separating the often overlapping and competing communities of physical medicine, rehabilitation, rheumatology and internal medicine.

TJ (Lord) Horder, a distinguished London physician and (Sir) Stanley Davidson, who served as a member of the Empire Rheumatism Council re-branded clinical rheumatology on a scientific basis alongside the evolving research disciplines in pathology and clinical pharmacology. The Empire Rheumatism Council, later known as the Arthritis and Rheumatism Council, also changed its emphasis from welfare to the promotion of scientific research and medical education, while developing charities focused on the welfare of patients with rheumatic disorders instead.

The link with General Medicine, the dissolution of the link with Physical Medicine and Rehabilitation, the growth of clinical science and the increasing sophistication of therapeutics have all influenced the change in paradigm. For example, it was not until 1953 that 'Rheumatoid Arthritis' was in the title of any article in UK and not until 1958 did a systemic rheumatic disease feature at all. As regards therapeutics, salicylates, corticosteroids and the early NSAIDs featured intermittently in clinical reports. Clinical trials were rare in the 1950s, but large clinical series were commonly reported, such as 1723 cases of meniscectomy (Wynn et al, 1958).

2.3 Aetiological debate

Despite the notable advances in knowledge regarding progression of rheumatoid arthritis, its cause remains elusive. In fact, there probably is not an exact cause for it. Researchers now are debating whether rheumatoid arthritis is one disease or several different diseases with common features. It appears to be a multi-factorial disease in which there are important genetic and environmental influences. There are no reports of clustering in space or time that would support an infectious cause. Jobanputra (Jobanputra et al, 1995) studied and suspected such infectious agents, as mycobacteria, Epstein-Barr virus and parvovirus as causal agents, but without any conclusive or convincing evidence. Sex hormones are implicated since there is an increased incidence in women and RA mostly improves in pregnancy, and relapses post-partum. Nulliparous women, women in the post-partum period, and women who have an early menarche have a greater risk of developing RA (Silman, 1998).While environmental stressors are likely to be involved, no definite environmental factors that precipitate disease onset have been identified. Current research is focused on elucidating the complex interactions of genetic, environmental, hormonal and auto-immune pathways. It becomes more evident that these factors nourish the immunopathogenesis on the initial stages of this disease and continue to fuel its maintenance and progression.

2.3.1 Stress theories

One of the oldest of explanation was the stress hormone hypothesis championed by Hans Selye (Selye 1949 & 1950). Roughly, his contention was that hormones released by the body, especially those released by the jacket of the adrenal glands, cause an adverse reaction to the joint tissues when they are released in excessive amounts, or in the wrong ratios under the conditions of environmental or psychological stress. His concept was generalised and only mentioned rheumatoid arthritis as an unlikely possibility. The theory had some plausibility since arthritis can be produced by injecting deoxycorticosterone, which is a potassium excreting hormone, into a patient with Addison's disease or reproduced in similar animal studies (Selye, 1944). The dramatic effect that cortisone has on arthritis was demonstrated first in 1948 by Edward C. Kendall and Philip S. Hench at the Mayo Clinic in Rochester, Minnesota. Their discovery stemmed from the astute clinical observation that a woman with severe RA felt much better during pregnancy. They found what was responsible. It was a hormone from the outer part (the cortex) of the adrenal glands that they called 'cortisone'. On September 21, 1948, Hench gave a synthesised version of cortisone developed by Kendall to a patient with arthritis and it became the first 'miracle drug' due to its powerful anti-inflammatory and other effects. In 1950 they shared the Nobel Prize in physiology for their discoveries relating to the hormones of the adrenal cortex. The question of whether patients with rheumatoid arthritis might have a defective hypothalamo-pituitary-adrenal axis was first raised then. It was initially hypothesised that this was due to an impaired ability of RA patients to synthesise sufficient amounts of endogenous glucocorticoids, but intensive investigations over the next few decades failed to reveal any significant defects in HPA axis activity in RA patients. The literature review provided no compelling evidence for significant differences in either basal or stress-stimulated HPA axis activity in RA patients compared with healthy individuals. However, Jessop and Harbuz (1999) did highlight an inherent defect, which resided in the inability of RA patients to mount an appropriately enhanced glucocorticoid response to increased secretion of proinflammatory cytokines such as interleukin (IL)-1, IL-6 and tumour necrosis factor (TNF) - α. 'In other words', they concluded, 'the HPA axis response in RA is defective precisely because it is normal'. Following an insulin-induced hypoglycaemia, which tests the HPA axis at all levels, there were no observed differences in serum cortisol responses between patients with active RA

and patients in remission (Demir et al, 1999). This study did not include non-RA subjects as controls, and there was no ACTH response to hypoglycaemia in either test group, suggesting a possible methodological problem. Although the HPA axis in RA is defective because its activity is not increased in response to inflammatory cytokines, as might be predicted from observations of increased corticosterone in rodent models of inflammation (Harbuz, 2002), the current evidence suggest that the HPA axis is not materially different in RA compared with normal healthy subjects under most experimental conditions (Jessop, Harbuz, 2005). Stress theories did not always emphasize steroid hormones. Histamine was suggested as possibly being involved by two University of Utah scientists, Chemist Henry Eyring and Anatomist Thomas F. Dougherty in 1955 (Eyring and Dougherty, 1955). Their theory stated that stress sets off a destructive chain reaction among the body cells with histamine acting as a destructive agent. Each cell is in a membrane envelope and, as long as the membrane is relatively impermeable, the cell functions normally. Under stress, however, the membrane starts to deteriorate. Histamine, which is normally present inside the cell when the cell is healthy, is violently released and stimulated by the cell breakdown. It attacks the disintegrating cell, which swells and bursts, liberating still more histamine to attack neighbouring cells. Over long periods of stress, the spreading destruction can lead to serious illness and may be present in every fatal illness, including cancer.
Supporting evidence of histamine hyperproduction comes from the study by Permin and colleagues (Permin et al, 1981). They found that basophilocytes from patients with rheumatoid arthritis responded to leukocyte nuclei from normal persons with histamine release and recorded 3.5 times as much histamine production in arthritics after the challenge than normally expected. A role of histamine in RA is also supported by the findings from the same study of clinical improvement during treatment with H1 and H2 antihistamines in six of 12 patients with RA in active phase, whereas four showed definite deterioration.

2.3.2 Autoimmune hypothesis

The most popular current hypothesis is the autoimmune hypothesis. Many do not even regard this concept as a hypothesis, but as a proven theory, as investigations into the autoimmune hypothesis are well funded. When rheumatoid arthritis presents, the immune system overcompensates and acts, attacking the joints and the body in general. The same thing occurs with other autoimmune diseases; the immunological mechanisms that manifest in these diseases have been identified, but there is still no explanation as to why this occurs.
Immunopathogensis of RA is multifactorial. Evidence suggests that an interaction between an unknown exogenous or endogenous antigen via antigen presenting cells and CD4 T helper cells are involved in the induction of the immune response in RA. Subsequent recruitment and activation of monocytes and macrophages occurs with the secretion of pro-inflammatory cytokines, in particular TNF-α and IL-1 into the synovial cavity. The release of these cytokines mediates tissue destruction by activation of chondrocytes and fibroblasts which release collagenases and metalloproteinases with resultant cartilage loss and bone erosion. B lymphocyte dysregulation, resulting in the production of rheumatoid factor and other auto-antibodies, as well as in the formation of immune complexes and the release of destructive mediators, also contribute to this process. Rheumatoid factor, an autoimmune response to IgG is a key feature of RA. High levels are relatively specific for RA but rheumatoid factor may also occur in other chronic diseases and is absent in around 30% of patients with established RA. Other auto-antigens have been proposed but as yet no single antigen has been incriminated (Jobanputra, 1992). Ankylosing spondylitis and rheumatoid

arthritis share many common features. However the presence of rheumatoid factor, histologically classic rheumatoid nodules, and the histocompatibility cell wall antigen (HLA-B27) helps distinguish one from the other. A much higher association of antigen HLA-B27, which is a known immune factor with the disorders in the arthritic group, such as Reiter's syndrome and ankylosing spondilitis (López-Larrea et al, 1998), has tended to reinforce evidence for autoimmune aetiology of RA.

The hypothesis that rheumatoid arthritis is an allergy is in the same general category as the autoimmune hypothesis. Such a hypothesis has the advantage, not shared by the autoimmune hypothesis directly, of advancing an environmental factor, which is almost certainly involved. The wide geographical variations virtually ensure this. There is evidence from several well documented case reports (Buchanan et al, 1991) that occasional patients with rheumatoid arthritis may develop an aggravation of their arthritis, as a result of allergy to some ingredient in their diet. A variety of foodstuffs have been implicated including milk and milk products, corn and cereals. Total fasting results in an improvement in rheumatoid arthritis, but appears to be mediated by diminution in production of chemical mediators of inflammation, rather than by elimination of a dietary allergen. According to Buchanan (Buchanan et al, 1991), there is conflicting evidence from the studies that used various intestinal probes, that patients with rheumatoid arthritis may have a 'leaky' intestinal mucosa, allowing the food allergens to be more easily absorbed. Clinical therapeutic trials of exclusion diets have employed the standard strategy of the double-blind randomised method. However, this presupposes that patients entered into such a study are capable of improvement with dietary manipulation. Since this is often not the case, a more appropriate method would be to employ the 'intensive research design', also known as 'single case experiment' and 'N of 1' study. The hypothesis pointing towards 'masked food intolerance' is an attractive theory, but one that is extremely difficult to prove in practice.

2.3.3 Genetic basis of Rheumatoid Arthritis

Support for a genetic predisposition for rheumatoid arthritis has come from the studies reporting rheumatoid arthritis clusters in families. Formal genetic studies have confirmed this familial aggregation and genetic influence is estimated at 50 to 60% (Ollier et al, 1999). Studies in monozygotic twins have shown a concordance rate of 15% - 30% and a relative risk of 3.5 for rheumatoid arthritis developing in monozygotic versus dizygotic twins of affected cases. A high prevalence rate of 5% - 6% has been described in some Native American populations, suggesting a higher genetic burden of rheumatoid arthritis risk genes. Differences in the prevalence rates in other ethnic groups are rather small and are partially explained by differences in disease ascertainment.

Interactive genetic effects are suspected to modulate the impact of individual disease-risk genes and are likely to contribute to the low penetrance. Genetic risk factors not only determine susceptibility for the disease but also correlate with the disease severity and phenotype, providing the unique opportunity to use genetic markers as prognostic tools in the management of rheumatoid arthritis. A measure used to estimate the genetic component to the disease is the coefficient of familial clustering, λs, defined as the ratio of the prevalence in affected siblings to the population prevalence. For rheumatoid arthritis, λs ranges from 2 to 12 in first-degree relatives of patients, depending on the published data (Dieudé & Cornélis, 2005). Although clearly supporting the influence of the genetic factors, this λs is rather low compared with other autoimmune diseases or common genetic diseases, leaving considerable room for any environmental or stochastic events in the pathogenesis of the disease. In part, λs may be rather low because rheumatoid arthritis is a heterogeneous syndrome that includes several genetically semi-homogeneous subsets.

The genetic system studied most thoroughly is the major histocompatibility complex (MHC). In the initial studies, rheumatoid arthritis was shown to be associated with human leukocyte antigen (HLA)-DR4 (Stastny et al, 1978). The association studies in different ethnic populations support the concept that HLA-DRB1 alleles, expressing a particular sequence motif are over-represented among people with rheumatoid arthritis (Ollier et al, 1999). This sequence polymorphism is characterized by a glutamine or arginine at position 70, a lysine or alanine at position 71, and an alanine at position 74. Alleles with a negatively charged amino acid at any one of these positions are not associated with the disease. MHC genes are not the only germline-encoded genes influencing susceptibility to rheumatoid arthritis. Female sex clearly increases the risk, and female patients develop a different phenotype of the disease than do male patients. However, no sex-linked genes have been identified as disease-risk genes. Several consortiums have started genome-wide searches, using affected sibling pairs (Seldin et al, 1999). Eventually, the candidate gene approach may be more sensitive for identifying risk genes, in particular when considering the heterogeneity of the disease severity and phenotype. The recent definition of single nucleotide polymorphisms throughout the human genome has increased significantly the feasibility of this approach. Studies of T-cell receptor (TCR) and immunoglobulin genes have not been revealing; several cytokine polymorphisms, including tumour necrosis factor (TNF)-α and interferon (IFN)- γ were described to influence disease severity, but studies are needed to confirm this hypothesis.

2.4 Diagnostic considerations

Reliable measurement is often a prerequisite of effective intervention, or at least of enabling clinical trials. Rheumatoid arthritis is diagnosed from a constellation of clinical and laboratory or radiographic abnormalities. Diagnosis may be obvious in some but in others it may be more difficult and require a period of clinical observation. Classification criteria for RA have been devised. The 1987 revised criteria for the classification of rheumatoid arthritis (Arnett et al, 1988) are shown in TABLE 1.4; it superseded The American Rheumatism Association criteria of1958. These criteria were derived from a group of typical patients who had been diagnosed with RA and had well-established disease. They have limited utility in routine practice and most clinicians diagnose RA without formal reference to such criteria, and many patients do not meet formal criteria at least early in disease (Harrison et al, 1998). Criteria 1 through 4 must have been present for at least 6 weeks. Rheumatoid arthritis is defined by the presence of 4 or more criteria, and no further qualifications (classic, definite, or probable) or list of exclusions are required. In addition, a "classification tree" schema is presented which performs equally as well as the traditional (4 of 7) format. The newer criteria demonstrated 91-94% sensitivity and 89% specificity for RA when compared with non-RA rheumatic disease control subjects. Criteria were also developed as an algorithm and these are more readily met in clinical practice (Emery et al, 1997).

Two diagnostic tests are included in the criteria: rheumatoid factor and X-ray changes. Rheumatoid factor (RF), measured in routine blood samples, is a circulating IgM autoantibody that is directed against IgG molecules. In established disease, IgM- RF can be detected with a sensitivity of 60-70% and a specificity of 80-90% (Van Gaalen et al, 2004). Another antibody against the cyclic citrulline protein (CCP) specific for RA was discovered later. In a meta-analysis published in 2007 it was found that anti-CCP antibody displays sensitivities comparable to that of RF (approximately 80%) but with superior specificity (98%) (Nishimura et al, 2007). Early in disease radiographs may show soft tissue swelling and reduced bone density around affected joints. Later there may be evidence of joint damage such as joint erosions (focal loss of bone and cartilage often near the joint margin) or a reduced joint space (indicating diffuse cartilage loss). With continued joint damage there may be extensive joint destruction, features of joint deformity or instability, and bony ankylosis. With advanced joint damage surgical intervention such as joint replacement arthroplasty, joint fusion or osteotomy may be necessary. At an earlier stage surgical treatment such as removal of synovial tissues (synovectomy) or other soft tissue procedures such as tendon release or repair may also be necessary.

Criterion	Definition
1. Morning stiffness	Morning stiffness in and around the joints, lasting at least 1 hour before maximal improvement
2. Arthritis of 3 or more joint areas	At least 3 joint areas simultaneously have had soft tissue swelling or fluid (not bony overgrowth alone) observed by a physician. The 14 possible areas are right or left PIP, MCP, wrist, elbow, knee, ankle, and MTP joints
3. Arthritis of hand joints	At least 1 area swollen (as defined above) in a wrist, MCP, or PIP joint
4. Symmetric arthritis	Simultaneous involvement of the same joint areas (as defined in 2) on both sides of the body (bilateral involvement of PIPs, MCPs, or MTPs is acceptable without absolute symmetry)
5. Rheumatoid nodules	Subcutaneous nodules, over bony prominences, or extensor surfaces, or in juxtaarticular regions, observed by a physician
6. Serum rheumatoid factor	Demonstration of abnormal amounts of serum rheumatoid factor by any method for which the result has been positive in <5% of normal control subjects
7. Radiographic changes	Radiographic changes typical of rheumatoid arthritis on posteroanterior hand and wrist radiographs, which must include erosions or unequivocal bony decalcification localized in or most marked adjacent to the involved joints (osteoarthritis changes alone do not qualify)

* For classification purposes, a patient shall be said to have rheumatoid arthritis if he/she has satisfied at least 4 or these 7 criteria. Criteria 1 through 4 must have been present for at least 6 weeks. Patients with 2 clinical diagnoses are not excluded. Designation as classic, definite, or probable rheumatoid arthritis is not to be made.

Table 1.4 1987 Criteria for the Classification of Acute Arthritis of RA

Among additional diagnostic tests are acute-phase reactants – the erythrocyte sedimentation rate (ESR) and C-reactive protein (CRP) level that correlate with the degree of synovial inflammation. They are useful for following the course of inflammatory activity in an individual patient. Other abnormalities include hypergannaglobulinemia, thrombocytosis, and eosinophilia. These occur more often in patients with severe disease, high RF titer, rheumatoid modules, and extra-articular manifestations.

2.5 Trends in pharmacological and biological therapy

In more recent years, a number of new exciting therapeutic options have become available, especially with the development of the biologic drugs, thus causing evolution of rheumatological science to spiral. This trend reflects the application of knowledge obtained from advancements in understanding of disease pathogenesis and underlying molecular mechanisms. This therapeutic philosophy has drawn on the model of oncology, with early diagnosis and aggressive treatment. While this has been in parallel with and to an extent dependent upon, sophisticated new imaging techniques such as MRI, clinicians have thought along these lines for many years (Emery, Gough, 1991).A number of these therapies are outlined below, including the various biological modifiers, in particular, anti-tumour necrosis factor-α agents and interleukin-1 (IL-1) receptor antagonists, which have been developed in recognition of the role of pro-inflammatory cytokines in RA. Also notable, is the current interest centering on the development and trials with B cell depletion therapies, specifically rituximab, in patients with RA. This demonstrates acknowledgment for a more significant role for B cells in the aetiology of RA, in contrast to the long held view that RA was a predominantly T cell mediated disease. The main categories of medications used to treat RA considered below.

2.5.1 Nonsteroidal Anti-Inflammatory Drugs (NSAIDs)

It has been shown that NSAIDs cause quite distinct and severe biochemical damage during drug absorption (uncoupling of mitochondrial oxidative phosphorylation proving to be most important) which results in increased intestinal permeability. All commonly used NSAIDs, apart from aspirin and nabumetone, are associated with increased intestinal permeability in man. Whilst reversible in the short term, it may take months to improve following prolonged NSAID use (Bjarnason et al, 1993). Avoiding NSAIDs is advisable in patients with inflammatory bowel disease (Kane et al, 2001).

2.5.2 Disease Modifying Antirheumatic Drugs (DMARDs)

DMARDs are used with NSAIDs and/or prednisone to slow joint destruction caused by RA over time. Examples of these drugs are methotrexate, injectable and oral gold, penicillamine, azathioprine, chloroquine, hydroxychloroquine, and sulfasalazine. DMARDs, particularly methotrexate, have been the standard for aggressively treating RA. Recently, studies have shown that the most aggressive treatment for controlling RA may be the combination of methotrexate and another drug, particularly biologic response modifiers (Olsen, 2006). The dual drug treatment seems to create a more effective treatment, especially for people who may not have success with or who have built up a resistance to, methotrexate or another drug alone. It appears that these combination drug therapies might become the new road to follow in treating RA. Oral corticosteroids, or steroids, are powerful anti-inflammatory drugs that are used to quickly reduce inflammation. These drugs include prednisone and prednisolone and are most often used in combination with DMARDs, which significantly enhances the benefits of DMARDs.

2.5.3 Biologic response modifiers

"Biologics" directly modify the immune system by inhibiting cytokines or B and T immune cells, which contribute to inflammation. Two types of agents can be used to eliminate circulating TNF: recombinant soluble receptors and monoclonal antibodies to TNF. There are three agents that were originally approved for patients with RA which inhibit the action of TNF-α; – infliximab, etanercept and adalimumab. Two additional novel TNF antagonists, Certolizumab pegol and Golimumab have recently been indicated for patients with RA for the treatment of moderate to severe, active RA in adult patients when the response to conventional DMARDs including methotrexate, has been inadequate.

Etanercept, a soluble TNF receptor, is labeled for use in monotherapy and combination therapy with methotrexate for arthritis (NICE guidelines, 2002). The TNF- α blocking agent infliximab is labelled for use in combination with methotrexate for the treatment of RA (NICE guidelines, 2002). Adalimumab is a recombinant human IgG1 monoclonal antibody that binds TNF-α, thereby precluding binding to its receptor. Enthusiastic support for early intervention with TNF-⟨ inhibitors for patients with RA comes with a strong safety message. Although infusion reactions and other AEs are infrequent, they may be very serious in some patients, in particular when complications associated with opportunistic infections occur. Certolizumab pegol, which targets TNF-α with a different mechanism of action than widely used biologics, was initially investigated for Crohn's disease but has now been shown to be effective for rheumatoid arthritis. There have been three significant clinical trials demonstrating the efficacy of certolizumab pegol in active rheumatoid arthritis; two with combination methotrexate and one with monotherapy (Ruiz et al, 2011). Significant improvements were observed at 24 weeks and at 52 weeks with the approved dose of 200 mg certolizumab pegol. The most common adverse events with certolizumab pegol 200 mg were: upper respiratory tract infections, hypertension and nasopharyngitis (Ruiz et al, 2011). Golimumab is a humanized inhibitor of Tumor necrosis factor-alpha, recently approved for the treatment of RA. Recent Cochrane systematic review (Singh et al, 2010), identified four Randomised Control Trials with 1,231 patients treated with golimumab and 483 patients treated with placebo. The authors concluded that Golimumab-treated patients were significantly more likely to achieve remission, low disease activity and improvement in functional ability compared to placebo (all statistically significant). No significant differences were noted between golimumab and placebo regarding serious adverse events, infections, serious infections, lung infections, tuberculosis, cancer, withdrawals due to adverse events and inefficacy and deaths.

2.5.4 Interleukin 1 receptor antagonists

Interleukin 1 is a pro-inflammatory cytokine produced by stimulated monocytes, macrophages and some specialised synovial lining cells. IL-1 receptor antagonist competes with IL-1 for binding to the receptor, subsequently down regulating IL-1 actions. By stimulating the release of matrix metalloproteinases and increasing bone resorption by effects on osteoclasts, IL-1 has been shown to have a significant role in RA pathogenesis, particularly in regards cartilage and bone erosion. Mice deficient of IL-1 receptor antagonist, demonstrate the development of inflammatory arthritis similar to RA (Horai et al, 2000). In addition, patients with RA have been shown to have lower IL-1 receptor antagonist levels than anticipated for the level of IL-1 in the joint (Arend et al, 1998). It was hypothesized that addressing this imbalance, with a recombinant IL-1 receptor antagonist could be beneficial in RA and anakinra was thus developed for this purpose (Fleischmann et al, 2003). Anakinra is administered by daily subcutaneous injection. The recombinant humanized anti-IL-6 receptor antibody tocilizumab is an innovative drug for the treatment of rheumatoid arthritis. Tocilizumab is generally well tolerated and efficacious in patients refractive to conventional DMARD therapies (Ohsugi, Kishimoto, 2008).

2.5.5 Abatacept

Abatacept selectively modulates the co-stimulatory signal required for full T cell activation. The agent, which binds to CD80 and CD86 on antigen-presenting cells, blocking the engagement of CD28 on T cells and thus preventing T cell activation, acts earlier in the inflammatory cascade than do other biologic therapies by directly inhibiting the activation of T cells and the secondary activation of macrophages and B cells. Abatacept is administered in a 30min infusion. Kremer provided data that originated from his clinical trial (Kremer et al, 2005), demonstrating that the combination of abatacept and methotrexate improves the signs and symptoms, physical functioning, and quality of life of patients with active RA.

2.5.6 B cell depletion therapy

Contrary to the long held view that RA is a predominantly T cell mediated disease, the important role of B cells in disease aetiology is supported by development and trials with B cell depletion therapies notably rituximab. B cells contribute to the pathogenesis of RA via a number of proposed mechanisms including; presentation of antigen complexes with IgG to T cells, and T cell independent generation of TNF-α by tissue macrophages after stimulation by oligomeric IgG rheumatoid factor (RF) immune complexes (Fleischmann et al, 2003). In addition, the ability of IgG RF B cells to self perpetuate due to secretion of own antigen, provided rationale for the proposal that elimination of the RF B cell clones may result in prolonged disease remission (Edwards et al, 1999).

2.5.7 Protein-A immunoadsorption therapy

Immunoadsorption is increasingly used to treat antibody-mediated autoimmune diseases. In its very basic form, it is a therapy that filters blood to remove antibodies and immune complexes that promote inflammation. Recent introduction of staphylococcal protein A (Prosorba) column, as an intervention for treatment-resistant, moderate to severe rheumatoid arthritis has prompted increased requests for this therapy by physicians and patients alike. The basis for the salutary effects of staphylococcal protein A immunoadsorption remains obscure. Because the column becomes saturated after removal of only ~1 gm of IgG, its efficacy clearly is not based on quantitative immunoglobulin depletion. Instead, an immunomodulatory effect is believed to occur, resulting from alterations in circulating immune complexes (Kiss, 2000). Column treatment appears to reduce the population of small molecular weight circulating immune complexes. These circulating immune complexes may interfere with antigen presentation to T-helper cells, thus blocking the formation of "protective" antibodies involved in immune clearance (Kiss, 2000). Circulating immune complexes may also inhibit the formation of anti-idiotypic antibodies, which down-regulate autoantibody responses. Felson et.al. studied the efficacy of SPA column treatment in comparison to a control group who received apheresis without column plasma perfusion (i.e., a sham arm) in a randomized double-blind study and his trial (Felson et al, 1999) reported that staphylococcal protein A column therapy was efficacious in patients with RA with 31.9% of 47 patients in the SPA group experiencing improvement in comparison to 11.4% in the control group (P=0.019). However, it appears that appropriate patient selection is essential. In general, it is recommended that such patients should be refractory to standard modes of therapy, and a risk versus benefit versus cost metric should be carefully considered.

3. Burden of illness

In economic terms, arthritis accounts for a substantial proportion of the overall economic burden of illness in society (Goetzel et al, 2004). The burden of illness is more evident in the more numerous musculo-skeletal conditions, including back pain and osteoathritis, where there has been documented limited therapeutic progress leading to a much bigger global impact on national health and social and economic spending. Further, the less readily pathologically classifiable disorders, such as chronic pain syndromes and disability itself, remain areas of unmet need and huge economic impact.

Some evidence indicates that comorbid depression interacts with physical illness to amplify the expected level of disability associated with physical disability (Katon et al, 2002). Hansen et al (2002) demonstrated that mentally disordered medical inpatients use health care more heavily than patients without mental health problems, even after adjusting for medical disease severity. Depression is one of the major challenges facing clinical medicine. Unipolar depression was ranked fifth among the leading causes of disability worldwide in 2000 and projections indicate that by 2020 it will be ranked second only to ischemic heart disease (Murray et al, 1997). In addition to negative health consequences, depression may contribute to unemployment, loss of work productivity, and increased health care costs in persons with arthritis (Li et al, 2006). The association between these two conditions has particular relevance in the elderly population, where a substantial proportion of the burden of depression is related to chronic physical illnesses, including arthritis, which has an attributable risk of 18.1% (95% confidence interval, 9.9-25.6%) (Dunlop et al, 2004). It is unclear whether indirect costs exceed direct medical costs overall, although it appears that patients and families, rather than health care services, incur a majority of the economic costs early in disease.

Norbert Schmitz and his team (2007) recently examined the synergistic effect of depression and chronic conditions on disability. The results of this population-based study demonstrated that arthritis/rheumatism represented one of the leading disability category at 16, 8%, second only to "back problems" group. The presence of depression substantially increased the number of disability days, e.g. depression increased the Odds Ratio for functional disability from 2.1 in chronic conditions to 6.3 in chronic conditions with comorbid depression.

3.1 Psychiatic morbidity in Rheumatoid Arthritis

Medical illness and major depression co-occur at high levels in epidemiological and clinical settings. Thus, while the prevalence of depression in nonmedical populations is estimated to be between 5% and 10% in primary care (Simon et al, 2002) and at 8 – 15% in hospital-based studies (Hansen et al, 2001), it is clear that medical diagnosis increases the risk for depression. Rheumatoid arthritis is associated with significant psychiatric morbidity that is often perceived, as surprisingly high. For example, Wells et al (1988) reported a lifetime psychiatric prevalence rate of 64% and a recent 6 months prevalence rate of 42% in patients with arthritis drawn from a community sample. Depression is one of the most common psychiatric conditions found in patients with arthritis: between 14% and 46% of patients with rheumatoid arthritis also fulfil the diagnostic criteria for depression (Zaphiropoulos et al, 1974; Frank et al, 1988; Creed et al, 1990; Hawley et al, 1993; Katz et al, 1993; Abdel-Nasser et al, 1998; Soderlin et al, 2000).

Patients are very likely to have difficulty with depression while managing their arthritis. In contradiction to the needs of this patient group, all of the above cited studies demonstrate that depression is universally associated with disability and that the detection of mental disorders and the rates of psychiatric referral and treatment are extremely low.

Depression includes a spectrum of disorders that vary in severity and associated disability. Patients with a history of major depression typically have a chronic course that requires comprehensive assessment, effective monitoring and management. Chronic depression may exist independently of, but can also be exacerbated by, disease flare -ups and other illness-related obstacles. Moderate to severe depression can adversely affect health outcomes and quality of life in a manner similar to that of other chronic medical conditions. In addition, depression may contribute to inflammation, interfere with medical adherence, and thus compromise medical treatment and management. In this regard, a longitudinal study by Ang et al (2005) found that clinical depression resulted in a 2-fold increase in the likelihood of early mortality in a cohort of patients with RA followed over a 12-year period. All of these factors heighten the importance of detecting and managing depression in patients with arthritis. When rheumatologists do not recognise depression, the risks to patients, their families, and the health care system can be severe.

In light of the above findings, the article by Sleath et al (2008) provides evidence of a significant clinical problem in the care of patients with RA. Although depression in primary care has been well studied, no studies have examined whether rheumatologists and RA patients discuss depression during medical visits. This study by Sleath et al, included 200 RA patients from four rheumatology clinics with eight participating doctors. Patient visits were audiotaped and patients were interviewed after their medical visits using a questionnaire to measure their mental status. The results showed that almost 11% of the patients in the study had moderately severe to severe symptoms of depression and that those who were rated as being more restricted in their normal activities were significantly more likely to have these symptoms. Furthermore, only 1 in 5 of the patients who showed symptoms discussed depression with their rheumatologists and they were always the ones to bring up the topic. Even when depression was brought up, it was often not discussed at any length. Several important findings stand out in this research. First, the authors found that patients who were rated by their rheumatologists as having worse functional status were more than twice as likely to have moderately severe to severe depression. Second, only 19% of the depressed patients had the opportunity to discuss their depression during medical visits. Third, when depression was addressed, the patient initiated the discussion each time. Not once during 200 office visits did a rheumatologist bring up the topic of depression to the patient. Because the study focused only on moderately severe to severe depression, the prevalence of minor depression was not assessed. Many more patients could have been afflicted with less severe forms of depression in the sample. Lastly, when patients visit their rheumatologists, their main focus is their RA, yet such chronic diseases can greatly impact a patient's psychosocial well-being. For these reasons the authors suggest that it is important for rheumatologists to consider addressing both the RA and the depression when they see their patients. The authors note that some physicians may not feel comfortable discussing depression with their patients and advocate the use of brief depression screening questionnaires before the patient's visits in order to identify problems early on.

The prevalence of anxiety has been less well studied in this population (Soderlin et al, 2000; VanDyke et al, 2004), though there is some evidence that anxiety may be even more common than depression (El-Miedany et al, 2002), a conservative estimates of the prevalence of co-existing somatic disorders and phobias, according to Hansen's study was 12.9%.

Psychiatric syndromes have significant implications for patients with rheumatoid arthritis: individuals with both arthritis and depression report increased functional disability (Vali et al, 1998) and increased levels of arthritis-related pain (Fifield et al, 1998), compared to individuals with arthritis alone. The importance of depression is further underlined by Timonen et al (2003), who reported that 90% of females with rheumatoid arthritis who committed suicide had suffered from a depressive disorder prior to suicide. It is known that the combination of depression and physical illness is associated with small increase in suicide risk, but it increases where pain is a significant part of clinical picture, especially in the elderly.

3.2 Coping

Coping has been shown to have a strong association with response and adjustment to chronic illness, including arthritis, (Jensen et al, 1991; Becker et al, 2000) and as such play an important role in mediating the impact of disease activity. Coping is a general concept used to describe the cognitive, emotional and behavioural reactions to the challenging and distressing situations and events. The two questions in relation to coping styles have received rigorous attention: first, how an individual copes with the stresses of having a chronic illness, and second, why individuals faced with essentially the same stressful events may vary so significantly in their ability to adjust. A tentative answer to the two questions posed lies in realisation that just as competent immune system heals by altering bodily equilibrium, so do adaptive coping mechanisms reduce stress by influencing subjective perception of one's condition. Different coping strategies are not in themselves good or bad and all may serve a useful function at various times of illness and in particular circumstances. Active and passive coping refer to the degree of internal and external control, respectively, that a patient relies on to manage the consequences of a disease. Research generally concludes that, overall, strategies involving denial, catastrophizing, avoidance of activity and wishful thinking are less positive for individuals' well being than problem-focused or avoidance-orientated coping. Coping effectiveness is defined by its outcome and usually measured by the level of distress, health-related disability, or other symptomatology. To illustrate this point Brown and Nicassio (Brown & Nicassio, 1987) studied a sample of 361 rheumatoid arthritis patients and found that passive coping was associated with greater pain, disability and depression, whereas active coping was associated with less pain, disability and depression.

Within the broader classification system that categorises coping strategies as operating principally along an engagement (e.g., approach, confrontive) versus disengagement (e.g., avoidance, escape) continuum (Carver et al., 1989; Krohne, 1996; Tobin et al., 1989), a number of specific coping strategies have been identified.

3.2.1 Emotion-focused coping strategies

Essentially, there are conscious and intentional cognitive strategies that originate in an attempt to combat emotional distress, such as distraction, 'shutting down' and passive avoidance on one hand, looking for sympathy, turning to religious faith and positive reappraisal on the other. Endler and Parker (1990) describe emotion-orientated coping as comprising emotional reactions that are self-orientated but that may actually increase stress levels since they fail to actively reduce stress and may instead heighten the negative emotional component of the stress experience. Examples of such maladaptive reactions include blaming oneself for being too emotional, worrying about what one is going to do, or getting angry.

3.2.2 Problem-focused coping strategies or task-orientated coping

There are the ways in which individuals consciously seek social support and elicit help from others: direct action, confrontation, planning and information seeking are all examples of this group. It involves using a problem-solving approach to eliminate stressors. For example, perceiving a demanding schedule as being stressful and deciding to use time management skills as a means to prioritise one's demands would be an example of task-orientated coping.

3.2.3 Avoidance-orientated coping

The coping strategies that are based on distraction and social diversion are characterised here. This coping style involves turning away from the stressors, possibly by ignoring it, psychologically distancing oneself from it, or engaging in another task. An avoidance coping style may not effectively eliminate stress since this style of coping does not actively reduce stress. However, engaging in substitute tasks may be beneficial as a means of temporarily removing oneself from stress until a patient is more able to actively face stress issues and implement a task-orientated coping style (Endler & Parker, 1990). Recent research findings have suggested that the use of an avoidance-orientated coping style may serve a protective function for individuals that are in situations in which they are not able to control the stressor that they are faced with (Simon-Thomas et al, 2001). For example, children that were exposed to the stressor of parental argument (stressor that they cannot control) were found to be protected/ buffered from the effects of inter-parental conflict on child internalising behaviours if they engaged in avoidance-orientated coping. Thus, depending upon the nature of the stressor, avoidance-orientated coping may be seen as either maladaptive or adaptive.

3.2.4 Adaptive involuntary coping strategies

Defence mechanisms reduce conflict and cognitive dissonance during sudden changes in reality caused by the illness. If such changes are not adjusted for they can result in disabling anxiety and depression. Adaptive defences operate in a hierarchical way: trough distortion or denial (immature defence level), repression, intellectualisation and reaction formation (intermediate defences), or at a higher adaptive level through self-assertion, affiliation, sublimation and humour.

3.2.5 Coping hierarchy

With the advent of measures that sought to investigate the nature, structure, and correlates of coping, theoreticians and researchers alike have begun to shift their views to focus more on the hierarchical nature of coping. Three broad levels have been implicated: (a) coping styles that reflect global, dispositional, macroanalytic tendencies (e.g., monitoring-blunting, vigilance-avoidance, approach-avoidance); (b) coping strategies or modes that reflect an intermediate level in this hierarchy, and are typically indicated by summative scores on coping scales (e.g., confrontation, seeking social support, planful problem solving); and (c) coping acts or behaviors that reflect specific, situation-determined, microanalytic responses that are often indicated by individual item endorsement on a coping scale (Endler & Parker, 1990; Krohne, 1996; Schwarzer & Schwarzer, 1996).

The literature on coping with chronic illnesses and disabilities has, likewise, generated much insight into the nature and structure of coping efforts directed at diffusing or removing the stress engendered by the associated trauma, loss, and pain. Results from these and other studies strongly suggest that coping plays a significant role during the process of psychosocial adaptation to both sudden and gradual onset of chronic illnesses and disabilities. More specifically, these results indicate that: (a) a wide range of coping efforts has been employed by persons with disabilities to deal with the stresses engendered by their conditions; (b) these numerous efforts, both problem-solving and emotional-focused coping, as well as engagement- and disengagement- type coping have been found to be adaptive; (c) different coping efforts assume different roles and are, therefore, differentially employed to regulate stressful emotions and solve problems during the adaptation process; (d) coping efforts have played both a direct role (i.e., are directly linked to measures of psychosocial adaptation to disability) and a mediator role (i.e., act as mediators between sociodemographic variables, personality attributes, disability-related factors, environmental conditions, and outcomes of psychosocial adaptation); and (e) different disabling conditions imply different functional (e.g., mobility, manipulation, fatigue, cognitive) limitations, medical courses and prognostic indicators (e.g., deteriorating, unpredictable, stable), related health problems, treatment modalities, and psychosocial reactions. Individuals cognitively appraise the situation in terms of its personal significance, and then look at the resources and options they have available. This notion helps to appreciate the variability in individual coping reactions. The coping strategies adopted by an individual are quite unique; they include the way one perceives threatening experiences and reacts to stressful events, how one manages ones emotions and how one attempt to solve problems.

3.2.6 Age and gender differences

The effectiveness of coping strategies across the lifespan has been another area of clinical interest. Contrary to suggested belief that individuals become less efficient at coping with the demands of life as they get older, research into success of coping revealed immunity to the age process. Thus, in a recent study investigating age variance in coping across a broad range of stressors in a sample of more than 2,000 men ranging in age from the late 40s to over 90, there were no significant age differences in the reporting of negative emotional states in response to stressors, nor perceived efficacy in coping (Dunkin & Amano, 2005).

In relation to gender differences, women appear to report positive and negative affects more vividly than men. In one study (Diener et al, 1999), gender accounted for 13 percent of the variance of the intensity of reported emotional experiences. There is also considerable evidence that women are more likely to use formal helping systems than are other groups, especially men and people of colour. One recent study addressed the natural coping systems of male and female students in largely young, Euro-American sample (Slattery et al, 2002).

They found significant gender-specific pattern in the use of coping strategies and their perceived effectiveness. The authors reported that females were significantly more likely than males to seek appropriate help and try to solve the problem, but also to use eating, cleaning, shopping, crying and praying. Interestingly enough, males were more likely to report using sex and masturbation in their attempt to cope than females. Both sexes described avoiding others, doing nothing, and ignoring the problem as least helpful.

3.2.7 Cultural aspects of coping

Cultural aspects of coping emerge as a new dimension in the ethnically diverse world today. Native Americans, for example, tend to turn to spiritual leaders and extended family (informal helping system) rather than to formal helping systems such as therapists (LaFramboisie, 2000). Similar findings have been reported for African Americans and Hispanic cultures (Sue & Sue, 1997); in England the Government's race equality strategy (Department of Health UK, 2003) have illustrated how local African community avoid statutory care systems and try to contain problems in their homes long beyond the expected point of seeking outside help. This could be a result of natural difficulty with disclosing problems or sharing emotions in this group or inadequacy of existing services to address their psychological needs. In his timely review Brendan Kelly (Kelly, 2003) highlighted that globalisation and large-scale social changes could induce a wave of 'anomie'in migrants, that is in essance a breakdown of social values (Durkheim, 1947). For Durkheim, in 1897 anomie arised more generally from a mismatch between personal or group standards and wider social standards, or from the lack of a social ethic, which produced moral deregulation and an absence of legitimate aspirations. For migrants living in a state where societal standing is compromised and social ties are broken, anomie becomes a nurtured condition that has detrimental effects on their coping capacity.

3.3 Illness perception

Patients do not respond to treatment in a predictable manner and show a wide variation in perception of causation. Individual preconceptions determine help seeking, compliance and treatment outcome, yet clinicians rarely explore these issues. Early exploration of illness perceptions may enhance health behaviour and maximise the impact of intervention.

Lay illness representations often diverge from the clinician's understanding of the presenting problem and strongly influence treatment behaviour. Perception of the significance of decline in social functioning, including some losses in valued activities, which an individual regards as being important, e.g. visiting the family, going away on holiday is an important factor that only recently has been emphasised by Katz & Yelin (1995). In their 4-yr longitudinal study they found that patients' perception of a decline in valued activities by 10% was followed by a seven-fold increase in depression over the subsequent year. The self-regulation model (Leventhal et al, 1980) suggests that the cognitive and emotional aspects of illness perception guide the response to illness and determine the effectiveness of coping. Furthermore, five components of illness perception have been recognised: the identity of the illness (i.e., the symptoms and their labels); the perceived consequences of the illness; the illness's causation; its likely time line and the potential for control and cure (Lau et al, 1989).

Studies investigating the relationship between illness perceptions and coping show that the way affected people deal with their illness has great influence on their physical and psychological wellbeing. Much of this work has focused on the health and wellbeing of chronically ill patients with musculoskeletal illnesses such as rheumatoid arthritis. Scharloo and colleagues (Scharloo et al, 1998) presented data showing that patients with rheumatoid arthritis, chronic obstructive pulmonary disease and psoriasis achieve significantly better functioning when cope by seeking social support and believe in controllability and curability of the disease. Support from family and close companions can help to increase individual's sense of control of their symptoms, as this kind of empowerment helps people act on their own behalf in relation to their dealings with RA (Delzell, 2011).

4. Conclusion

While today we celebrate the advances in clinical science and in therapeutics, the enigmatic nature of RA still gives way to conceptualisation disparity. Indeed, despite some significant gains in the areas of immunopathology and genetics, Landré Beauvais' first clinical description of rheumatoid arthritis in 1800 encompasses most of what we know about this disease today. Where no single factor can provide a satisfactory explanation of a disorder in question, the biopsychosocial approach helps to position the multiple layers of existing knowledge in relation to it. Laboratory studies of inflammation and genetics provide the scientific basis of mainstream treatments, although the speciality still lacks good clinical and laboratory markers for making prognosis in each individual case.

In conclusion, our predecessors are to be congratulated for providing a platform for future developments. There are compelling data to suggest that the combination of earlier use of disease modifying treatments, attention to coexisting conditions and patient's coping and illness perception, that are considered to be important contributing factors in the relationship between physical and psychological factors in RA. The evolution and refinement of the newer therapies will allow more patients to realistically strive for disease remission and return of function in the near future. Rheumatologists of tomorrow are to be encouraged to carefully sift through the complex information generated during assessment process and to focus clinical and therapeutic developments where they can best be translated into better care for those with this taxing disease.

5. References

Abdel-Nasser AM, Abd El Azim S, Taal E, El-Badawy SA, Rasker JJ, Valkenburg HA. Depression and depressive symptoms in rheumatoid arthritis patients: an analysis of their occurrence and determinants. Br J Rheumatol 1998; 37: 391-7.

Alexander F. Psychosomatic Medicine. New York: Norton; 1950.

Alexander F, French T, Pollack GH. Psychosomatic Specificity. Chicago: University of Chicago Press; 1968.

Arend WP, Malyak M, Guthridge CJ, Gabay C. Interleukin-1 receptor antagonist: role in biology. Annu Rev Immunol 1998; 16: 27- 55.

Arnett F, Edworthy S, Bloch D. The American Rheumatism Association 1987 revised criteria for the classification of rheumatoid arthritis. Arthritis Rheum 1988; 31:315-324.

Ang DC, Choi H, Kroenke K, Wolfe F. (2005) Comorbid depression is an independent risk factor for mortality in patients with rheumatoid arthritis. J Rheumatol 32:1013–9.

Appelboom T, de Boelpaepe C, Ehrlich GE, Famaey JP. Rubens and the question of antiquity of rheumatoid arthritis. JAMA1981 Feb 6; 245(5): 483-6.

Becker N, Sjogren P, Bech P, et al: Treatment outcome of chronic non-malignant pain patients managed in a Danish multidisciplinary pain centre compared to general practice: a randomised controlled trial. Pain 2000; 84:203-211.
Bechterev VM. Ankylosing rigidity of the spine as a distinct condition (in Russian). Vrach ("Physician"), St Petersburg; 1892.
Bjarnason I, Hayllar J, Macpherson A, et al. Side effects of nonsteroidal antiinflammatory drugs on the small and large intestine in humans. Gastroenterology 1993; 104:1832-1837.
Boyle AC. The scientific approach. Rheumatology 1954;2: 75-80
Brown GK and Nicassio PM. Development of a questionnaire for the assessment of active and passive coping strategies in chronic pain patients. Pain1987; 31: 53-64.
Calin A. "Ankylosing spondilitis". Clinics in Rheumatic Diseases 1985; 11: 41–60.
Cannon DS, Tiffany ST, Coon H, Scholand MB, McMahon WM, Leppert MF. The PHQ-9 as a brief assessment of lifetime major depression. Psychol Assess 2007; 19: 247-51.
Cornelis F. Susceptibility genes in rheumatoid arthritis. In: Goronzy JJ, Weyand CM (eds). Rheumatoid Arthritis. Basal, Switzerland: Karger, 2000; pp 1-16.
Creed F, Murphy S, Jayson MV. Measurement of psychiatric disorder in RA. J Psychosom Res 1990; 34: 79-87.
Davis, J.M., Wang, Z., Janicak, P.G. (1993) Psychopharmacol. Bull., 29, 175-81.
Dequeker J. Arthritis in Flemish paintings (1400-1700). Br Med J. 1977 May 7;1(6070):1203-5.
Delzel E. Friends for life. Arthritis Foundation 2011; May 97-99.
Dequeker J, Rico H. Rheumatoid arthritis-like deformities in an early 16th-century painting of the Flemish-Dutch school. JAMA.1992 Jul 8;268(2):249-51.
Demir H, Kelestimur F, Tunc M, Kirnap M, Ozugul Y. Hypothalamo-pituitary-adrenal axis and growth hormone axis in patients with rheumatoid arthritis. Scand J Rheumatol 1999;28:41–6.
Department of Health UK. Delivering race equality. A framework for action. London: Department of Health; 2003
Dickens C, Creed F. The burden of depression in patients with rheumatoid arthritis. Rheumatology 2001; 40:1327–30.
Diener E, Sue EM, Lucas RE, Smith HL. Subjectiuve well-being: three decades of progress. Psychol Bull. 1999;125:276-302.
Dieppe P (1988). "Did Galen describe rheumatoid arthritis?". Annals of the Rheumatic Diseases 47: 84–87.
Dieudé P and Cornélis F. Genetic basis of rheumatoid arthritis. Joint Bone Spine. Volume 72, Issue 6, December 2005, 520-526.
Doll R. The scientific approach. Rheumatology 1954;2:85-9.
Dunbar F. Emotions and Bodily Changes. New York; 1954.
Dunkin JJ & Amano SS. Psychological Changes with Normal Aging. In: Kaplan & Saddock's comprehensive textbook of psychiatry - 8th ed. Philadelphia; 2005.
Dunlop DD, Lyons JS, Manheim LM, Song J, Chang RW. Arthritis and heart disease as risk factors for major depression: the role of functional limitation. Med Care 2004; 42: 502-11.
Durkheim E, in Simpson G trans. The Division of Labor in Society. Glencoe, IL: Free Press, 1949.

Edwards JCW, Cambridge G, Abrahams VM. Do self-perpetuating B lymphocytes drive human autoimmune disease? Immunology 1999; 97: 1868– 96.

El-Miedany YM, El-Rasheed AH Is anxiety a more common disorder than depression in RA? Joint Bone Spine 2002; 69: 300-6.

Emery P, Gough A. Why early arthritis clinics? Rheumatology 1991;30:241-4.

Emery P, Symmonds D. What is early rheumatoid arthritis? Definition and diagnosis. Balliere's Clinical Rheumatology 1997; 11:13-26

Endler N, Parker D. The multidimensional assessment of coping: a critical evaluation. J Pers Soc Psychol 1990; 58: 844–54.

Entezami P, Fox DA, Clapham PJ, Chung KC. Historical perspective on theetiology of RA.. Hand Clin. 2011 Feb;27(1):1-10.

Eyring H., Dougherty T. F, "Molecular Mechanisms in Inflammation and Stress,". Am. Scientist(1955), 43, 457.

Espinosa-Morales R, Escalante A. Diagnostic confusion caused by hepatitis C: hemochromatosis presenting as rheumatoid arthritis. J Rheumatol 1998; 25(12):2459-63.

Felson D, Lavalie MP, et al. The Prosorba® column for treatment of refractory rheumatoid arthritis: a randomized, double-blind, SHAM-controlled trial. Arthritis Rheum. 1999; 42: 2153-59.

Fifield J, Tennen H, Reisine S, McQuillan J. Depression and the long-term risk of pain, fatigue, and disability in patients with rheumatoid arthritis. Arthritis Rheum 1998; 41: 1851-7.

Fleischmann RM, Schechtman J, Bennett R, Handel ML, Burmester GR, Tesser J, Modafferi D, Poulakos J, Sun G. Anakinra, a recombinant human interleukin-1 receptor antagonist (r-metHuIL-1ra), in patients with rheumatoid arthritis: a large, international, multicenter, placebo-controlled trial. Arthritis Rheum 2003; 48: 927–34.

Folkman S, Lazarus RS. An analysis of coping in a middle-aged community sample. J Health Soc Behav 1980; 21: 219–39.

Frank RG, Beck NC, Parker JC, Kashani JH, Elliott TR, Haut AE, et al. Depression in RA. J Rheumatol 1988; 15: 920-5.

Garrod AB. Treatise on nature and treatment of gout and rheumatic gout. London: Walton and Moberly, 1859.

Gillespie C, Nemeroff CB. Corticotropin-Releasing Factor and the Psychobiology of Early-Life Stress. Current Directions in Psychological Science, 2007, Volume 16 Issue 2, Pages 85 - 89

Goetzl RZ, Long SR, Ozminkowski RJ, Hawkins K, Wang S, Lynch W. Health, absence, disability, and presenteeism cost estimates of certain physical and mental health conditions affective U.S. employers. J Occup Environ Med 2004; 46: 398-412.

Hansen MS, Fink P, Frydenberg M, Oxhoj M, Sondergaard L and Munk -Jorgensen. P. Mental disorders among internal medical inpatients: prevalence, detection, and treatment status. J Psychosom Res 2001; 50:199-204

Hansen MS, Fink P, Frydenberg M, Oxhoj. Use of Health Services, Mental Illness, and Self-Rated Disability and Health in Medical Inpatients. Psychosomatic Medicine (2002); 64(4):668-675

Harbuz MS, Jessop DS. Is there a defect in cortisol production in rheumatoid arthritis? Rheumatology 1999;38:298–302.

Harbuz M. Neuroendocrinology of autoimmunity. Int Rev Neurobiol 2002;52:133–61.

Harrison B, Symmons D, Barret E, Silman A. The performance of the 1987 ARA classification criteria for rheumatoid arthritis in a population based cohort of patients with early inflammatory polyarthritis. J Rheumatol 1998; 25:2324-2330.

Horai R, Saijo S, Tanioka H, Nakae S, Sudo K, Okahara A, Ikuse T, Asano M, Iwakura Y. Development of chronic inflammatory arthropathy resembling rheumatoid arthritis in interleukin 1 receptor antagonist-deficient mice. J Exp Med 2000; 191: 313– 20.

Hurwicz M, Berkanovic E. The stress process in rheumatoid arthritis. J Rheumatol1993; 20: 1836–44.

Jensen M, Turner J, Romano J, Karoly P. Coping with chronic pain: a critical review of the literature. Pain 1991 Dec; 47(3):249-83.

Jessop DS, Richards LJ, Harbuz MS. Effects of stress on inflammatory autoimmune disease: destructive or protective? Stress 2005

Jobanputra P. Cellular responses to human chondrocytes: absence of allogeneic responses in the presence of HLA-DR and ICAM-1. Clin Exp Immunol 1992; 90:336-3

Jobanputra P, Davidson F, Graham S, O'Neill H, Simmonds P, Yap L. High frequency of parvoirus B19 in patients tested for rheumatoid factor. BMJ 1995; 311:1542.

Kane, S. Nonsteroidal anti-inflammatory drugs are associated with an increased risk of disease activity in inflammatory bowel disease. Evidence-Based Gastroenterology: Volume 2(1)February 2001pp 20-21

Katon W, Ciechanowski P: Impact of major depression on chronic medical illness. J Psychosom Res (2002);53:859-63

Katz PP, Yelin EH. Prevalence and correlates of depressive symptoms among persons with RA.. J Rheumatol 1993; 20: 790-6.

Kannabikh Y. History of Psychiatry (in Russian). Russ. Ed., Moscow 1925; 492.

Kelly BD. Globalisation and psychiatry. Advances in Psychiatric Treatment 2003; vol. 9, 464-474.

Kiss, JE. Use of Staphylococcal Protein A (SPA) Immunoadsorption in Rheumatoid Arthritis and Immune Thrombocytopenic Purpura , August 2000, Transfusion Medicine Update, Institute For Transfusion Medicine.

Kremer JM, Westhovens R, Leon M, Di Giorgio E, Alten R, Steinfeld S, Russell A, Dougados M, Emery P, Nuamah IF, et al.: Treatment of rheumatoid arthritis by selective inhibition of T-cell activation with fusion protein CTLA4Ig. N Engl J Med 2003, 349:1907-1915.

Krohne, H W. Handbook of Coping.1996, New York: Wiley.

Kvein TK. Epidemiology and burden of illness of rheumatoid arthritis. Pharmacoeconomics 2004; 22(2 Suppl): 1-12

LaFramboise TD. Implications of research with Native American adolescents: For current and future practice. Washington, D. C. Symposium at the annual meetings of the American Psychological Association publication 2000.

Lefebvre JC, Keefe FJ. Memory for pain: The relationship of pain catastrophizing to the recall of daily rheumatoid arthritis pain. Clin J Pain 2002; 18:56–63.

Leventhal H, Meyer D, Nerenz D: The common sense representation of illness danger. In Medical psychology. Volume 2. Edited by: Raceman S. Elmsford, NY: Pergamon; 1980.

Levesque J, Eugene F, Joanette Y, et al. Neural circuitry underlying voluntary suppression of sadness. Biol Psychiatry 2003;53:502–510

Li X, Gignac MA, Anis AH. The indirect costs of arthritis resulting from unemployment, reduced performance, and occupational changes while at work. Med Care 2006; 44: 304-10.

López-Larrea C, González S, Martinez-Borra J. The role of HLA-B27 polymorphism and molecular mimicry in spondylarthropathy. Mol Med Today 1998 Dec;4(12):540-9.

Murray, C.J., Lopez, A.D. (1997) Lancet, 349, 1498-1504.

NICE guidelines, 2002. Assessment report for etanercept and infliximab for rheumatoid arthritis.

Nishimura K, Sugiyama D, Kogata Y, Tsuji G, Nakazawa T, Kawano S, et al. Meta-analysis: Diagnostic Accuracy of Anti-Cyclic Citrullinated Peptide Antibody and Rheumatoid Factor for Rheumatoid Arthritis. Ann Intern Med 2007;146:797-808.

Ohsugi Y, Kishimoto T. The recombinant humanized anti-IL-6 receptor antibody tocilizumab, an innovative drug for the treatment of rheumatoid arthritis. Expert Opin Biol Ther. 2008 May;8(5):669-81. PubMed PMID: 18407769.

Ollier W, Winchester R. The germline and somatic genetic basis for rheumatoid arthritis. In: Theofilopoulos AN (ed). Genes and Genetics of Autoimmunity. Basel, Switzerland: Karger, 1999; pp 166-193.

Olsen, N. Alternatives to methotrexate for infliximab combination therapy in rheumatoid arthritis, Nature Clinical Practice Rheumatology (2006) 2, 472-473

Parke A.L and Buchanan W.W. Sjögren's syndrome: History, clinical and pathological features. Inflammopharmacology Volume 6, Number 4 / December, 1998: 271-287

Permin H, Stahl P, Skov S, Norn A, Geisler R et al. Possible Role of Histamine in Rheumatoid Arthritis. Treatment with Cimetidine and Mepyramine Allergy (1981) 36 (6), 435–436

Ruiz GV, Jobanputra P, Burls A, Cabello JB, Gálvez Muñoz JG, Saiz Cuenca ES, Fry-Smith A. Certolizumab pegol (CDP870) for rheumatoid arthritis in adults. Cochrane Database Syst Rev. 2011 Feb 16;(2):CD007649. Review.

Scharloo M, Kaptein AA, Weinman J, Hazes JM, Willems LN, Bergman W, Rooijmans HG. Illness perceptions, coping and functioning in patients with rheumatoid arthritis, chronic obstructive pulmonary disease and psoriasis. J Psychosom Res 1998 May; 44(5):573-85.

Schwarzer, R., & Schwarzer, C. A critical survey of coping instruments. In M. Zeidner & N. S. Endler (Eds.), Handbook of coping: Theory, research and applications 1996:pp. 107-132. New York: Wiley.

Seavey WG, Kurata JH, Cohen RD. Risk factors for incident self-reported arthritis in a 20 year followup of the Alameda County Study Cohort. J Rheumatol 2003; 30: 2103-11.

Seldin MF, Amos CI, Ward R, Gregerson PK. The genetics revolution and the assault on rheumatoid arthritis. Arthritis Rheum 1999;42:1071-1079.

Selye H et al 1944 Hormonal production of arthritis. Journal of the American Medical Association 124; 201

Selye H 1949 Further studies concerning the participation of the adrenal cortex in the pathogenesis of arthritis. British Medical Journal 2; 1129

Selye H 1950 The Physiology and Pathology of Exposure to Stress, 1st edition. Acta inc Montreal.

Short CL. The antiquity of rheumatoid arthritis. Arthritis Rheum. 1974 May-Jun; 17(3): 193-205.

Silman A. Epidemiology and rheumatic diseases. In: Maddison P, Isenberg D, Woo P, Glass D, editors. Oxford Textbook of Rheumatology. Oxford: Oxford University Press, 1998: 811-828.

Simon GE, Goldberg DP, Von Korff M, Ustun TB. Understanding cross-national differences in depression prevalence. Psychol Med. 2002;32(4):585-594.

Simon-Thomas, J., Kamman, T.J., Silverman, P.S., & Rothman, W. Child Coping Moderates the Effects of Interparental Conflict on Child Adjustment. Poster session presented at the Society for Research in Child Development Biennial Meeting, Minneapolis, Minnesota, (2001) 19-22.

Singh JA, Noorbaloochi S, Singh G. Golimumab for rheumatoid arthritis. Cochrane Database Syst Rev. 2010 Jan 20;(1):CD008341. Review.

Slattery JM, Kromer AM, Kifer S, Miller C. Gender-specific use of natural coping strategies and their perceived effectiveness. Boston: Eastern Psychological Association annual meeting publication 2002.

Sleath B, Chewning B, de Vellis BM, Weinberger M, de Vellis RF, Tudor G, Beard A. Communication about depression during rheumatoid arthritis patient visits Arthritis Care and Research 2008Volume 59 Issue 2: 186-191

Soderlin MK, Hakala M, Nieminen P. Anxiety and depression in a community-based rheumatoid arthritis population. Scand J Rheumatol 2000; 29: 177-83.

Stastny P. Association of the B-cell alloantigen DRw4 with rheumatoid arthritis. N. Engl J Med 1978; 298:869-871.

Still GF. On a form of joint disease in children. Med Chir Trans 1897; 80:47–59.

Timonen M, Villo K, Hakko H, Sarkioja T, Ylikulju M, Meyer-Rochow VB, et al. Suicides in persons suffering from rheumatoid arthritis. Rheumatology (Oxford) 2003; 42: 287-91.

Turner CD 1955 General Endocrinology, 2nd edition. WB Saunders Co. Philadelphia

Vali FM, Walkup J. Combined medical and psychological symptoms: impact on disability and health care utilization of patients with arthritis. Med Care 1998; 36: 1073-84.

VanDyke MM, Parker JC, Smarr KL, Hewett JE, Johnson GE, Slaughter JR, et al. Anxiety in RA. 2004;51: 408-12.

Van Gaalen FA, Linn-Rasker SP, Van Venrooij WJ, et al. Autoantibodies to cyclic citrullinated peptides predict progression to rheumatoid arthritis in patients with undifferentiated arthritis: a prospective cohort study. Arthritis Rheum 2004;50:709-15.

Wynn Parry CB, Nichols PJR, Lewis NR. Meniscectomy: a review of 1,723 cases. Rheumatology 1958;4:201-15

Zaphiropoulos G, Burry HC. Depression in rheumatoid arthritis. Ann Rheum Dis 1974; 33: 132-5.

12

Sexual Health and Intimate Relationships in Rheumatoid Arthritis

Kristina Areskoug Josefsson[1] and Ulrika Öberg[2]
[1]Lund University, Samrehab, Värnamo Hospital,
[2]Futurum – Academy for Healthcare
Sweden

1. Introduction

The aim of this chapter is to describe how rheumatoid arthritis (RA) can affect sexual health and intimate relationships negatively and to explore some possible ways to improve sexual health for persons with RA. To introduce the subject the chapter will begin with a short introduction to the term sexual health and how chronic illness can affect sexual health. Thereafter follows a description of how RA affects sexual health and intimate relationships, current research in this field by the authors, suggestions on how to improve sexual health and intimate relationships for persons with RA, and finally new research in the area and conclusions.

2. Background

According to World Health Organization (WHO) (World Health Organization 2006) sexual health is a state of physical, emotional, mental and social well-being in relation to sexuality. Sexual health incorporates a positive and respectful approach to sexuality and sexual relationships, and includes the possibility of having pleasurable and safe sexual experiences, free of coercion, discrimination and violence. To have a good sexual health is not only absence of sexual diseases, but is connected to self-esteem, intimate relationships and general quality of life. Sexuality has a multidimensional nature consisting of biologic, affective, cognitive and motivational parts. During the lifespan, sexuality is an integrated part of life. A good sexual health is to many people an important factor in order to achieve a desired quality of life, but the essence of what is good sexual health differs between individuals. A description of what a good sexual health is can also differ during the lifespan for the same person due to life circumstances. According to a recent study one of the two main predictors of global life satisfaction is satisfaction with sexual life (Tasiemski, Angiaszwili-Biedna, and Wilski 2009). A person´s sexual health affects their intimate relationship. A poor sexual health can also affect the person's view of the possibilities of finding a partner to share an intimate relationship with.

Chronic illness affects the patient physically, psychologically, socially and in their relationship with their partner.. The impact of a chronic disease on sexual health can be due to indirect factors influencing sexual function such as altering self image, fatigue, pain and dependency (Basson and Schultz 2007). Sexual health is one of the domains that can be affected by chronic illness, such as RA. Effects of chronic conditions on sexual health is often under diagnosed (Bitzer et al. 2007), which can prolong or worsen the difficulties. Sexual health is included in the International Classification of Functioning, Disability and Health (ICF) (*International Classification of Functioning, Disability and Health.* 2001) within two separate areas, sexual functions (body functions) and intimate relationships (activity and participation). The ICF core sets for rheumatoid arthritis (Stucki et al. 2004) acknowledge both areas as important since they can be affected by the disease. However, since sexual health is a complex and broad field there are other components of the ICF, such as pain, sleep, physical functions, psychological functions etc., that are of importance when exploring sexual health. The importance of sexual health is at the same level for persons with a chronic disease as for healthy persons (Kedde et al. 2010) Therefore sexual health must be acknowledged by health care professionals. This is especially important since people with decreased sexual pleasure due to physical impairment can experience a decreased overall wellbeing which can be very distressing (Hull 2008).

The prevalence of RA is approximately 0.5-1% and the disease affects the life of the persons with RA in many different areas during life. There is a gender division for RA, with more women than men getting the disease (Englund et al. 2010). RA is characterised by joint swelling, joint tenderness and destruction of synovial joints (Aletaha et al. 2010). It is a chronic inflammatory disease and common symptoms are pain, fatigue, limited function, and decrease in physical capacity. The criteria for RA were revised in 2010 in order to increase focus on earlier stages of the disease (Aletaha et al. 2010). The most important treatment outcomes for persons with RA are reduction of pain, disability, fatigue and improved general wellness (Carr et al. 2003). All of these outcomes are connected to sexual health. The commonality of sexual health problems for persons with RA makes it assumable that sexual health is addressed routinely by health professionals within rheumatology and in patient reported outcome measurements. However, neither standard patient reported outcome measurements nor communication about sexual health is common within the field of rheumatology. Commonly used patient reported outcome measurements for RA such as Stanford Health Assessment Questionnaire (HAQ) (Fries et al. 1980) and Arthritis Impact Measurement Scales 2 (AIMS2) (Meenan et al. 1992) do not include questions about sexual health and intimate relationships. In the revised version of the HAQ, the Multi-Dimensional Health Assessment Questionnaire (MD-HAQ) one simple question about effect on sexuality by the disease is included (Pincus, Sokka, and Kautiainen 2005). If the MD-HAQ was used more often it might enhance the communication about sexual health in the clinical situation. Unfortunately MD-HAQ is only available in a few languages which limits the use of the instrument both in research and clinical work.

Generic outcome measurements are often used for patients with RA, such as Short Form 36 (SF 36) (Ware and Sherbourne 1992) and the EQ5D (EuroQol--a new facility for the measurement of health-related quality of life. The EuroQol Group 1990). These instruments are also lacking questions concerning sexual health. The lack of inclusion of sexual health and intimate relationships in the patient reported outcome measurements is a principal reason why the subject rarely is brought up in clinical meetings between persons with RA and health professionals. By using patient report outcome measures that include sexual health for patients with RA the communication about sexual health between health professionals and patients might be easier to start and perhaps increase.

Earlier research concerning communication about sexual health issues with persons with RA, indicates that this rarely appears in the meeting between the person with RA and health professionals (Abdel-Nasser and Ali 2006; Akkas 2010; Josefsson and Gard 2010; Hill, Bird, and Thorpe 2003; Rkain et al. 2006). Possible reasons for this will be discussed further in this chapter. Persons with RA can also be unaware of the fact that their reduced sexual health can be due to RA and therefore patient information about sexual health and RA is important. Ways of informing patients are by using material that often is available from organizations for persons with RA, both on-line and/or by leaflets. There are also on-line help-lines for persons with RA, where questions about sexual health have been presented (Richter et al. 2011). It is possible that further use of such information including sexual health might assist the communication concerning sexual health between partners and perhaps also between persons with RA and health professionals.

3. How does RA affect sexual health and intimate relationships?

Sexual health difficulties due to RA can include decreased sexual arousal, decreased sexual desire and decreased satisfaction (Abdel-Nasser and Ali 2006; Karlsson, Berglin, and Wallberg-Jonsson 2006). The reasons for reduced sexual health often include both psychological and physical components. These factors can be experienced in combination or separately and they might change during the course of the disease. Psychological responses to chronic illness can include feelings of loss of independence, disrupted self-image, depression and anxiety (Basson and Schultz 2007). The physical components can include pain, fatigue, reduced functional ability, reduced strength and mobility (Hill, Bird, and Thorpe 2003). Both the psychological and the physical factors interrupt and affect sexual health in several ways. Problems before sexual activities can be due to decreased sexual arousal and/or negative body image (Gutweniger et al. 1999). Decreased sexual desire is reported for 50-60% of patients with RA (Abdel-Nasser and Ali 2006). Sexual health difficulties during sexual activities can be pain and/or decreased mobility. After sexual activities, persons with RA can experience sexual health problems such as decreased satisfaction and increased pain. There can also be an altering of the sexual activities such as wanting to reach orgasm quickly, because prolonged sexual activity increases both pain and fatigue (Elst et al. 1984).

Intimate relationships can be affected negatively by RA and there has been some studies concerning the situation of the partner of a person with RA according to the persons with RA (Rkain et al. 2006; Matheson, Harcourt, and Hewlett 2010; Bermas et al. 2000). Factors that can influence the intimate relationship of a person living with a chronic illness are: if the partner reacts negatively to illness; fear of rejection from the partner; lack of information about sexual rehabilitation; and if there is a cultural belief that persons with illness should not be engaged in sexual activities (Basson and Schultz 2007; Clayton and Ramamurthy 2008). There is also research showing that RA has a negative impact on the sexual relationship according to spouses of individuals with RA (van Lankveld et al. 2004; Lapsley et al. 2002). Reasons for this can be psychological distress and the need for social support within the relationship.

There is some research concerning how various medical treatments affect sexual health, but it is far from complete. Therefore there is limited information concerning the effect of common medication for RA on sexual health. Corticostereoids are often used for persons with RA and they can cause weight gain and "moon face" (i.e. edematous appearance of the face), which can be perceived as ugly and unpleasant by the person taking the medication (Clayton and Ramamurthy 2008). Feelings of being unattractive affect sexual health negatively. Another common medication for persons with RA are non steroidal anti-inflammatory drugs (NSAIDs). NSAIDs have a negative effect on sexual desire and sexual arousal (Clayton and Ramamurthy 2008). There is a lack of research concerning the effects of newer Disease Modifying Anti Rheumatic Drugs (DMARDs) on sexual health. However, older DMARDs, such as methotrexate and sulphasalazine, have a known negative effect on erection (van Berlo et al. 2007).

Negative impact on sexual health is common for persons with RA. Previous research has shown that sexual health is decreased for 36-70% of persons with RA (Areskoug-Josefsson and Oberg 2009). Studies have been performed in different cultural contexts, but the problems remain similar, e.g. decreased sexual satisfaction, pain during sexual activities and diminished sexual desire (Yoshino and Uchida 1981; Abdel-Nasser and Ali 2006; van Berlo et al. 2007; van Lankveld et al. 2004; Josefsson and Gard 2010). These problems affect individuals with RA in Europe, U.S.A., Asia and Africa (Yoshino and Uchida 1981; Abdel-Nasser and Ali 2006; van Berlo et al. 2007; Rkain et al. 2006; Hill, Bird, and Thorpe 2003). Persons with RA often experience a change in the importance of sexual health during the lifespan since the importance decreases with increased age (Helland, Dagfinrud, and Kvien 2008; Hill, Bird, and Thorpe 2003; Abdel-Nasser and Ali 2006; van Berlo et al. 2007).

Decreased satisfaction with sexual life has been shown to be persistent during the first two years of RA, which indicates that the problems remain even after control of disease activity has been achieved (Karlsson, Berglin, and Wallberg-Jonsson 2006). Karlsson et al also showed that persons living with RA for a longer period of time had worse sexual health. The reasons for a decrease in sexual health also include fatigue, pain, stiffness, limited physical capacity, joint mobility and depression (Kraaimaat et al. 1996; Yoshino and Uchida 1981; Helland, Dagfinrud, and Kvien 2008; le Gallez 1993). Several of the mentioned symptoms occur in combination which can further increase the difficulties. An example of this is decreased functional ability, reduced hip mobility and fatigue, which all have a negative effect on sexual health because they contribute to fatigue (Ibn Yacoub et al. 2011). The different symptoms due to RA that have a negative impact on sexual health will be described briefly.

Pain is the major reason why persons with RA seek medical care, and pain is strongly associated with functional status, anxiety, depression (Sokka 2005) and quality of life (Garip, Eser, and Bodur 2010). The experiences and the intensity of pain can differ during different stages of the disease, but for many persons with RA chronic pain is an everyday problem. Chronic pain can in itself lead to decrease of sexual health, and sexual activities can increase pain (Ruehlman, Karoly, and Taylor 2008). Thereby persons with high levels of pain might avoid sexual activities in order to lessen the risk of exacerbating their pain. The avoidance of sexual activities can be shown as less amount of sexual activities, or shortening the sexual activity time wise, as well as a complete avoidance of engagement in sexual activities.

Concerning joint mobility, whilst it is mainly hip mobility that is problematic for women with RA during sexual intercourse (Abdel-Nasser and Ali 2006), involvement of other joints can also affect a person´s sexual life. For example, inflammatory joints in the hands and limited hand function can reduce the ability to caress one´s partner. Pain in the hands can lead to avoidance of holding hands, which can limit the romantic side of an intimate relationship. The enjoyment of being caressed can also be reduced due to pain when being touched (Josefsson and Gard 2010). Hugging can also be difficult if there is inflammation or decreased joint mobility in the shoulders. Those limitations are rarely discussed when discussing sexual health, but it is important to acknowledge that a good sexual health includes more than sexual intercourse.

Many persons with RA consider morning stiffness to be problematic and the level of morning stiffness is correlated with pain and physical capacity (Khan et al. 2009). Morning stiffness in itself can be problematic for intimate relationships if a person prefers to engage in sexual activities in the morning when fatigue can be less troublesome.

A major consequence of RA is limited physical capacity, which is connected to a number of symptoms including pain, limited mobility, stiffness and fatigue. Another reason for limited physical capacity among persons with RA might be the attitude towards physical activities for persons with RA. Until a few decades ago persons with RA were recommended not to engage in physical activities (Reinseth et al. 2010), and this inactivity decreased their physical capacity even further.

Having to cope with a chronic disease, and its´ consequences, can cause low mood, anxiety and depression. All of these symptoms can be present for persons with RA and can affect their sexual health negatively. Depression is often associated with increased fatigue, pain and anxiety (Gettings 2010). Persons with RA can experience reduced psychological wellbeing, even if they are not suffering from depression, due to the effects of RA on their daily life.

Fatigue has been shown to affect quality of life as well as psychosocial aspects of life for persons with RA. Fatigue interferes with a person´s ability to perform daily activities of life and this symptom is present in 40-80% of persons with RA (Ibn Yacoub et al. 2011). Among persons with RA, many of them believe that reduction of fatigue should be a major treatment aim (Pollard, Choy, and Scott 2005). There is a link between disease activity and fatigue, showing that persons in remissions have reduced feelings of fatigue according to their score on fatigue scales (Ibn Yacoub et al. 2011). However, the effect of the biologics on fatigue induced by RA is small (Chauffier et al. 2011), indicating that the problem of fatigue remains despite the development of this new class of drugs.

Many persons with RA also have secondary Sjögren´s syndrome (Coll et al. 1987), a chronic disease that can decrease a person´s sexual health both indirectly and directly. Indirect effects can be connected with increased fatigue (Ibn Yacoub et al. 2011). Direct negative effects on sexual health are due to Sjögren's syndromes effects on exocrine glands, which leads to vaginal and mouth dryness. Thus persons with Sjögren´s syndrome can feel discomfort when kissing and can also experience problems with painful intercourse (Tristano 2009). This, of course, affects sexual health negatively. In a majority of the research about RA and sexual health, the prevalence of Sjögrens syndrome in the investigated group is not reported, which must be seen as a limitation of these studies.

4. Current research

In order to explore women's experiences of sexual health when living with RA and their experiences of physiotherapy in this context, a research plan of four studies was prepared. Two of the completed studies are discussed in this chapter.

The first study was a qualitative interview study. The study consisted of interviews with ten women with RA on their views of how their sexual health was affected by RA and how their sexual health could be improved (Josefsson and Gard 2010). The subjects ("informants") varied in age (42-66 years old), illness duration (2-31 years) and HAQ levels (0-2.13). The material from the interviews was analysed with a phenomenological approach according to Giorgi (Giorgi 1985; Giorgi 2000). This model of analyses contains the following steps:

1. Reading through the material to get a general sense of the whole statement.

2. Re-reading of the material to discriminate meaning units from a holistic perspective and to focus on the experience of sexual health when living with RA.
3. Going through the meaning units and expressing deepened insight contained in them more directly.
4. Synthesizing of the transformed meaning units into a consistent statement regarding the subjects' experience.

The following themes emerged from the analysis of the material: Sexual health - physical and psychological dimensions; and, Impacts of RA and Possibilities to increase sexual health - does physiotherapy make a difference?

The informants' view of sexual health showed individual views but all the informants believed sexual health to be complex and composed of several different physical and psychological factors. Described factors, such as, caresses, feelings of closeness and attractiveness, and affectionate attitudes towards the partner, as well as sexual activities and sexual intercourse were included in their view of sexual health. This broad perception of sexual health by the informants is in line with the definition of sexual health by WHO (Defining sexual health. Report of a technical consultation on sexual health, 28-31 January 2002, Geneva 2006).

"Sexual health is close companionship, to be there for each other. Sexual health is also touching each other in a loving way."

The informants also included feelings that arise in sexual situations and intimate relationships into their description of sexual health.

"Sexual health is being together and caring for someone. Sexual health gives happiness and joy."

Some of the informants described their views of what sexual health is and at the same time how it was affected by RA. Sexual health was limited for some of the informants, for example, parts of what they described as sexual health was accepted (e.g. closeness) and other parts were rejected (e.g. sexual intercourse).

They also believed that their view of sexual health and its importance changed during the lifespan. This could be due to other changes in life and to age.

"You do revalue things. I wouldn´t have answered the same way 10 years ago as I do now."

An example of specific sexual problems mentioned by the informants was the difficulties that can come after having joint surgery.

"But then it was my first hip replacement, well... It was so hard to come back after that, because I was so afraid that something would happen. I was so lucky, so I had both hips done at the same time."

The results of this study show that the informant's sexual health was negatively affected by RA due to pain, fatigue, decreased joint mobility and anxiety. Experienced negative emotions due to RA included anger, frustration, and fear of being abandoned by the partner. Fear of being left by the partner might be considered as a threat and cause anxiety, which can further decrease sexual health.

"And then it´s like this, if somebody touches me, it hurts."

The informants also linked RA to decreased sexual arousal and sexual satisfaction.

"The arousal is gone and then you know that it is going to hurt when you try (to have intercourse). It first feels good, but then you know it is going to hurt and you think, should I tell, should I not? And afterwards it will hurt even more."

"The sexual satisfaction is not like before. Definitely not. I don´t know what has happened."

The problems with sexual health due to RA also affected the informants´ intimate relationship with their partner. Some of the informants thought that their relationships had changed, but that they had a mutual understanding with their partner about how RA had affected their sexual life. While others felt that their relationships suffered due to the sexual health problems. That sexual health should be free of coercion is stated by WHO and was not thought by the authors to be an issue for this group of informants, but still there were mentions of feelings of pressure to have sexual intercourse and also a direct mention that physical force should not be involved in sexual activities and that sexual activities should be voluntary. Perhaps coercion within intimate relationships for women with RA is more common than for other women and this is a field for future research.

"I´m tired. And then it is all of the medication that lowers the sexual arousal so much. I have talked to my husband about it. That it is like, nothing. And still, I feel sorry for my husband… you have to do it just so he won´t get hysterical. Yes, it has changed."

A majority of the informants had experienced several of those problems. The informants thought that improving sexual health could be done by removing or decreasing the mentioned problems.

"Take away the tiredness!"

"If I didn´t have the pain."

Suggestions on how this could be done were improved partner communication and physiotherapy.

"So I think it is up to each person, but I´m sure that a lot of people would want someone to talk to. Except the partner, that you might not dare to talk with. Or you might think is embarrassing. If you have a conversation with someone about your sexual life, perhaps it is easier to come home and talk to your partner after that."

Physiotherapy was considered to improve sexual health via pain reductive treatment, and exercise interventions by improving physical function, joint mobility, and fatigue. Physiotherapy for persons with RA is often directed towards increasing the level of physical activity and it is important that physiotherapists appreciate that, according to patient's feedback, this can also be used to improve sexual health.

"Physiotherapy is good to be able to keep mobile and strong and to give feelings of satisfaction. By physical exercise you feel pleased with your body. Otherwise you lose your desire…"

Experiences of positive feelings during physiotherapy and how those positive emotions can be of importance and enhance the effects of the physiotherapy interventions have been investigated (Gard 2000) but needs further exploration before being adopted for routine clinical use.

The results of the study lead to the conclusion, that physiotherapy can play an active role in improving sexual health for patients with RA according to the informants.

To further increase knowledge of the impact of RA on sexual health and how physiotherapy could affect it, a larger, second study was performed to complement the interview study (Josefsson & Gard, in print). This study was based on a new questionnaire, which was derived from the themes in the interview study and from earlier studies in the field (Josefsson and Gard 2010; Hill, Bird, and Thorpe 2003). Both men and women were included in this study so that possible gender differences could be explored. The results of this study show that a large majority of the patients agreed that there were strong connections between sexual health and pain, stiffness, fatigue, and physical function. Body image was affected by RA, but the study showed that the person's body image could be positively as well as negatively influenced after the diagnosis of RA. Most other studies have only shown a negative influence on body image of RA (Gutweniger et al. 1999). Although one study showed that body image did not affect sexual relationships for persons with RA (le Gallez 1993). The differences concerning the effect on body image by RA indicates that further research should be performed to increase knowledge of the phenomena. The sexuality of both the partner and the patient was affected by RA and the level of strain on the partnership caused by RA was similar in this study to results found in other studies, where for example 35% experienced that RA had to put a strain on their partnership in the study by Hill et al (Hill, Bird, and Thorpe 2003; Matheson, Harcourt, and Hewlett 2010). This study also concluded that health professionals and their RA patients did not communicate about sexual health, which supports previous research in this field (Ryan and Wylie 2005; Hill, Bird, and Thorpe 2003). This result stresses the importance of having a strategy in order improve communication concerning how to bring up sexual health in meetings between patients and health professionals. Additionally, health professionals need to be trained in dealing with sexual issues and communication about sexual health (Ryan and Wylie 2005) and they need to be aware of how they can assist patients in improving their sexual health. Physiotherapists also need to be aware that, in order to give best possible care, they should recognize that pain, fatigue, decreased joint mobility and impaired physical capacity can affect the sexual health of RA patients.

5. How can sexual health be improved for persons with RA?

There is very little evidence that the inflammatory process of RA influences the ability to engage in sexual activities, instead the problems appear to occur due to the symptoms of the disease, such as fatigue and pain. In order to investigate possible methods for improving sexual health in persons with RA, a literature review was performed by Areskoug-Josefsson & Oberg (2009). The review showed that research aiming to improve sexual health for patients with RA is scarce and only a few studies include specific recommendations. These recommendations were physiotherapy and improved communication. Communication concerning sexual health needed to be improved both between partners and between patient and health professionals. If patients with RA and health professionals communicate about sexual health, the health professionals get a broader view of how the disease affects the patient's life. Health professionals might think that persons with chronic diseases have more important subjects to discuss than their sexual health, but this must be the choice of the patient and not of the health professional. Health professionals could also inform the persons with RA that optimal treatment of the disease may reduce the sexual difficulties (Perdriger, Solano, and Gossec 2010). It is not always easy for persons with chronic illness to verbalise their sexual problems and it is important that health professionals acknowledge this and have skills in communication about sexual health (Kedde et al. 2010). Improved communication about sexual health often includes giving information such as how sexual health can be affected by RA, and how sexual health can be improved. Information, communication and physiotherapy should not be used as single interventions to improve sexual health, but in combination, in order to cover the full scope of the problem (Fig 1).

5.1 Treatment models

All members of rehabilitation teams should be involved in discussing and working towards improving sexual health with RA patients (Haboubi and Lincoln 2003; Couldrick, Gaynor, and Cross 2010; Post et al. 2008). The studies performed by the authors show that physiotherapists are important for improving sexual health in RA patients, and the authors believe that each of the various team members should be involved to provide the best possible care for patients. All of the health care professionals that are involved in the care of a person with RA, have different competencies that in different ways can improve sexual health for persons with RA, depending on the type of sexual health problem that the individual has. The treatment models that will be brought up in this chapter are the role of physiotherapy to improve sexual health and increased communication and information about sexual health issues.

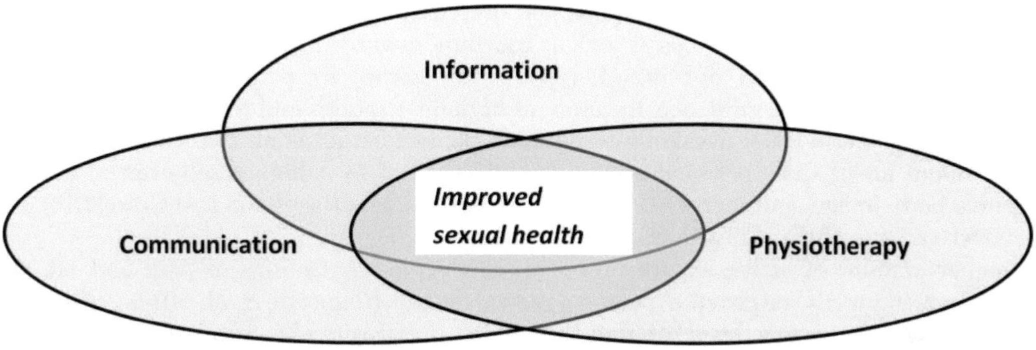

Fig. 1. Improvement of sexual health

5.1.1 The role of physiotherapy

In order to improve sexual health via physiotherapy the interventions must be individually assessed and the needs of the interventions can change during the disease. A person that has had RA for several years might have more joint difficulties and functional limitations, than a person with newly diagnosed RA. Physiotherapy is usually directed towards improving activities of daily living, dealing with specific symptoms, such as pain or limited joint mobility, and sexual relations should be included in this context (Hewlett et al. 2005). Physiotherapy for persons with RA often consist of mobility exercises, pain reductive treatment and physical activities. Those interventions are often combined and changed over time in order to have optimal effect. Included in physiotherapy interventions is information about joint protection and how to achieve a healthy life style. Due to lack of research there is limited evidence as to whether many physiotherapy interventions have a beneficial effect(Vliet Vlieland 2007). However, regular physical exercise and encouragement to increase physical activity have been proven to be effective in decreasing symptoms in persons with RA (Brodin et al. 2008). The described positive outcomes of regular physical activities are improved physical function including increased muscle strength and endurance, aerobic fitness, and joint range of motion, as well as reduction of pain and fatigue (Cairns and McVeigh 2009; Cooney et al. 2011). For example, RA patients who exercise on a regular basis have less fatigue and disabilities compared to non-exercisers (Lee et al. 2006). Those positive effects of physical activities and regular exercise can enhance sexual health since the mentioned outcomes are affecting sexual health (Hill, Bird, and Thorpe 2003; Josefsson and Gard 2010). Physical activities can be coached directly by the physiotherapist in 2-3 sessions/week or by homebased programs where coaching is done by phone or by follow-up visits at the physiotherapy clinic (Brodin et al. 2008).
Pain is a prioritized outcome for persons with RA and pain often affects sexual health negatively. Physiotherapy interventions aimed at pain reduction are common. The evidence of interventions such as TENS, acupuncture and massage is scarce due to few studies and

their poor methodological quality (Casimiro et al. 2002; Ying and While 2007; Cameron 2002). Despite the lack of evidence these interventions might be used and evaluated on the individual level with the aim to reduce pain. The interventions can also be aimed at improving sexual health; TENS could for example be used during sexual activities to reduce pain, but this also needs further research.

The level of physical activity can affect sexual health, since increased physical activity can improve the amount of sexual intimacy (Bortz and Wallace 1999; Post et al. 2008). Introduction of physical activities as well as coaching towards increased physical activity is a basic, but important part, of physiotherapy. Physiotherapy for persons with RA has been shown to improve self-confidence, the amount of daily activities and reduce and depression (Kavuncu and Evcik 2004; Areskoug-Josefsson 2006; Neuberger et al. 2007). When a person is confident about their physical ability this is reflected in a higher self-esteem, a more positive body image, and increased feelings of attractiveness (Josefsson and Gard 2010). All of which can affect sexual health in a positive way.

A higher amount of active leisure time activities decreases feelings of pain and fatigue, which can indirectly improve a person´s sexual health (Reinseth et al. 2010). And, not surprisingly, a person´s level of daily activities are positively correlated with sexual functioning (Monga et al. 1998), which implies the importance of encouraging persons with RA to adopt an active life in order to improve their sexual health. The level of physical fitness is also related to the level of sexual activities (Bortz and Wallace 1999), which is another indicator that it is important to involve physiotherapists and their expertise of coaching towards physical activity in rehabilitation for persons with RA. Physiotherapists regularly coach persons with RA towards being more physically active and to continue with physical activity after onset of the disease (Brodin et al. 2008), but the relation between sexual activity levels and physical activity levels shows that physical activity coaching should be done not only to improve physical fitness but also to improve sexual health.

Physiotherapy can also increase the choice of possible sexual intercourse positions by increasing joint mobility and muscle strength, and the patient's knowledge of their physical abilities. Different exercise positions that are involved in physiotherapy programs can inspire persons with RA to try new positions during sexual activities and encourage new sexual fantasies (Josefsson and Gard 2010). Examples of this could be exercises performed on all fours or exercises involving stabilization of pelvic region. Different coital positions put different levels of strain on joints and muscles. It is of value for physiotherapist to have a basic knowledge about this and to be able to answer questions of how joints and muscles are affected during sexual activities. Another key time for physiotherapists to work on and communicate about issues concerning sexual health is when patients have had joint surgery. Hip replacement surgery can of course affect positions during sexual activity. Similarly, shoulder surgery can affect hugging and caressing, as well as coital positions. Depending on the patient's preferences in their sexual life, their need for advice and their wish to communicate about sexual health differs, but the physiotherapist needs to be able to use their professional expertise concerning musculoskeletal issues, pain reduction and exercise interventions in order to provide the best care and information on sexual health matters.

6. Communication about sexual health

Knowledge and openness about sexual health issues are important for rheumatology health professionals (Helland et al. 2011) and must be attained if good communication about sexual health is to be established with RA patients. In order to do so the experiences and views of the persons with RA on how health professionals should communicate about sexual health need to be brought forward. When communicating about sexual issues the views of the persons with RA on possible ways to improve sexual health are important, since sexual health is a sensitive subject on which to communicate. The health professionals must be sensitive to how and if the person with RA wishes to discuss sexual health during clinical encounters. If knowledge and competence in communication about sexual health is lacking for health professionals, it is likely that sexual health will not be brought up, even if the person with RA wants to discuss it. The communication problems between health professionals and persons with chronic illness concerning sexual health have been brought forward in earlier research (McInnes 2003; Haboubi and Lincoln 2003). Health professionals within the field of rheumatology rarely have expertise in the field of sexual health, which can make them unsure of how it should be included in their professional role and if/how they should communicate about sexual health. However, it is important to find ways to communicate about sexual health, since ignoring these concerns may damage sexual health for persons with RA.

There are several possible reasons for the lack of discussion of sexual health by health professionals, such as: the sensitivity of the subject; the health professionals can be unsure on how to bring up the subject; being unsure of how they can support persons with RA having sexual health problems; and believing that somebody else in the health care team is responsible for discussing sexual health with patients (Couldrick, Gaynor, and Cross 2010; Stausmire 2004; Ryan and Wylie 2005; Bitzer et al. 2007). There can also be more practical reasons like lack of time or lack of privacy during the meeting between the patient and the health professional (Britto et al. 2000). One study (Haboubi and Lincoln 2003) examined the possible differences between different health care professionals concerning their ability to address sexual health with their patients. This study showed that all of the health professionals had similar reluctance in addressing the subject, but that physiotherapists and occupational therapists were the least likely to discuss sexual health with their patients (Haboubi and Lincoln 2003). The patients themselves might be unwilling to discuss sexual health, especially if they do not think that the health care professionals can offer any support (McInnes 2003; Bitzer et al. 2007). Additionally, they might believe that the onus is on the health professional to bring up the subject (Post et al. 2008). A way to show that sexual health is an accepted subject to discuss in clinical encounters is to have information leaflets about the subject in the waiting room.

Patient preferences regarding whom they wish to communicate with about sexual health differ. A common choice is the nurse or the rheumatologist, but the personality of the health professional, and the feeling as to whether the subject is "allowed" is more important than the profession (Areskoug & Gard, unpublished). Earlier research (Taylor and Davis 2006) shows that patients prefer the health professionals to bring up the subject of sexual health first. Health professionals might also have pre-conceived opinions that can make communication about sexual health more difficult. For example, health professionals are more reluctant to discuss sexual health with patients from ethnic minority groups, non-heterosexual patients and older age patients (Couldrick, Gaynor, and Cross 2010; Gott et al. 2004). Most RA patients are initially diagnosed with RA in later life, which might be a reason why sexual health is not generally discussed with this group of patients. Research into health professional students has shown that they have a high level of discomfort concerning communication about sexual issues, which shows that it is not easier for younger or more recently educated health professionals to deal with this than it is for older, more established health professionals (Weerakoon et al. 2004).

There are gender differences showing that men have higher levels of sexual activity, interest in sex and better quality sex lifes, and that those gender gaps increase with age (Lindau and Gavrilova 2010). However a recent study of patients with RA showed that male gender was associated with a larger negative impact on sexual activity (Helland, Dagfinrud, and Kvien 2008), which indicates that this field needs further exploration. There are of course several other factors influencing sexual health and the perspective of gender on sexual health is complex (Vanwesenbeeck 2009), but most individuals with RA are women and the subject of sexual health needs to be discussed with a gender perspective since there are differences concerning how RA affects the sexual health of women and men. As examples, women often experience that feelings of intimacy are more important than sexual arousal (Basson and Schultz 2007), and women often have more joint pain during sexual activities (van Berlo et al. 2007). One possible reason for the increased pain for women during sexual activities could be differences in strain on joints in intercourse positions, but the reasons for this need further investigation. There are also gender differences concerning sexual satisfaction, with females with RA having lower sexual satisfaction than men with RA (Majerovitz and Revenson 1994). For younger women with RA, pregnancy can be an issue that needs to be discussed, since pregnancy can cause a remission of symptoms but this positive effect relapses in 90% cases within 6 months post-partum (Gerosa et al. 2008; Ostensen 1999). It is necessary to have strategies of how to deal with both men´s and women´s sexual health within the rheumatological team and to acknowledge the gender differences. There are also differences in the use of coping strategies between men and women with chronic pain. Women are more prone to use coping strategies such as ignoring and self talk and traditional coping strategies does not seem to be relevant for men concerning chronic pain and sexual functioning (Ruehlman, Karoly, and Taylor 2008). Those gender differences should be taken into consideration when communicating about sexual health with persons with RA.

There might be sexual health problems that are more difficult to discuss than others, for example fear of being left by the partner or feeling forced to have sexual activities. Therefore it is important to have knowledge of one´s limitations as a professional and to acknowledge when further expertise is needed in order to aid the person with RA.

6.1 Information

Information on the internet as well as patient-online-helplines can be of use. Several national organizations for persons with arthritis offer information about how intimate relationships and sexual life can be affected by RA. A recent investigation into a patient online helpline showed that 10% of the questions concerned sexual and reproductive issues (Richter et al. 2011). And for most RA patients a wide concept of sexual health, including social functioning and an emotional perspective, is more important than a more mechanical description of disease consequences on sexual health (Couldrick, Gaynor, and Cross 2010).

The following websites contains useful information about sexual health, intercourse positions and intimate relationships for persons living with RA. They are written in an informative and open manner and are a useful resource for RA patients and their partners.

http://www.arthritiscare.og.uk/PublicationsandResources/Relationshipsemotions

http://www.cks.nhs.uk/patient_information_leaflet/arthritis_sexuality_arc
The website below contains information for persons who have had hip replacement surgery and gives information about recommended intercourse positions after hip replacement, as well as information about which positions should be avoided.
http://www.ranawatorthopaedics.com/faq-hip.html

6.2 Communication models

Studies of health professional's attitudes towards discussing sexual health with their patients often show that they feel uneasy and that they lack training in how to bring up sexual health issues with their patients (Couldrick, Gaynor, and Cross 2010). To be able to communicate about sexual health in a respectful and open way it is fundamental to have established a trusting relationship with the patient and to know one´s own ability and limitations concerning issues of sexual health and intimate relationships. In order to ease and improve communication about sexual health, a communication model can be useful. In this section two different models will be introduced, the PLISSIT and the Recognition Model. Both models can be useful for health professionals working with persons with RA.

The **PLISSIT model** has been used when discussing sexual health with patients with various physical and mental diseases. The PLISSIT model provides a graded counseling approach that allows health professionals to deal with sexual issues at their own level of comfort and competence (Annon 1974). The model includes four steps:

P-Permission: This step is the introduction of sexual health into the communication between the healthcare professional and the patient. Examples of permission giving could be having leaflets with information about how RA affects sexual health and intimate relationships in the waiting room. A permission giving attitude can also be shown by using the following question: "It is common that persons with RA experience difficulties with their sexual health. Would you like some information about this?" or "Many persons with RA experience concerns on how RA affects their sexual life. Do you have any questions or concerns about this?" By asking if the person with RA wants information or has questions about sexual health issues, it gives the person with RA the possibility to decline to discuss the subject if they wish to do so. Therefore this might be a more relaxed way to start the conversation, than with direct questions, such as: "Has your disease affected your sexual life? In what way?"

LI- Limited Information: Information can be given about how the RA affects sexual health and about treatments that can increase sexual health. This could be done by handing out information leaflets or by providing information verbally about how your specific professional expertise can be of assistance. In this step it is important to have learnt what type of information the patient is interested in, instead of giving information that the health professional think is relevant.

SS – Specific Suggestions: This is a step with a problem solving approach. Suggestions might include: reading written material about sexuality and how it is affected by RA; taking pain medication before sexual activities; or advice on coital positions. The type of solutions that can be discussed in this step depends on the expertise of the health professional. For example, the physiotherapist can inform about positions that are less strenuous to the joints, the occupational therapist can give advice on planning daily activities in life (including sexual activities), and the rheumatologist can give advice concerning medication.

IT – Intensive Therapy: This level requires special training and is usually performed by a psychiatrist, psychologist or counselor.

This model also shows when the health professional needs to refer the patients to colleagues with more experience concerning sexual health, since the different steps clearly shows how far the discussion has reached. As a standard, persons with psychosexual problems should be referred to a psychosexual therapist, and persons with relationships difficulties should be referred to a counselor. For many patients the permission-step and the limited information-step is sufficient to improve their sexual health (McInnes 2003). There is an extension of the PLISSIT-model, the EX-PLISSIT which includes reflection to raise self-awareness to challenge assumptions and requires review of all interactions with patients (Taylor and Davis 2006).

The core of the **Recognition Model** is the recognition that disabled persons have sexual needs and desires (Couldrick, Gaynor, and Cross 2010). The Recognition Model identifies the existing skills among health professionals that can be used to promote and protect sexual health for persons with disabilities and is intended to be used by multi-professional teams. The step of recognition is important, especially if the health professionals´ expertise is within disability, rather than sexual health. The Recognition model also aids in what is included in each professional role when it comes to addressing sexual health issues.

The steps in the Recognition model might overlap and it is important that the team ensures that all steps are included in the service given by the team around the patient. Sexual health issues should be employed with persons that express their sexuality in a different ways, not only with those persons that seem to be relevant, such as younger persons living in relationship with a partner of the opposite sex. Examples of persons expressing their sexuality in other ways can be persons who have chosen not to be sexually active or persons, persons having several partners or persons attracted to the same sex.

The following steps are described in the Recognition Model (Couldrick, Gaynor, and Cross 2010):

1. Recognition of the service user as a sexual being. This step requires patient centeredness and acknowledgement of the patient as a sexual being, with sexual needs and desires. All team members should be able to have a positive approach to direct questions of sexual health asked by the patient. If the team has a specific person with expertise in sexual health issues, a referral to this person could be done for example like this: "I understand you have sexual concerns that you wish to discuss. It is not my area of expertise, but I can ask my colleague to speak with you."
2. Provision of sensitive, permission giving, strategies such as indirect questions, and printed information. An example of an indirect question that can be used is the following: "Some persons also have questions about sex. If you have anything you wish to ask, I am happy to discuss your concerns." The aim of this step is to invite persons to speak about sexual issues if they wish and still respect their privacy.
3. Exploration of the sexual problem/concern. This step includes exploring what issues are of importance to the patient. For some it might be issues of fatigue or pain and for others it might be maintaining an intimate sexual relationship. Other questions may concern how soon sexual intercourse can be resumed after hip replacement. This step of exploration is essential to give the appropriate advice and information to the person with RA.

The first three steps can be performed by all team members.

1. Address issues that fit within the team´s expertise and boundaries. This step includes the specific competencies of different professionals, for example the occupational

therapist can assist in fatigue management and enabling meaningful activities, and the physiotherapist can use their skills in managing pain and addressing biomechanical issues. In order to simplify the different roles and competencies in the teams, a useful question is:" What can your profession offer in the field of sexual health that cannot be offered by other health professions?" This step includes analysis of sexual concerns, planning of treatment and setting goals.

2. Referral on, when necessary. This step demands that the team members have knowledge of wider resources that might be of use to the patient.
   Psychosexual counseling by a sexologist can be an option when expert advice or intensive therapy is needed. Research concerning psychosexual counseling for persons with chronic physical illness is scarce, but the results of the available studies are promising (Kedde et al. 2010).

7. New research

The field of sexual health and intimate relationships is moving forward within rheumatology. Advances include self-strategies and cognitive behavioural therapy within physiotherapy as ways to improve sexual health (Helland et al. 2011; Breton, Miller, and Fisher 2008). The self-strategies showed great variety including postponing sexual activities during flares, ignoring restrictions, adapting positions, using alternative locations, using painkillers, initiating less strenuous sexual activities, engaging in sexual activities despite lack of desire and being creative during the sexual act. The efficacy of the strategies is not researched and further knowledge is needed in this field. The initial results from cognitive behavioural therapy to improve sexual health are promising (Breton, Miller, and Fisher 2008), but needs further investigation. Research on ways of coping with RA are also of interest in relation to sexual health, since the decrease in sexual health seems to be persistent during the disease.

8. Future research

Areas that need to be further researched within the field of sexual health and RA include:

- gender specific research; what are the differences between men and women in how RA affects sexual health? Which methods are most appropriate for improving sexual health in men with RA and in women with RA?
- the effects of disease modifying medication on sexual health
- the effects of physical activity and improved fitness on the sexual health of RA patients
- how to improve communication concerning sexual health between patients and health professionals
- which physiotherapy interventions are most effective for improving sexual health.

9. Conclusion

Sexual health and intimate relationships need further attention among health professionals, since many individuals with RA have decreased sexual health which can affect their intimate relationships negatively, and thereby decrease their general wellbeing and overall happiness. Each profession has a professional expertise that can assist RA patients in this field. Optimal treatment of RA can decrease sexual health problems for persons with RA, since the difficulties are often connected with clinical disease activity. In order to give holistic care to persons with RA it is important to have a strategy within the rheumatological team on how to communicate and address problems concerning sexual health, and to acknowledge the need to protect, support and restore the sexual health of RA patients. To enhance the communication of sexual health there are useful communication models that are appropriate to rheumatological care.

10. Acknowledgment

We would like to acknowledge Futurum- the Academy for Healthcare, County Council, Jönköping, Sweden, for funding the authors' research in sexual health and RA.

11. References

Abdel-Nasser, A. M., and E. I. Ali. 2006. Determinants of sexual disability and dissatisfaction in female patients with rheumatoid arthritis. *Clin Rheumatol* 25 (6):822-30.

Akkas, Y. Nakas, D. Kalyoncu, U. 2010. Factors Affecting the Sexual Satisfaction of Patients with Rheumatoid Arthritis and Ankylosing Spondylitis *Sexuality and Disability* 28 (4):223-232.

Aletaha, D., T. Neogi, A. J. Silman, J. Funovits, D. T. Felson, C. O. Bingham, 3rd, N. S. Birnbaum, G. R. Burmester, V. P. Bykerk, M. D. Cohen, B. Combe, K. H. Costenbader, M. Dougados, P. Emery, G. Ferraccioli, J. M. Hazes, K. Hobbs, T. W. Huizinga, A. Kavanaugh, J. Kay, T. K. Kvien, T. Laing, P. Mease, H. A. Menard, L. W. Moreland, R. L. Naden, T. Pincus, J. S. Smolen, E. Stanislawska-Biernat, D. Symmons, P. P. Tak, K. S. Upchurch, J. Vencovsky, F. Wolfe, and G. Hawker. 2010. 2010 Rheumatoid arthritis classification criteria: an American College of Rheumatology/European League Against Rheumatism collaborative initiative. *Arthritis Rheum* 62 (9):2569-81.

Annon, J.S. 1974. *The Behavioural Treatment of Sexual Problems: Brief Therapy*. Honolulu: Kapiolani Health Services.

Areskoug-Josefsson, K., ed. 2006. *Welchen Einfluss hat Physiotherapie auf die soziale Inklusion von Menschen mit rheumatoider Arthritis?* Edited by W. Bautz, Harms, J., Ulbricht-Thiede, S., *Europäische Anregungen zu Sozialer Inklusion*. Berlin: Frank & Timme Gmbh Verlag für wissenschaftliche Literatur.

Areskoug-Josefsson, K., and U. Oberg. 2009. A literature review of the sexual health of women with rheumatoid arthritis. *Musculoskeletal Care* 7(4):219-26.

Basson, R., and W. W. Schultz. 2007. Sexual sequelae of general medical disorders. *Lancet* 369 (9559):409-24.

Bermas, B. L., J. S. Tucker, D. K. Winkelman, and J. N. Katz. 2000. Marital satisfaction in couples with rheumatoid arthritis. *Arthritis Care Res* 13 (3):149-55.

Bitzer, J., G. Platano, S. Tschudin, and J. Alder. 2007. Sexual counseling for women in the context of physical diseases: a teaching model for physicians. *J Sex Med* 4 (1):29-37.

Bortz, W. M., 2nd, and D. H. Wallace. 1999. Physical fitness, aging, and sexuality. *West J Med* 170 (3):167-9.

Breton, A., C. M. Miller, and K. Fisher. 2008. Enhancing the sexual function of women living with chronic pain: a cognitive-behavioural treatment group. *Pain Res Manag* 13 (3):219-24.

Britto, M. T., S. L. Rosenthal, J. Taylor, and M. H. Passo. 2000. Improving rheumatologists' screening for alcohol use and sexual activity. *Arch Pediatr Adolesc Med* 154 (5):478-83.

Brodin, N., E. Eurenius, I. Jensen, R. Nisell, and C. H. Opava. 2008. Coaching patients with early rheumatoid arthritis to healthy physical activity: a multicenter, randomized, controlled study. *Arthritis Rheum* 59 (3):325-31.

Cairns, A. P., and J. G. McVeigh. 2009. A systematic review of the effects of dynamic exercise in rheumatoid arthritis. *Rheumatol Int* 30 (2):147-58.

Cameron, M. 2002. Is manual therapy a rational approach to improving health-related quality of life in people with arthritis? *Australas Chiropr Osteopathy* 10 (1):9-15.

Carr, A., S. Hewlett, R. Hughes, H. Mitchell, S. Ryan, M. Carr, and J. Kirwan. 2003. Rheumatology outcomes: the patient's perspective. *J Rheumatol* 30 (4):880-3.

Casimiro, L., L. Brosseau, S. Milne, V. Robinson, G. Wells, and P. Tugwell. 2002. Acupuncture and electroacupuncture for the treatment of RA. *Cochrane Database Syst Rev* (3):CD003788.

Chauffier, K., C. Salliot, F. Berenbaum, and J. Sellam. 2011. Effect of biotherapies on fatigue in rheumatoid arthritis: a systematic review of the literature and meta-analysis. *Rheumatology (Oxford)* Epub ahead of print.

Clayton, A., and S. Ramamurthy. 2008. The impact of physical illness on sexual dysfunction. *Adv Psychosom Med* 29:70-88.

Coll, J., A. Rives, M. C. Grino, J. Setoain, J. Vivancos, and A. Balcells. 1987. Prevalence of Sjogren's syndrome in autoimmune diseases. *Ann Rheum Dis* 46 (4):286-9.

Cooney, J. K., R. J. Law, V. Matschke, A. B. Lemmey, J. P. Moore, Y. Ahmad, J. G. Jones, P. Maddison, and J. M. Thom. 2011. Benefits of exercise in rheumatoid arthritis. *J Aging Res* 2011:681640.

Couldrick, L. , S. Gaynor, and V. Cross. 2010. Proposing a new sexual health model of practice for disability teams: the Recognition Model. *Int J Ther Rehabil* 17 (6):290-298.

Defining sexual health. Report of a technical consultation on sexual health, 28-31 January 2002, Geneva. 2006. In *Sexual health document series*, edited by W. H. Organization. Geneva.

Elst, P., T. Sybesma, R. J. van der Stadt, A. P. Prins, W. H. Muller, and A. den Butter. 1984. Sexual problems in rheumatoid arthritis and ankylosing spondylitis. *Arthritis Rheum* 27 (2):217-20.

Englund, M., A. Joud, P. Geborek, D. T. Felson, L. T. Jacobsson, and I. F. Petersson. 2010. Prevalence and incidence of rheumatoid arthritis in southern Sweden 2008 and their relation to prescribed biologics. *Rheumatology (Oxford)* Aug;49 (8):1563-9.

EuroQol--a new facility for the measurement of health-related quality of life. The EuroQol Group. 1990. *Health Policy* 16 (3):199-208.

Fries, J. F., P. Spitz, R. G. Kraines, and H. R. Holman. 1980. Measurement of patient outcome in arthritis. *Arthritis Rheum* 23 (2):137-45.

Gard, G. Lundvik Gyllensten, A. 2000. The importance of emotions in physiotherapeutic practice. *Physical Therapy Reviews* 5:155-160.

Garip, Y., F. Eser, and H. Bodur. 2010. Health-related quality of life in rheumatoid arthritis: comparison of RAQoL with other scales in terms of disease activity, severity of pain, and functional status. *Rheumatol Int* 31 (6):769-72.

Gerosa, M., V. De Angelis, P. Riboldi, and P. L. Meroni. 2008. Rheumatoid arthritis: a female challenge. *Womens Health (Lond Engl)* 4 (2):195-201.

Gettings, L. 2010. Psychological well-being in rheumatoid arthritis: a review of the literature. *Musculoskeletal Care* 8 (2):99-106.

Giorgi, A. 2000. Concerning the application of phenomenology to caring research. *Scand J Caring Sci* 14 (1):11-5.

Giorgi, Amadeo, ed. 1985. *Phenomenology and Psychological research.* Pittsburgh, U.S.A.: Duquesene University Press.

Gott, M., E. Galena, S. Hinchliff, and H. Elford. 2004. "Opening a can of worms": GP and practice nurse barriers to talking about sexual health in primary care. *Fam Pract* 21 (5):528-36.

Gutweniger, S., M. Kopp, E. Mur, and V. Gunther. 1999. Body image of women with rheumatoid arthritis. *Clin Exp Rheumatol* 17 (4):413-7.

Haboubi, N. H., and N. Lincoln. 2003. Views of health professionals on discussing sexual issues with patients. *Disabil Rehabil* 25 (6):291-6.

Helland, Y., H. Dagfinrud, and T. K. Kvien. 2008. Perceived influence of health status on sexual activity in RA patients: associations with demographic and disease-related variables. *Scand J Rheumatol* 37 (3):194-9.

Helland, Y., I. Kjeken, E. Steen, T. K. Kvien, M. I. Hauge, and H. Dagfinrud. 2011. Rheumatic diseases and sexuality: Disease impact and self management strategies. *Arthritis Care Res (Hoboken).*

Hewlett, S., Z. Cockshott, M. Byron, K. Kitchen, S. Tipler, D. Pope, and M. Hehir. 2005. Patients' perceptions of fatigue in rheumatoid arthritis: overwhelming, uncontrollable, ignored. *Arthritis Rheum* 53 (5):697-702.

Hill, J., H. Bird, and R. Thorpe. 2003. Effects of rheumatoid arthritis on sexual activity and relationships. *Rheumatology (Oxford)* 42 (2):280-6.

Hull, T.H. 2008. Sexual pleasure and wellbeing. *Journal of Sexual Health* 20 (1-2):133-145.

Ibn Yacoub, Y., B. Amine, A. Laatiris, F. Wafki, F. Znat, and N. Hajjaj-Hassouni. 2011. Fatigue and severity of rheumatoid arthritis in Moroccan patients. *Rheumatol Int.*

International Classification of Functioning, Disability and Health. 2001. Edited by W. H. Organization. Geneva.

Josefsson, K. A., and G. Gard. 2010. Women's experiences of sexual health when living with Rheumatoid Arthritis - an explorative qualitative study. *BMC Musculoskelet Disord* 11:240.

Karlsson, B., E. Berglin, and S. Wallberg-Jonsson. 2006. Life satisfaction in early rheumatoid arthritis: a prospective study. *Scand J Occup Ther* 13 (3):193-9.

Kavuncu, V., and D. Evcik. 2004. Physiotherapy in rheumatoid arthritis. *MedGenMed* 6 (2):3.

Kedde, H., H. B. Van De Wiel, W. C. Schultz, W. M. Vanwesenbeek, and J. L. Bender. 2010. Efficacy of sexological healthcare for people with chronic diseases and physical disabilities. *J Sex Marital Ther* 36 (3):282-94.

Khan, N. A., Y. Yazici, J. Calvo-Alen, J. Dadoniene, L. Gossec, T. M. Hansen, M. Huisman, R. Kallikorm, R. Muller, M. Liveborn, R. Oding, E. Luchikhina, A. Naranjo, S. Rexhepi, P. Taylor, W. Tlustochowich, A. Tsirogianni, and T. Sokka. 2009. Reevaluation of the role of duration of morning stiffness in the assessment of rheumatoid arthritis activity. *J Rheumatol* 36 (11):2435-42.

Kraaimaat, F. W., A. H. Bakker, E. Janssen, and J. W. Bijlsma. 1996. Intrusiveness of rheumatoid arthritis on sexuality in male and female patients living with a spouse. *Arthritis Care Res* 9 (2):120-5.

Lapsley, H. M., L. M. March, K. L. Tribe, M. J. Cross, B. G. Courtenay, and P. M. Brooks. 2002. Living with rheumatoid arthritis: expenditures, health status, and social impact on patients. *Ann Rheum Dis* 61 (9):818-21.

le Gallez, P. 1993. Rheumatoid arthritis: effects on the family. *Nurs Stand* 7 (39):30-4.

Lee, E. O., J. I. Kim, A. H. Davis, and I. Kim. 2006. Effects of regular exercise on pain, fatigue, and disability in patients with rheumatoid arthritis. *Fam Community Health* 29 (4):320-7.

Lindau, S. T., and N. Gavrilova. 2010. Sex, health, and years of sexually active life gained due to good health: evidence from two US population based cross sectional surveys of ageing. *BMJ* 340:c810.

Majerovitz, S. D., and T. A. Revenson. 1994. Sexuality and rheumatic disease: the significance of gender. *Arthritis Care Res* 7 (1):29-34.

Matheson, L., D. Harcourt, and S. Hewlett. 2010. 'Your whole life, your whole world, it changes': partners' experiences of living with rheumatoid arthritis. *Musculoskeletal Care* 8 (1):46-54.

McInnes, R. A. 2003. Chronic illness and sexuality. *Med J Aust* 179 (5):263-6.

Meenan, R. F., J. H. Mason, J. J. Anderson, A. A. Guccione, and L. E. Kazis. 1992. AIMS2. The content and properties of a revised and expanded Arthritis Impact Measurement Scales Health Status Questionnaire. *Arthritis Rheum* 35 (1):1-10.

Monga, T. N., G. Tan, H. J. Ostermann, U. Monga, and M. Grabois. 1998. Sexuality and sexual adjustment of patients with chronic pain. *Disabil Rehabil* 20 (9):317-29.

Neuberger, G. B., L. S. Aaronson, B. Gajewski, S. E. Embretson, P. E. Cagle, J. K. Loudon, and P. A. Miller. 2007. Predictors of exercise and effects of exercise on symptoms, function, aerobic fitness, and disease outcomes of rheumatoid arthritis. *Arthritis Rheum* 57 (6):943-52.

Ostensen, M. 1999. Sex hormones and pregnancy in rheumatoid arthritis and systemic lupus erythematosus. *Ann N Y Acad Sci* 876:131-43.

Perdriger, A., C. Solano, and L. Gossec. 2010. Why should rheumatologists evaluate the impact of rheumatoid arthritis on sexuality? *Joint Bone Spine* 77 (6):493-5.

Pincus, T., T. Sokka, and H. Kautiainen. 2005. Further development of a physical function scale on a MDHAQ [corrected] for standard care of patients with rheumatic diseases. *J Rheumatol* 32 (8):1432-9.

Pollard, L., E. H. Choy, and D. L. Scott. 2005. The consequences of rheumatoid arthritis: quality of life measures in the individual patient. *Clin Exp Rheumatol* 23 (5 Suppl 39):S43-52.

Post, M.W.M., W. L. Gianotten, L. Heijnen, E. J. Lambers, Hille R., and M. Willems. 2008. Sexological competence of different rehabilitation disciplines and effects of a discipline-specific sexological training. *Sexuality and Disability* 26 (1):3-14.

Reinseth, L., T. Uhlig, I. Kjeken, H. S. Koksvik, J. F. Skomsvoll, and G. A. Espnes. 2010. Performance in leisure-time physical activities and self-efficacy in females with rheumatoid arthritis. *Scand J Occup Ther* E-pub ahead of print.

Richter, J. G., A. Becker, H. Schalis, T. Koch, R. Willers, C. Specker, R. Monser, and M. Schneider. 2011. An ask-the-expert service on a rheumatology web site: Who were the users and what did they look for? *Arthritis Care Res (Hoboken)* 63 (4):604-11.

Rkain, H., F. Allali, I. Jroundi, and N. Hajjaj-Hassouni. 2006. Socioeconomic impact of rheumatoid arthritis in Morocco. *Joint Bone Spine* 73 (3):278-83.

Ruehlman, L. S., P. Karoly, and A. Taylor. 2008. Perceptions of chronic pain's interference with sexual functioning: The role of gender, treatment status, and psychosocial factors. . *Sexuality and Disability* 26 (3):123-136.

Ryan, S., and E. Wylie. 2005. An exploratory survey of the practice of rheumatology nurses addressing the sexuality of patients with rheumatoid arthritis. *Musculoskeletal Care* 3 (1):44-53.

Sokka, T. 2005. Assessment of pain in rheumatic diseases. *Clin Exp Rheumatol* 23 (5 Suppl 39):S77-84.

Stausmire, J. M. 2004. Sexuality at the end of life. *Am J Hosp Palliat Care* 21 (1):33-9.

Stucki, G., A. Cieza, S. Geyh, L. Battistella, J. Lloyd, D. Symmons, N. Kostanjsek, and J. Schouten. 2004. ICF Core Sets for rheumatoid arthritis. *J Rehabil Med* (44 Suppl):87-93.

Tasiemski, T., N. Angiaszwili-Biedna, and M. Wilski. 2009. Assessment of objective and subjective quality of life in people with rheumatoid arthritis - preliminary study. *Ortop Traumatol Rehabil* 11 (4):346-59.

Taylor, B., and S. Davis. 2006. Using the extended PLISSIT model to address sexual healthcare needs. *Nurs Stand* 21 (11):35-40.

Tristano, A. G. 2009. The impact of rheumatic diseases on sexual function. *Rheumatol Int* 29 (8):853-60.

van Berlo, W. T., H. B. van de Wiel, E. Taal, J. J. Rasker, W. C. Weijmar Schultz, and M. H. van Rijswijk. 2007. Sexual functioning of people with rheumatoid arthritis: a multicenter study. *Clin Rheumatol* 26 (1):30-8.

van Lankveld, W., G. Ruiterkamp, G. Naring, and D. J. de Rooij. 2004. Marital and sexual satisfaction in patients with RA and their spouses. *Scand J Rheumatol* 33 (6):405-8.

Vanwesenbeeck, I. 2009. Doing gender in sex and sex research. *Archives of Sexual Behaviour* 38 (6):883-898.

Ware, J. E., Jr., and C. D. Sherbourne. 1992. The MOS 36-item short-form health survey (SF-36). I. Conceptual framework and item selection. *Med Care* 30 (6):473-83.

Weerakoon, P., M. K. Jones, R. Pynor, and E. Kilburn-Watt. 2004. Allied health professional students' perceived level of comfort in clinical situations that have sexual connotations. *J Allied Health* 33 (3):189-93.

Vliet Vlieland, T. P. 2007. Non-drug care for RA--is the era of evidence-based practice approaching? *Rheumatology (Oxford)* 46 (9):1397-404.

World Health Organization. 2006. Defining sexual health. Report of a technical consultation on sexual health. In *Sexual health document series*. Geneva: World Health Organisation.

Ying, K. N., and A. While. 2007. Pain relief in osteoarthritis and rheumatoid arthritis: TENS. *Br J Community Nurs* 12 (8):364-71.

Yoshino, S., and S. Uchida. 1981. Sexual problems of women with rheumatoid arthritis. *Arch Phys Med Rehabil* 62 (3):122-3.

13

Association of Cardiovascular Disease with the Metabolic Syndrome in a Predominantly Male Cohort with Rheumatoid Arthritis

G.S. Kerr[1] et al.*
[1]*Washington DC Veterans Affairs Medical Center and Georgetown University, Washington, DC USA*

1. Introduction

Despite the therapeutic advances in RA that have led to reduced pain, joint destruction and disability, as many as 50% of patients are at risk of death from a cardiovascular event (Maradit-Kremers et al., 2005; Stevens et al., 2005). Inexplicable by the usual traditional risk factors, the accelerated atherosclerosis (Gaonzalez-Gay et al., 2005) has been postulated to result from the increased systemic inflammatory burden of rheumatoid disease (Del Rincon et al., 2001; Gabriel et al., 1999; Kremers & Gabriel, 2006; McEntegart et al., 2001).

The metabolic syndrome (MetS) is a composite diagnosis, combining phenotypic features that portend an increased risk for cardiovascular disease (CVD). The syndrome consists of visceral obesity, atherogenic dyslipidemia, hypertension, and impaired fasting glucose/glucose tolerance test or overt diabetes mellitus (DM) (National Cholesterol Education Program, 2001). Studies have reported the presence of MetS to be associated with an approximate 2- fold increased risk for incident cardiovascular morbidity and mortality (Lakka et al., 2002), a 2.1 fold increase for initial stroke (Najarian et al., 2006), and 3.5 fold increased risk for Type II DM (Lorenzo et al., 2003). The complex interplay of genetic and environmental factors, insulin resistance and inflammation, are all believed to contribute to the pathogenesis of the syndrome.

The overall prevalence of MetS in the US population, as evaluated by the National Health and Nutrition Examination Survey (NHANES III), is 23.1%, and increases with age to as high as 44% in those 65 years or older (Ford et al., 2002). Several studies have established an increased prevalence of insulin resistance and increased risk for CVD in RA patients (Dessein et al., 2002a, 2002b). However, there are few reports regarding MetS in RA, and the

---

* I. Sabahi[1], J.S. Richards[1], T.R. Mikuls[2], B.V. Rangan[3], A. Reimold[3], G.W. Cannon[4], D. Johnson[5] and L. Caplan[6]
[2]*Omaha Veterans Affairs and University of Omaha, Omaha, NE, USA*
[3]*Dallas Veterans Affairs and University of Texas Southwestern, Dallas, TX, USA*
[4]*George E. Wahlen Veterans Affairs and University of Utah, Salt Lake City, UT, USA*
[5]*Jackson Veterans Affairs and University of Mississippi, Jackson, MS, USA*
[6]*Denver Veterans Affairs and University of Colorado, Denver, CO, USA*

existing data reflect variations in the populations studied (Crowson et al., 2011; Karvounaris et al., 2007). Data from Europe and the US have shown associations between the syndrome and the inflammatory burden of RA.

Most data on RA, including reports related to MetS and CVD, are comprised mainly of females. The few reports on RA in males indicate a more severe course of disease, and worse outcome (Ford et al., 2002; Janghorbani et al., 1993; Jawaheer et al., 2006; Mikuls et al., 2011). Further, elderly males more often have comorbid diseases such as diabetes mellitus and hypertension that places them at even greater risk for CVD.

Therefore we sought to examine the prevalence and relationship of MetS to RA disease burden and CVD in a primarily elderly, male RA cohort.

2. Patients and methods

2.1 Study population

Study patients enrolled in the ongoing Veterans Affairs Rheumatoid Arthritis (VARA) Registry prior to January 2009 were included in the study. The characteristics of this population have been previously described (Mikuls et al., 2007). Briefly, VARA is a multi-center chronic disease registry initiated in 2003 now including collection sites at VA Medical Centers across the U.S. The current study included participants from VA sites in Dallas, Denver, Jackson, Omaha, Salt Lake City, and Washington, DC. Rheumatoid arthritis (RA) patients with disease onset after age 18 years who fulfill American College of Rheumatology (ACR) classification criteria for RA (Arnett et al., 1988) are invited to enroll. Participating sites prospectively collect and archive clinical and laboratory observations associated with RA during routine visits and standard of care. VARA has been approved by the Institutional Review Board (IRB) and VA Research and Development Committee at each participating site. All subjects provide written consent for a single blood draw and ongoing review of their electronic medical records.

2.2 Metabolic syndrome definition

The NCEP/ATPIII criteria (National Cholesterol Education Program, 2001) for MetS were modified so that a body mass index (BMI) of ≥ 30 kg/m^2 replaced waist/hip circumference. Because waist and hip measurements are not routinely available on study subjects, BMI was used as a surrogate for waist-to-hip circumference with the following rationale: a) weight and annual height measurements are routinely obtained on all our patients, b) data support BMI to be as accurate as waist circumference in identifying individuals for risk of CVD (Farin et al, 2006), c) BMI is included in the WHO definition for MetS (World Health Organization [WHO], 1999) and there appears to be at least modest levels of agreement between BMI and waist-to-hip ratio in both men and women (Balkau et al., 2006), and d) to obviate the varied cut off points for waist circumference for different ethnic groups (Alberti et al., 2005). Additionally, documented prior use of disease specific medications were used as surrogates for the other three MetS components. Hence MetS was defined as presence of ≥ 3 of 4 criteria (BMI ≥ 30 kg/m^2, anti-hypertensive, lipid lowering, and/or diabetes agents) (Grundy et al., 2005).

2.3 Clinical measures

RA disease severity was assessed by rheumatoid factor (RF) positivity, duration of disease, presence of radiographic changes suggestive of RA (based on ACR criteria) and nodules at enrollment. Disease activity was assessed at the time of the most recent clinic visit by erythrocyte sedimentation rate (ESR), C-reactive protein (CRP), total swollen and tender joint count (0-28 joints), patient global well-being 100 mm visual analog scale, modified health assessment questionnaire (MD-HAQ, 0-3) and three-variable Disease Activity Score (DAS28-3v; a composite measure based on swollen/tender joint counts and ESR) (Bawa et al., 2005; Prevoo et al., 1995). The three-variable DAS was used in place of a four variable DAS to minimize the impact of missing data from patient global scores.

Disease-modifying anti-rheumatic therapy (DMARD), biologic treatments, and prednisone use were also recorded at the most recent visit. DMARD agents included methotrexate, sulfasalazine, hydroxychloroquine, and leflunomide; biologic treatments included anti-tumor necrosis factor (adalimumab, etanercept, infliximab), anti-signal 2 inhibitor (abatacept) and anti-CD20 (rituximab) agents. Patient report of ever or never smoking was tabulated, and subjects were categorized based on a history of CVD (documentation of prior coronary artery disease, myocardial infarction, angina, cerebrovascular event, transient ischemic attack, or peripheral vascular disease).

2.4 Statistical analysis

Descriptive statistics were used to define the group. Group comparisons, based on the presence/absence of MetS, were performed using Chi-square for categorical variables and a one-way ANOVA for continuous data. Odds ratios (OR) and 95% confidence intervals were used to assess the association of MetS with prevalent CVD and were calculated using multivariable logistic regression, adjusting for age, sex, smoking status (ever vs. never), and the current use of DMARDs and/or biologic therapies. Given the reported anti-inflammatory effect of select lipid lowering agents (statins) in RA, we performed a subanalysis in subjects with MetS to examine the association of statin use with measures of disease activity. All analyses were performed using SAS (SAS Inc, Cary, NC).

3. Results

Six-hundred seventy-one patients were included in this study (Table 1). The study cohort included 53 (7.9%) women, had a mean age of 65.4 years [SD10.8], and a mean disease duration of 13.7 years [SD 11.5]. The majority were Caucasian (n = 543, 80.9%). Four hundred and twelve (61.4%) had radiographic changes consistent with RA, and 312 (46.5%) had nodules. Approximately 58.3% were on a traditional DMARD at their most recent clinic visit, while an additional 25.8% were receiving a combination of a biologic agent with a traditional DMARD. Fifty three percent of the study cohort was receiving prednisone.

The mean DAS28 was 3.2 [SD 1.3] and CRP was 1.3 [SD 1.9] mg/dl. The majority (78.8%) were either previous or current smokers. One-hundred eighty-nine subjects satisfied the modified criteria for MetS, corresponding to a prevalence of 28.2% (95 % CI 24.7-31.7). There were no significant differences in subject demographics, measures of disease severity or activity, use of biologic agents or DMARDS, prednisone use, or smoking status in RA subjects with MetS compared to those without MetS (Table 1). In a subanalysis of subjects with and without MetS, there were no significant differences in measures of disease activity in those taking statins compared to individuals not taking statins (data not shown). As expected, disease components of MetS were far more common in those with the syndrome in comparison to those without MetS (Figure 1). Of note, a BMI that exceeded 30 kg/m^2 was present in only one-third of study patients, but comprised 66% of MetS patients and only 20% of individuals without MetS. The use of anti-hypertensive and lipid lowering agents were nearly universal among those meeting criteria for MetS, with over 95% use. Logistic regression analysis revealed MetS to be associated with an approximately three-fold risk of CVD (OR=2.9; 95% CI 1.95-4.34), after adjusting for age, sex, DMARD / biologic use, and smoking status (Table 2). There was no increased CVD risk with individual components of the metabolic syndrome.

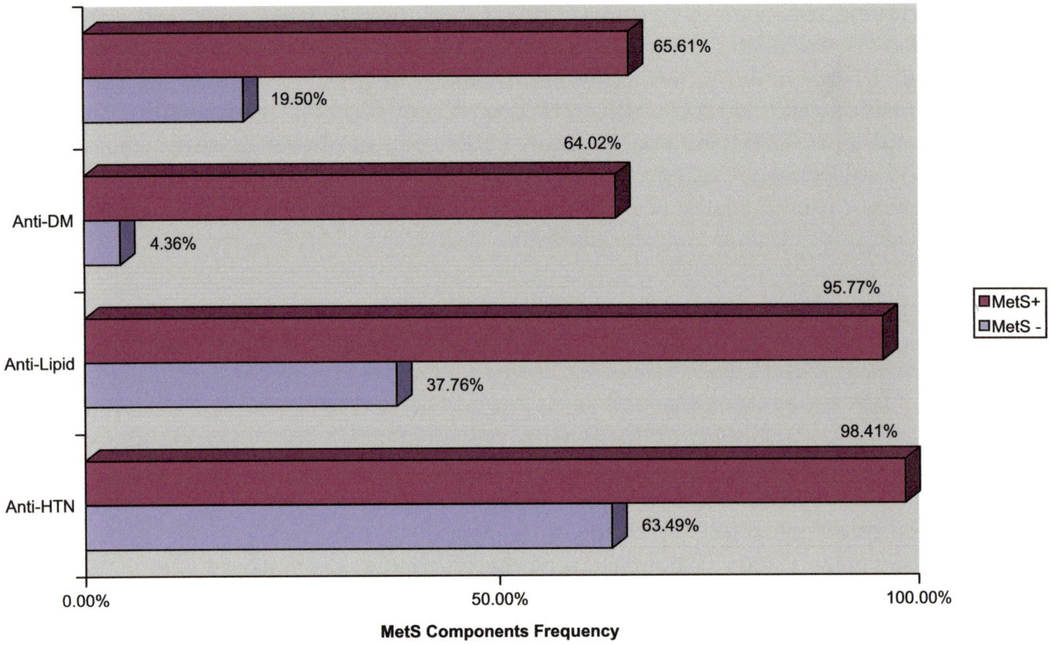

MetS= Metabolic Syndrome
BMI = Body Mass Index
Anti-DM = Treatment for diabetes with insulin and/or oral hypoglycemic medications
Anti-Lipid = Treatment for dyslipidemia with cholesterol lowering medications
Anti-HTN = Treatment for high blood pressure with medications

Fig. 1. MetS Components Frequency in VARA cohort

4. Discussion

In our cohort, the prevalence of MetS was 28.2% and had significant association with CVD. The few existing studies that have examined the relationship of RA with MetS primarily involved women, and indicated increased mortality from CVD among those satisfying criteria for MetS. Men with RA have more extra-articular disease and a greater overall mortality (Janghorbani et al., 1993; Jawaheer et al., 2006; Mikuls et al., 2011). In general, there is a disproportionate individual impact of MetS, CVD, and RA in men. Our findings provide data previously lacking regarding the frequency of MetS in older men with RA and its relationship with RA-specific factors and CVD co-morbidity.

In non-RA populations, MetS has been reported to increase the risk for CVD by two fold, and death by as much as 4 fold (Dekker et al., 2005; Lakka et al., 2002). In a Finnish cohort of men aged 42 to 60 years of age, MetS was found in only 14.3%, but with a 2.9 to 4.3 greater risk of death from coronary heart disease (Lakka et al., 2002). In a population-based cohort

	VARA Cohort *% (n), mean [SD]*		
	% (Number)	MetS Absent	MetS Present
Variables	(N=671)	78% (482)	28% (189)
Age	65.35 [SD 10.75]	65.23 [SD11.43]	65.66 [8.79]
Female	7.9 (53)	9.8 (47)	3.2 (7)
Caucasian	80.6 (543)	80.3 (387)	82.5 (156)
African American	14.6 (98)	15.4 (74)	12.7 (24)
Erosions present	61.4 (412)	63.9 (308)	55 (104)
Disease Duratio	13.74 [SD 11.5]	14.08 [SD 11.61]	12.89 [SD 11.21]
Nodules present	46.5 (312)	47.5 (229)	43.9 (83)
RF Positive	88.4 (593)	89 (429)	86.8 (164)
DAS28(3v)†	3.20 [SD 1.34]	3.21 [SD 1.33]	3.18 [SD 1.38]
CRP	1.29 [SD 1.87]	1.37 [SD 1.98]	1.09 [SD 1.53]
DMARDS	58.3 (391)	56.2 (271)	63.5 (120)
DMARDS+Biologic*	25.8 (173)	26.4 (127)	24.3 (46)
Prednisone	43.5 (292)	46.7 (225)	35.5 (67)
Ever Smoke	78.8 (529)	78.7 (379)	79.4 (150)

P values not statically significant for all variables
Veteran **A**ffairs **R**hematoid **A**rthritis Registry
MetS = Metabolic Syndrome DMARDS=Disease-Modifying Anti-Rheumatic Drugs
*Biological Agents (mainly anti-tumor necrosis factor) †Disease Activity Score, 28 joints
SD = Standard Deviation

Table 1. Demographics and Parameters of Disease Severity and Activity of Veterans Affairs Rheumatoid Arthritis Patients with and without the Metabolic Syndrome

Variables	*OR*	*95% C.I.*		*P value*
		Lower	Upper	
MetS Present	2.91	1.95	4.34	<0.001
DMARDS	2.27	1.47	3.50	<0.001
Age	1.04	1.02	1.07	<0.001
Ever Smoking	1.67	0.99	2.82	0.05
Gender (male)	0.38	0.11	1.29	0.12
DMARDS+Biologic*	1.06	0.66	1.72	0.80

DMARDS (Disease Modifying Anti-rheumatic drugs)
*Biologic Agents (mainly anti-tumor necrosis factor)
CI = Confidence Interval

Table 2. Multivariable Logistic Regression Model examining the association of Metabolic Syndrome with Cardiovascular Disease in VARA cohort

of 615 men aged 50 to 75 years, the prevalence of MetS varied from 17% - 32% when assessing the agreement in the various definitions of MetS (Dekker et al., 2005). When using NCEP-ATPIII criteria, the hazard ratio for fatal and non-fatal CVD in men with MetS was 1.91 (1.31–2.79), compared to 1.68 (1.11–2.55) in the 749 women.

A similar risk for CVD occurs for RA patients with MetS, but these results are obtained from cohorts consisting primarily of female patients (Dessein et al., 2002; Karvounaris et al., 2007).

Further, as in the non-RA study cohorts, the definitions and criteria of both MetS and CVD varied. In one study, MetS, as defined by WHO criteria, was a better predictor of coronary calcification than NCEP-ATPIII criteria (Pandya et al., 2006). Though coronary calcification detection by electron beam computer tomography is a more sensitive means of detecting atherosclerosis than clinical diagnoses, the association with MetS achieved an odds ratio of 2.02, (95% CI: 1.03-3.97, $p=0.04$.), less than the 2.91 (95% CI: 1.95-4.34, $p<0.001$) in our cohort. In that study (Pandya et al, 2006), almost 50% of the patients had longstanding disease (median = 20 years), were younger than our cohort (median 59 years), and were majority female. The almost three-fold risk for CVD in our cohort was independent of anti-rheumatic treatment, smoking, age or gender. There was, however, a trend to increased risk with increasing age and DMARD therapy alone, the latter perhaps related to channeling bias or confounding by indication.

Given the notable comorbidity in our study population, and the historically age-matched prevalence of MetS in 44% of the US NHANES III population aged 65 years, our prevalence of 28% was unexpected. The limited data from other disease cohorts involving U.S. veteran populations report higher frequencies on the order of 50% (Meyer et al., 2006; Pandya et al., 2006). However, our results are similar to another US RA cohort, 40% of whom were male. The prevalence of MetS was approximately 26% as defined by NCEP-ATPIII criteria, and was almost half that of controls (Rodriguez-Pla et al., 2007). In that study, the difference in prevalence between RA and controls could not be explained by differences in physical activity. In contrast, in 200 similarly aged but primarily female RA patients, MetS occurred in 44% of patients at a similar rate to the age- and sex- matched controls, but used ATPIII criteria (National Cholesterol Education Program, 2001). Of the 53 men in the study, approximately 30% with MetS had coronary disease ($p=0.02$). Not only do differences in MetS classifications make comparisons amongst cohorts difficult, but the disparate muscle loss with fat retention that occurs in RA patients, affects BMI assessments. Rheumatoid cachexia, which is present in most (two-thirds) RA patients, doesn't merely involve fat "retention"; there is exacerbated fat gain. When body composition is assessed (i.e. % body fat), up to 80% of RA patients satisfy BMI criteria for obesity i.e. ≥27% for males, and ≥38% for females (Baumgartner et al., 1999). This prevalence of obesity in RA is not reflected by BMI because of the concomitant loss of muscle. Thus, for individuals with the same BMI, an RA patient will have, on average, 4.3% higher % body fat than a healthy, age- and sex-matched subject. Therefore, in RA patients, a BMI greater than $28kg/m^2$ has been proposed to define obesity, and may therefore lead to higher, and more accurate, estimations of MetS in RA cohorts. (Stavropoulos-Kalinoglou et al., 2007).

Our modified definition of MetS based on NCEP-ATPIII criteria though highly specific, may have lacked sensitivity by excluding otherwise eligible patients with discordance between waist-to-hip ratio and BMI, or those who had not received pharmacological treatment for component diseases. We recognize therefore that our prevalence estimate may have trended towards the conservative and underestimated the true impact of MetS in this population; an important concern given the strong association between MetS and CVD. However, of note is the rigor with which VA patients are screened and treated for diabetes mellitus, hypertension and hyperlipidemia based on adherence to select process indicators (Steven, 2004). Therefore it is likely that our use of medication is a reasonable surrogate for the select comorbidities of MetS. Surprisingly, our study found no significant risk of any of the individual components of MetS, and may indicate that traditional risk factors do not impart the same risk for CVD in RA as in the general population.

The role of adipose tissue and BMI in inflammatory disease is evolving as is its impact on response to disease-modifying therapies (Klaasen et al., 2011; Ouchi et al., 2011). Yet the association of MetS with RA disease activity and severity is equivocal. One study has reported an increase of nine-fold in odds ratio correlation between MetS and disease activity, but not with severity (Karvounaris et al., 2007). A relationship between MetS and disease activity and severity was not found in our cohort, but the mean disease activity was low and the effect of DMARD therapies on MetS is unknown. Aware that statin use may be more frequent in the context of MetS and of its potential anti-inflammatory and immunomodulatory effects, we explored but were unable to find an association between statin use and disease activity in RA patients with and without MetS.

There are limitations to our study. The use of BMI in place of waist-to-hip circumference may have limited the sensitivity of our criteria. However, the use of BMI in lieu of waist-to-hip circumference allows pragmatic application in clinical practice, and thereby easier identification of MetS. There is a reported positive correlation between BMI and CVD and increased CRP levels, and BMI is inversely related to functional status in inflammatory rheumatic diseases (Choi et al., 2002; Kremer & Reed, 2006). There was no difference in disease activity amongst the cohort, and the increased risk for CVD in RA patients with MetS was independent of disease activity. Whether a lower DAS score is found in RA patients with MetS, regardless of traditional or biologic DMARD, remains to be determined.

Strengths of the study include that it is of a well-characterized group of males with RA, a group that to date has been vastly underrepresented in clinical research. Moreover, the patients treated at these sites have equal access to medical care and RA therapies, hence providing the unique opportunity to explore disease related outcomes in a uniform health system. Although premature atherosclerosis occurs in RA independent of traditional risk factors, our findings indicate that it is the composite entity of the metabolic syndrome rather than its individual components that pose the risk for CVD. Optimum control of all individual components is required to minimize cardiovascular morbidity.

5. Acknowledgement

Jeffrey Huang, Research Assistant, for manuscript preparation and literature review.

6. References

Alberti KG, Zimmet P, Shaw J, for the IDF Epidemiology Task Force Consensus Group. The metabolic syndrome--a new worldwide definition. *Lancet* 2005;366:1059-1062.

Arnett FC, Edworthy SM, Bloch DA, et al. The American Rheumatism Association 1987 revised criteria for the classification of rheumatoid arthritis. *Arthritis and Rheum,* 1988 Mar;31(3):315-24.

Balkau B, Sapinho D, Petrella A, et al. D.E.S.I.R. Study Group. Prescreening tools for diabetes and obesity-associated dyslipidaemia: comparing BMI, waist and waist hip ratio. The D.E.S.I.R. Study. *Eur J Clin Nutr.* 2006 Mar;60(3):295-304.

Baumgartner et al., 1999, Am J Epidemiol 147:755-763

Bawa, S, Fowler L, Bradlow A. Comparison between DAS 28 4 Score & 3 Score- Would it influence patient eligibility for, or evaluation of response to Anti-TNF alpha? *British Society for Rheumatology Annual Meeting, 19-22 April 2005. Supplement 1:i99. 2005 March*

Choi HK, Hernan MA, Seeger JD, et al. Methotrexate and mortality in patients with rheumatoid arthritis: a prospective study. *Lancet*. 2002 Apr 6;359(9313):1173-7.

Chung CP, Oeser A, Solus JF, et al. Prevalence of metabolic syndrome is increased in rheumatoid arthritis and is associated with coronary atherosclerosis. *Atherosclerosis* 2008;196:756-763

Crowson CS, Myasoedova E, Davis JM 3rd, Matteson EL, Roger VL, Therneau TM, Fitz-Gibbon P, Rodeheffer RJ, Gabriel SE. Increased prevalence of metabolic syndrome associated with rheumatoid arthritis in patients without clinical cardiovascular disease. J Rheumatol. 2011 Jan;38(1):29-35.

Dekker JM, Girman C, Rhodes T, et al. Metabolic syndrome and 10-year cardiovascular disease risk in the Hoorn Study. *Circulation*. 2005;112:666–73.

Del Rincon ID, Williams K, Stern MP, et al. High incidence of cardiovascular events in a rheumatoid arthritis cohort not explained by traditional cardiac risk factors. *Arthritis Rheum*. 2001;44:2737–45.

Dessein PH, Joffe BI, Stanwix A, et al. The acute phase response does not fully predict the presence of insulin resistance and dyslipidemia in inflammatory arthritis. *J Rheumatol*. 2002;29:462–6.

Dessein PH, Stanwix AE, Joffe BI. Cardiovascular risk in rheumatoid arthritis versus osteoarthritis: acute phase response related decreased insulin sensitivity and high-density lipoprotein cholesterol as well as clustering of metabolic syndrome features in rheumatoid arthritis. *Arthritis Res*. 2002;4:R5.

Expert Panel on Detection, Evaluation, and Treatment of High Blood Cholesterol in Adults. Executive summary of the third report of the National Cholesterol Education Program (NCEP) Expert Panel on Detection, Evaluation, and Treatment of High Blood Cholesterol in Adults (Adult Treatment Panel III). *JAMA*. 2001;285:2486-2497.

Expert Panel on Detection, Evaluation, and Treatment of High Blood Cholesterol in Adults. Executive summary of the third report of the National Cholesterol Education Program (NCEP) Expert Panel on Detection, Evaluation, and Treatment of High Blood Cholesterol in Adults (Adult Treatment Panel III). *JAMA*. 2001;285:2486-2497

Farin HM, Abbasi F, Reaven GM. Comparison of body mass index versus waist circumference with the metabolic changes that increase the risk of cardiovascular disease in insulin-resistant individuals. *Am J Cardiol*. 2006;98(8):1053-6.

Ford ES, Giles WH, Dietz WH. Prevalence of the metabolic syndrome among US adults: findings from the third National Health and Nutrition Examination Survey. *JAMA*. 2002;287:356-359.

Gabriel SE, Crowson CS, O'Fallon WM. A comparison of two comorbidity instruments in arthritis. *J Clin Epidemiol*. 1999 Dec;52(12):1137-42.

Gonzalez-Gay MA, Gonzalez-Juanatey C, Martin J. Rheumatoid arthritis: a disease associated with accelerated atherogenesis. *Semin Arthritis Rheum*. 2005 Aug;35(1):8-17.

Grundy SM, Cleeman JI, Daniels SR, Donato KA, Eckel RH, Franklin BA, Gordon DJ, Krauss RM, Savage PJ, Smith SC Jr, Spertus JA, Costa F. Diagnosis and management of the metabolic syndrome: an American Heart Association/National Heart, Lung, and Blood Institute Scientific Statement. *Circulation* 2005;112:2735-2752.

Janghorbani M, Hedley AJ, Jones RB. Gender Differential in All-Cause and Cardiovascular Disease Mortality. *Int. J. Epidemiol.*1993;22:1056-1063

Jawaheer D, Lum RF, Gregersen PK, et al. Influence of male sex on disease phenotype in familial rheumatoid arthritis. *Arthritis Rheum. 2006 Oct;54(10):3087-94*

Karvounaris SA , Sidiropoulos PI, Papadakis JA, et al. Metabolic syndrome is common among middle-to-older aged Mediterranean patients with rheumatoid arthritis and correlates with disease activity: a retrospective, crosssectional, controlled, study. *Ann Rheum Dis.* 2007;66:28–33.

Klaasen R, Wijbrandts CA, Gerlag DM, Tak PP. Body mass index and clinical response to infliximab in rheumatoid arthritis. *Arthritis Rheum* 2011;63:359–64

Kremer JM , Reed G. Obesity is an Independent Contributor to Functional Capacity and Inflammation in Rheumatoid Arthritis and Psoriatic Arthritis. Presented at EULAR 2006 Meeting; June 21-24, 2006, Amsterdam, Netherlands.

Kremers HM, Gabriel SE. Rheumatoid arthritis and the heart. Curr Heart Fail Rep. 2006 Jun;3(2):57-63

Lakka HM, Laaksonen DE, Lakka TA, et al. The Metabolic Syndrome and Total and Cardiovascular Disease Mortality in Middle-aged Men. *JAMA.* 2002;288:2709-2716

Lorenzo C, Okoloise M, Williams K, et al. The metabolic syndrome as predictor of type 2 diabetes: the San Antonio Heart Study. *Diabetes Care.* 2003;26:3153-3159.

Maradit-Kremers H, Nicola PJ, Crowson CS, Ballman KV, et al. Cardiovascular death in rheumatoid arthritis: A population-based study. *Arthritis Rheum.* 2005 Mar; 52(3):722-32.

McEntegart A, Capell HA, Creran D, et al. Cardiovascular risk factors, including thrombotic variables, in a population with rheumatoid arthritis. *Rheumatology (Oxford).* 2001;40:640–4.

Meyer, J. Loh, C, Leckband SG, et al. Prevalence of the metabolic syndrome in veterans with schizophrenia. J. *Psychiatr Pract.* 2006 Jan;12(1):5-10

Mikuls TR, Fay BT, Michaud K, Sayles H, Thiele GM, Caplan L, Johnson D, Richards JS, Kerr GS, Cannon GW, Reimold A. Associations of disease activity and treatments with mortality in men with rheumatoid arthritis: results from the VARA registry. Rheumatology (Oxford). 2011 Jan;50(1):101-9.

Mikuls TR, Kazi S, Cipher Det al. The association of race and ethnicity with disease expression in male US veterans with rheumatoid arthritis. *J Rheum.* 2007 July;34(7):1480-1484

Najarian RM, Sullivan LM, Kannel WB, et al. Metabolic syndrome compared with type 2 diabetes mellitus as a risk factor for stroke: the Framingham Offspring Study. *Arch Intern Med.* 2006;166:106–11.

Ouchi N, Parker JL, Lugus JJ, Walsh K. Adipokines in inflammation and metabolic disease. *Nat Rev Immunol* 2011;11:85–97.

Pandya, P, Mathur S, Callahan P, et al. The prevalence of metabolic syndrome in veterans with chronic hepatitis C virus. *DDW,* May 21-24, 2006, Los Angeles.

Prevoo ML, Van 't Hof MA, Kuper HH, van Leeuwen MA, et al. Modified disease activity scores that include twenty-eight-joint counts. Development and validation in a prospective longitudinal study of patients with rheumatoid arthritis. Arthritis Rheum. 1995 Jan;38(1):44-48.

Rodriguez-Pla A, Giles JT, Blumenthal RS, Post W, Szklo M, Petri M, Gelber AC, Detrano R, Bathon JM. Decreased Prevalence of the Metabolic Syndrome in Rheumatoid Arthritis. *Arthritis Rheum* 2007; 56(9S):S416.

Stavropoulos-Kalinoglou A, Metsios GS, Koutedakis Y, Nevill AM, Douglas KM, Jamurtas A, van Zanten JJ, Labib M, Kitas GD. Redefining overweight and obesity in rheumatoid arthritis patients. *Ann Rheum Dis.* 2007 Oct;66(10):1316-21

Steven M. Comparison of Quality of Care for Patients in the Veterans Health Administration and Patients in a National Sample. *Ann Intern Med.* 2004 Dec;141:938-945.

Stevens RJ, Douglas KM, Saratzis AN, et al. Inflammation and atherosclerosis in rheumatoid arthritis. *Expert Rev Mol Med.* 2005 May 6;7(7):1-24.

World Health Organization. Definition, Diagnosis and Classification of Diabetes Mellitus and Its Complications: Report of a WHO Consultation. Geneva: World Health Organization. 1999.

14

Nontuberculous Mycobacterium Infections in Rheumatoid Arthritis Patients

Maiko Watanabe[1] and Shogo Banno[2]
[1]*Nagoya City University*
[2]*Aichi Medical University*
Japan

1. Introduction

Nontuberculous mycobacteria (NTM) are a large, diverse group of ubiquitous environmental organisms found in tap water, soil, dust, plants, animals, and food. NTM infection can cause various diseases, such as pulmonary disease (PD), which are most frequently observed in immunocompromised individuals. Diseases associated with NTM are particularly severe in those receiving tumor necrosis factor (TNF)-alpha (α) blockers, which predispose individuals to NTM infection. Experts generally agree that patients with active NTM disease should receive TNF-α blockers only if they are also receiving adequate therapy for NTM disease. On the other hand, the Japanese College of Rheumatology recommends that TNF-α blockers not be used in patients with active NTM infection, because NTM is resistant to most antimycobacterial drugs.

Bronchiectasis is one of the most frequent manifestations of NTM infection, not only in NTM-PD patients, but also in rheumatoid arthritis (RA) patients. It is difficult to distinguish the bronchiectasis associated with NTM-PD from that with RA on chest radiography or high-resolution computed tomography (HRCT). Due to the ease of NTM contamination from the environment, the diagnosis of NTM-PD is extremely difficult. The most recent American Thoracic Society (ATS) and Infectious Disease Society of America (IDSA) guidelines recommend diagnosing NTM-PD via a combination of clinical, radiographic, bacteriologic (two positive sputum cultures, or one positive bronchoalveolar lavage (BAL) culture or transbronchial biopsy), and histological criteria. In NTM-PD patients receiving TNF-α blockers, *Mycobacterium avium* was the most common etiologic organism, accounting for half of all NTM isolates (Winthrop et al., 2009). Recently, Kitada et al. (2008) established an enzyme immunoassay (EIA) for the serological diagnosis of *M. avium*-complex (MAC)-PD by examining the level of serum IgA antibody to the glycopeptidolipid (GPL) core, which is a MAC-specific antigen. Unlike bronchoscopy and sputum culture examinations, EIA kits are less invasive and provide more rapid diagnosis of MAC-PD.

In this chapter, we discuss the characteristics of NTM, relationship between NTM infections and RA patients, particularly those receiving TNF-α blockers, and diagnosis of MAC-PD with RA patients using the recently developed EIA kit.

2. NTM infections

2.1 Etiology of NTM infections

NTM are environmental organisms found in not only in natural and tap water, but also in soil, dust, plants, animals, and food (Falkinham, 1996, 2002; Jarzebowski & Young, 2005; Sugita et al., 2000; Tortoli, 2006). Presently, NTM consist of more than 130 species, with approximately 60 of these being suspected or known to cause disease. However, NTM infections are not transmitted between humans or between animals and humans (Cook, 2010). NTM infection can result in skin and pulmonary disease, lymphadenitis, gastrointestinal disease, and in severely immunocompromised individuals, disseminated disease (McGrath, 2010). Moreover, the progression of NTM infection to clinical disease requires one or more predisposing host conditions; NTM-PD typically occurs in patients who are not obviously immunosuppressed, but who nearly always have pre-existing abnormalities.

Notably, approximately 80% of patients with NTM disease are middle-aged or elderly women (Cook, 2010), and it is suspected that the high rate of NTM lung disease in postmenopausal women is due to their lower estrogen levels (Koh & Kwon, 2005). Other hypotheses for the higher disease rate in women include differences in the anatomy and physiology of the respiratory tract, combined with repeated infections by different strains over time (Chalermskulrat et al., 2002). Most female patients have underlying bronchiectasis that typically requires computed tomography (CT) examination for detection and that is associated with previous histories of lung infection or other, often obscure, underlying causes.

Chronic pulmonary manifestations of NTM infections, which are among the most common in NTM-PD patients, include chronic obstructive pulmonary disease (COPD), bronchiectasis, periostitis, *Mycobacterium tuberculosis* (TB) infection, cystic fibrosis, and pneumoconiosis. Patients receiving treatment with TNF-α blockers, or those with certain body characteristics (*e.g.*, pectus excavatum or scoliosis, particularly in postmenopausal women) are at higher risk for such manifestations, although NTM infection in individuals without risk factors is well reported (Griffith et al., 2007). Impairment of local immune function, including clearance of secretions, abnormal composition of airway surface liquid, and airway and mucosal damage due to chronic PD, may increase the propensity for NTM-PD (Morrissey, 2007). In addition, although a clear association exists between bronchiectasis and NTM disease (Cook, 2010), NTM infection also develops prior to the manifestation of bronchiectasis (Holling et al., 2002; Kubo et al., 1998; Moore, 1993; Primak et al., 1995). Thus, the observations in bronchiectasis patients suggest that bronchiectasis appears to be both a risk factor and a consequence of NTM infection (Barker, 2002).

2.2 Types of NTM-PD

Chest radiographs are not as sensitive as HRCT scanning for detecting abnormalities associated with NTM-PD (Kubo et al., 1998; Olivier, 1998; Swensen et al., 1994; Tanaka et al., 2001; Winttram & Weisbrad, 2002). CT can further characterize cavities and reveal associated bronchiectasis and pleural thickening (Ellisi & Hansell, 2002; Hartman et al., 1993). Three prototypical presentations of lung disease are reported in NTM-PD: (1) cavitary disease, (2) fibronodular bronchiectasis, and (3) hypersensitivity pneumonitis (HP) (Field & Cowie, 2006). The two former types are the most common manifestations observed in NTM-PD patients (Goo & Im, 2002).

1. Cavitary disease

This type of lung disease, which represents "a TB-like pattern" of disease, is quite similar to that associated with post-primary TB. Cavitary disease is often seen in older men with substantial smoking histories and chronic PD (*e.g.*, COPD, pneumoconiosis, prior TB, and sarcoidosis) (Bandoh et al., 2004; Christensen et al., 1981; Dhillon & Watanakunakorn, 2000; Fowler et al., 2006; Glassroth, 2008; Morita et al., 2005; Sonnenberg et al., 2000; Teosk & Lo, 1992; Wickremasinghe et al., 2005; Witly et al., 1994). Cavitary disease associated with NTM mostly occurs in the apical and posterior segments of the upper lobe, although multiple lung segments may be involved. Cavitations typically include thick walls and no air-fluid level, and are often associated with pleural thickening, which is more extensive than that seen in TB. However, pleural effusion and substantial lymph node enlargement are less common than in TB (Albelda et al., 1985; Christensen et al., 1981; Reich & Johnson, 1991; Woodring et al., 1987) (Fig. 1). The symptoms of NTM-induced cavitary disease include cough, fever, weight loss, weakness, haemoptysis, and respiratory insufficiency (Griffith et al., 2007; Piersimoni & Scarparo, 2008).

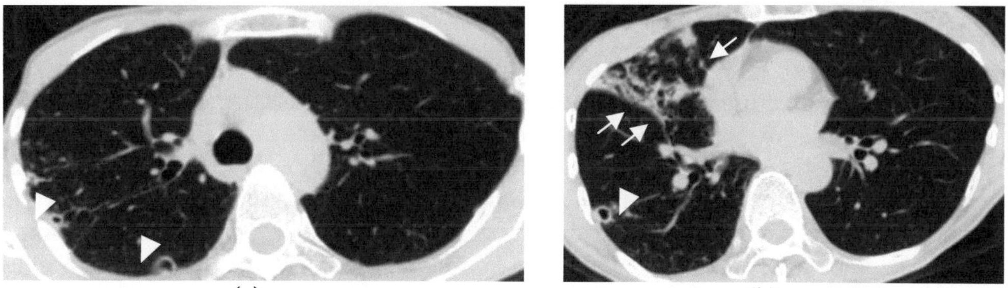

(a) (b)

Fig. 1. HRCT images of the lungs of a 63-year-old woman with MAC-PD. *M. avium* was detected in several sputum cultures. (a) Cavities with thick walls and no air-fluid level were seen in the right upper lobe (arrowheads) (b) Bronchiectasis with infiltration in the right middle lobe (arrows) and a cavity in the right lower lobe (arrowhead) were detected.

2. Fibronodular bronchiectasis

In fibronodular bronchiectasis, CT findings are characterized by small centrilobular nodules or tree-in-bud opacities, with cylindrical bronchiectasis typically detected in the same lobe (Han et al., 2003; Hartman et al., 2003; Moore, 1993; Obayashi et al., 1999; Primack et al., 1995; Swensen et al., 1994) (Fig. 2). Bronchiectasis is more commonly associated with NTM than in TB (Primack et al., 1995), with bilateral bronchiectasis and bronchiolitis occurring in one third of NTM patients, as detected by HRCT. However, the coexistence of bronchiectasis and bronchiolitis (*i.e.*, centrilobular nodules and mosaic pattern) is also highly suggestive of NTM infection (Koh et al., 2005). Typical HRCT findings are often observed in the right middle lobe or lingual, which are anatomically predisposed to impaired clearance of secretions, a condition referred to as "Lady Windermere syndrome" (Reich & Johnson, 1992). Fibronodular bronchiectasis is most common in elderly women without preexisting pulmonary conditions or histories of tobacco abuse, but who often have anatomic abnormalities of the chest (Chan et al., 2007; Daley & Griffith, 2002; Dhillon & Watanakunakorn, 2000; Field & Cowie, 2006; Iseman et al., 1991; Jarzembowski & Young, 2008, Okumura et al., 2008, Prince et al., 1989; Taiwo & Glassroth, 2010). The major symptom of fibronodular bronchiectasis is a persistent cough, and the disease can result in severe lung damage, although many patients experience a less aggressive, chronic course (Prince et al., 1989; Taiwo & Glassroth, 2010).

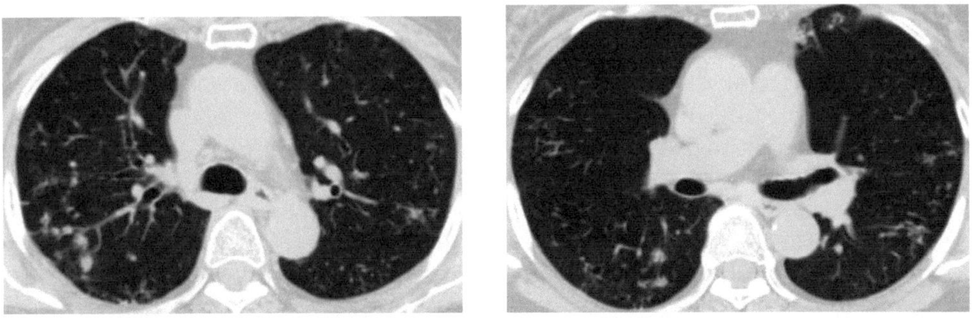

Fig. 2. HRCT images of the lungs of a 69-year-old woman with MAC-PD. Multiple diffuse, small, centrinodular nodules and tree-in bud opacities were seen in the all lobes.

3. Hypersensitive pneumonitis

The third presentation of lung disease in NTM-PD is HP, which has first recognized as having a presentation similar to hypersensitivity lung disease (Griffith et al., 2007). HP can occur after the use of hot tubs and medicinal baths (Khoor et al., 2001). The lung inflammation and infection associated with HP are thought to lead to unique pathological features that differ distinctly from those of other NTM lung diseases. It is unclear whether MAC antigens are solely responsible for triggering host responses or whether there are other hot-tub associated cofactors (organic or inorganic) or host predispositions that may be contributing to the disease process (Griffith et al., 2007).

2.3 Diagnosis and treatment of NTM

As NTM are ubiquitous environmental saprophytes often found in water supplies, it is difficult to determine whether the growth of NTM isolates from a patient specimen represents true disease and transient colonization of a nonsterile site, such as the lung, or is a result of laboratory contamination. Pseudo-outbreaks of NTM have been described as a result of contamination of hospital laboratories, water supplies, and instruments such as bronchoscopes (Gubler et al., 1992). Once the diagnosis of NTM infection has been made, a treatment of long duration of is typically required (Stout, 2006). As the risk of contamination of the sputum by environmental mycobacteria is high, the misattribution of the clinical significance of a positive detection would lead to a useless treatment for the patient (Tortoli, 2008).

The ATS/IDSA guidelines of 2007 set criteria for the diagnosis of NTM and recommend that the minimum evaluation of a patient suspected of having NTM-PD should include the following: (1) chest radiograph or, in the absence of cavitations, chest HRCT scan, (2) collection of three or more sputum specimens for acid-fast bacterium (AFB) analysis, and (3) exclusion of other disorders such as TB and lung malignancy. Furthermore, diagnosis of NTM pulmonary infection requires the fulfillment of both clinical and microbiological criteria. Clinically, it necessary that both of the following criteria are met: (1) pulmonary symptoms, nodular or cavity opacities on chest radiograph, or a HRCT scan showing multifocal bronchiectasis with multiple small nodules, and (2) appropriate exclusion of other diagnoses. Microbiologically, only one of the following criteria are required: (1) positive culture result from at least two separate expectorated sputum samples, (2) positive culture result from at least one bronchial wash or lavage, or (3) transbronchial or other lung biopsy with mycobacterial histopathologic features (granulomatous inflammation or AFB) and positive culture for NTM, or biopsy showing mycobacterial histopathologic features and one or more sputum or bronchial washings that are culture positive (Griffith et al., 2007).

NTM patients with multiple positive cultures for the identical NTM pathogen and cavitary PD or major areas of bronchiectasis usually require therapy (Cook, 2010). Treatment of NTM infection should include at least three effective drugs, such as macrolides, for a minimum of 12 months after sputum samples appear similar to negative controls. However, long-term treatment with macrolides can lead to resistance, which is most frequently due to 23S rRNA gene mutations at positions 2058-2059. It was reported that 76% of patients receiving macrolide monotherapy or macrolide plus a fluoroquinolone developed resistance, whereas resistance only developed in 4% of patients treated with a regimen of clarithromycin, etambutol, and a rifamycin (Griffith et al., 2006). Due to the long duration of treatment, side effects, and the impact of these factors on patient compliance, the treatment outcomes of NTM are variable and often poor (Glassroth, 2008; Piersimoni & Scarparo, 2008).

2.4 Mycobacterium avium complex

Mycobacterium avium complex (MAC) is the term used to describe a group of slow-growing, nonpigmented (although a yellow pigment may be produced in the absence of light) AFB (Griffith et al., 2007; Inderljed et al., 1993; Tortoli, 2006). MAC species are found worldwide, but are isolated more frequently in temperate regions, including the USA, Europe, Japan, and South Africa (Inderljed et al., 1993). MAC consists of at least two major mycobacterial species, *M. avium* and *M. intracellulare*, which cannot be differentiated on the basis of traditional physical and biochemical tests, and require specific DNA probes for identification. MAC is the most common cause of NTM infections and predominantly results in pulmonary or disseminated disease (Haverkort, 2003; Marin-Casabona et al., 2004; Thomsen et al., 2002). *M. avium* is the more important pathogen in disseminated disease, whereas *M. intracellulare* is the more common respiratory pathogen.

MAC-PD is predominantly observed in postmenopausal, non-smoking, Caucasian females (Griffith et al., 2007). In Japan, among 273 newly diagnosed MAC-PD cases between 1996 and 2002, 70.3% were female with a mean age of 63.2 years (Okumura et al., 2008). The HRCT findings of MAC-PD also exhibit all three forms of lung disease, as described for NTM-PD, namely cavitary disease, fibronodular bronchiectasis, and HP (Cappelluti et al., 2003; Embil et al., 1997; Glassroth, 2008; Kahana et al., 1997). Fibronoduar bronchiectasis caused by MAC is most frequently observed in women >60 years old, and compared to patients with other types of NTM infection, the lingual and right middle lobe tend to be more severely and progressively involved (Hollings et al., 2002; Kim et al., 2005; Kubo et al., 1998; Obayashi et al., 1999; Prince et al., 1989; Tanaka et al., 2001). In a recent clinical study, MAC was cultured from the sputum of 25% of the patients with fibronodular bronchiectasis, and MAC infection was documented in 50% of bronchoscopies, including BAL and transbronchial biopsies (Griffith et al., 2007). Although the cornerstones of MAC treatment are the macrolides clarithromycin, azithromycin, and ethambutol, MAC species are saprophytic and possess cell walls that are relatively impenetrable to an array of chemicals, endowing them with intrinsic resistance to many antimicrobials (Mdluli et al., 1998).

2.5 The role of TNF-α in NTM infection

Host defenses of the lung against NTM involve both anatomical and functional integrity of the airway system and specific cellular immune responses (Arend et al., 2009). Disorders of the cellular immune system are associated predominantly with disseminated NTM infection, and are also found in patients receiving immunosuppressive drugs for inflammatory disorders, such as TNF-α blockers. TNF-α blockers are also associated with an increased risk of TB, as well as susceptibility to other opportunistic infections by intracellular pathogens (Arend et al., 2009; Crum et al., 2005; Kaene, 2005, 2008). TNF-α is released by a variety of inflammatory cells in response to immune recognition of mycobacterial lipoarabinomannan. Interferon-γ and interleukin (IL)-12 control mycobacteria in large part through the up-regulation of TNF-α, which is predominantly produced by monocytes/macrophages (Ehlers et al., 1999; Gardam et al., 2003; Griffith et al., 2007). TNF-α binds to the macrophage membrane-bound TNF-α receptors 1 and 2 and acts through the intracellular nuclear factor–kappa B pathway to modulate gene expression (Griffith et al., 2007; Jacob et al., 2007; Mutlu et al., 2006). Intracellular signaling through TNF receptor 1 is essential for efficacious host defense against intracellular pathogens, such as *M. tuberculosis* (Bean et al., 1999; Pfeffer et al., 1993), whereas TNF receptor 2 plays only a minimal role in this process. TNF-α recruits and activates other inflammatory cells, and is essential for granuloma formation (Kindler et al., 1989), which has a crucial role in the control of infections due to intracellular pathogens, including *M. tuberculosis, Listeria monocytogens, Histoplasma capsuptum*, and NTM (Ehlers, 2005; Wallis, 2004). As TNF-α blockers interfere with granuloma formation, one of their side effects is increased susceptibility to mycobacterial disease (Keane et al., 2001; Marie et al., 2005; Wallis et al., 2004). As with TB, TNF-α blockers represent important, new, potent factors for predisposing individuals to NTM infections (Griffith, 2010). However, the incidence of NTM infections during treatment with TNF-α blockers, such as infliximab and etanercept, was several-fold lower than that of TB (Wallis et al., 2004). The risks underlying predisposition to NTM infections and those promoting progression of active NTM infection are unknown (Griffith et al., 2007).

2.6 Biologics used in RA patients and adverse side effects, including NTM infections

RA is a systemic autoimmune disorder characterized by chronic polyarticular synovial inflammation that often leads to irreversible joint damage, disability, and deformity. Joint inflammation is a result of the excessive production of pro-inflammatory cytokines, such as TNF-α, IL-1, and IL-6, by activated T cells and the stimulation of immunoglobulin production by B cells. Over the last two decades, numerous effective biotherapies have been developed to lower pro-inflammatory cytokine production. Prior to biotherapy, the incidence rate of infections in the RA population was nearly twice as high as that in matched non-RA controls. In post-marketing surveillance and observational studies of TNF-α blockers, serious NTM infections appear to be the most frequent adverse event, with a reported prevalence of 6%-18% and an incidence rate of approximately 6 per 100 patient-years, representing a two- to three-fold higher incidence in patients receiving TNF-α blockers compared with controls (Salliot et al., 2009).

Presently, nine biologics for treating RA are available: five TNF-α blockers (Infliximab (Remicade®), etanercept (Enbrel®), adalimumab (Humira®), certolizumab pegol (Cimzia®), golimumab (Simponi®), an anti-IL-1 therapy (anakinra (Kineret®)), an anti-CTLA4 therapy (abatacept (Orencia®)), an anti-CD20 therapy (rituximab (Rituxan® or Mabthera®)), and an anti-IL-6 therapy (tocilizumab (Actemura®)). TNF-α blockers include both soluble receptors that serve as decoy receptors competing with TNF receptors (etanercept) and monoclonal antibodies that target TNF receptors (infliximab, adalimumab, golimumab, and certolizumab pegol). Anakinra is an IL-1 receptor antagonist that targets IL-1, which is an important cytokine in RA pathogenesis. Rituximab is a monoclonal antibody that selectively targets the chimeric anti-CD20, which is found primarily on B-cells. Abatacept is a recombinant human fusion protein consisting of a monoclonal antibody against CTLA-4 and a domain of CTLA-4, and serves to down-regulate T-cell activation (Salliot et al., 2009).

According to the most recent meta-analysis of adverse effects of biologics based on randomized controlled trials, controlled clinical trials, and open-label extension studies, biologics as a group, after adjusting for dose, were associated with a statistically higher rate of total adverse events odds ratio (OR; 1.19) and withdrawals due to adverse events (OR 1.32), and an increased risk of TB reactivation (OR 4.68) compared to controls (Gauhar et al., 2007). Notably, TB reactivation with TNF-α blockers was drug specific, and the incidence in the biologic group was 0.149%, whereas that in control group was 0.030% (Gauhar et al., 2007). Although the risk of TB was analyzed in this report, the incidence of NTM infection was not described. However, several case reports have noted NTM-associated disease in patients receiving infliximab and etanercept (Marie et al., 2005; Mufti et al., 2005; Salvana et al., 2007; Winthrop et al., 2008), and infliximab has been statistically more increased infection ratio of mycobacterium species than etanercept (Wallis et al., 2004). There is less incidence of NTM with Infliximab than with etanercept, because infliximab binds both monomeric and trimeric forms of soluble TNF-α, whereas etanercept only binds the trimeric form. Moreover, etanercept binds less strongly to transmembrane TNF-α than infliximab (Keane, 2005; Wallis et al., 2004).

One reason for the few reports of NTM infections caused by TNF-α blocker administration may relate to the lack of evidence for a latent phase in NTM infections. In addition, NTM disease is generally insidious, occasionally difficult to diagnose, and is not required to be reported to health authorities. Furthermore, NTM infections can persist even after at least 12 months of TNF-α blocker therapy and are therefore often considered to be new infections. The generally lower pathogenicity of NTM species, as compared to *M. tuberculosis*, could further explain the lower frequency of TNF blocker-associated NTM disease (van Ingen et al., 2008). However, the frequency of NTM disease compared with TB reactivation was reported to be 5- to 10-fold higher in patients undergoing therapy with TNF-α blockers (Wallis et al., 2004). As there is no evidence for the existence of a latent phase in NTM disease, screening for NTM before initiating immunosuppressive treatment might be challenging, and is further complicated by the lack of specific tests for the detection of NTM infection. Chest radiography typically only detects diverse and partly species-specific patterns (Griffith et al., 2007); moreover, these features represent active NTM disease and cannot be used to identify early infection. Despite these difficulties, the number of NTM infections has recently exceeded that of TB (Winthrop et al., 2008), which may reflect improvements in the screening for latent TB infection (Arend et al., 2003; Beglinger et al., 2007; Carmona et al., 2005; Centers for Disease Control and Prevention, 2004; Keane & Bresnihan, 2008; Leding et al., 2005).

Among the new drug classes developed for anti-RA therapy, anti-IL-17 and anti-IL-23 antibodies are particularly significant to NTM infections, as they have important roles in all stages of the immune response against mycobacterial infection, from neutrophil recruitment in early phases to granuloma formation and maintenance in later stages (Lubberts, 2008;

McInnes & Liew, 2005). These two agents modify JAK-STAT signaling, which is an essential step in mycobacterial immunity, leading to increased susceptibility to mycobacterial disease in humans (Haverkamp et al., 2006). Metalloproteinase inhibitors are also likely to confer an increased risk of mycobacterial infection (van Ingen et al., 2008). Although NTM infection in patients receiving TNF-α blockers is relatively rare and its diagnosis can be difficult, the presence of infection should be evaluated because TNF-α blockers and new drugs for anti-RA therapy represent notable predisposing factors for potentially serious, even fatal, infections.

In a number of RA patients receiving TNF-α blockers, NTM-PD progressed despite aggressive antimycobacterial treatment (Winthrop et al., 2009). Etanercept therapy has been reported in association with fatal MAC-PD, fatal pulmonary *M. xenopi* infection (Maimon et al., 2007), *M. chelonae* endophthalmitis (Stewart et al., 2006), *M. xenopi* spinal osteomyelitis (Yim et al., 2004), and pulmonary *M. szulgai* infection (van Ingen et al., 2007). Due to the long duration and potential side effects of antibiotics, the treatment of NTM disease is difficult and the outcome is often disappointing (Griffith et al., 2007; Jenkins et al., 2008; van Ingen et al., 2007). Although the ATS recommendations consider active TB infection prior to completing a standard regimen of anti-TB therapy to be a contraindication for treatment with biologic agents, no information is available for NTM disease (Saag et al., 2008). The Japanese College of Rheumatology recommends that TNF-α blockers not be used in patients with active NTM infection, because NTM is resistant to most antimycobacterial drugs. On the other hand, expert opinion is that patients with active NTM disease should receive TNF-α blockers only if they are concomitantly receiving adequate therapy for the NTM disease (Griffith et al., 2007). American College of Rheumatology and European Urban Research Association don't restrict the use of TNF-α blockers in patients the NTM. By contrast, several reports on immune reconstitution inflammatory syndrome (IRIS) have been described for a variety of diseases in HIV patients, including MAC lymphadenitis and pulmonary and central nervous system tuberculosis. IRIS appears to be mediated by a recovering immune system upon the recognition of circulating antigens to which it previously mounted a minimal response (Shelburne & Hamill, 2003). While IRIS to TB associated with infliximab treatment has been described in HIV-uninfected individuals (Belknop et al., 2005; Garcia et al., 2005), no cases of IRIS to MAC have been reported for this subset of patients. However, concurrent low-dose treatment with TNF-α blockers might produce immunological regulation that is beneficial for this group of patients (Garcia et al., 2005), because the disruption of granuloma formation by TNF-α blockers could increase exposure of the bacteria to antimycobacterial drugs, resulting in improved infection outcomes (Wallis, 2005). Whether TNF-α blockers can be safely continued during antimycobacterial therapy remains unclear. It is also not evident when it would be safe to reinstitute anti-TNF-α therapy in NTM-infected patients (Winthrop et al., 2009). Therefore, TNF-α blockers should always be discontinued on diagnosis of NTM infection, but IRIS should be strongly suspected if clinical and radiologic deterioration occur during an appropriate time frame after cessation of these drugs (Salvana et al., 2007).

2.7 Pulmonary manifestations in RA

Extra-articular manifestations of RA include intrathoracic lesions; parenchymal pulmonary disease; interstitial lung disease (fibrosing alveolitis); rheumatoid nodules, cryptogenic organizing pneumonia, bronchiolotis obloterans and bronchiectasis; airway disease; cricoarytenoid arthritis and obstructive airway disease; pleural disease; pleural effusion, pneumothorax, and pleurisy; vascular disease (pulmonary hypertension and vasculitis), eosionophilic pneumonia, shrinking lung, and pulmonary amyloidosis (Anaya et al., 1995; Ganhar et al., 2007; Mori et al., 2008; Tanaka et al., 2004). It is reported that bronchial and bronchiolar changes, which include bronchiectasis, centrilobular nodules, or tree-in-bud opacities, are the most prevalent lung lesions in RA patients (Akira et al., 1999; Remy-Jardin et al., 1994). Rheumatoid PD, which includes bronchiolitis and bronchiectasis, develops in approximately 10% of RA patients. A genetic susceptibility to the development of bronchiectasis was identified for RA patients (Hillarby et al., 1993), and it has been proposed that the increased susceptibility of RA patients to pulmonary infections coupled with recurrent respiratory tract infections, which triggers immune reaction, may eventually lead to bronchiectasis and bronchiolectasis (Gauhar et al., 2007; Perez et al., 1998). Supporting this speculation, bronchiectasis was detected in HRCT scans in approximately 30% of RA patients, and represented one of the most frequent lung manifestations (Cortet et al., 1995; Hassan et al., 1995; Perez et al., 1998); however, clinically significant bronchiectasis is uncommon in RA, reportedly occurring in only 1%-3% of patients (Bryckaert et al., 1994; Shadick et al., 1994).

Bronchiectasis in RA predominantly involves the lower half of the bronchial tree (Manjunatha et al., 2010) (Fig. 3). Severe bronchiectasis typically occurs in female RA patients (Shadick et al., 1994), and the incidence of bronchiectasis in lifelong-nonsmoking RA patients with no pulmonary symptoms is 25% (Hassan et al., 1995). RA patients with bronchiectasis are 7.3 fold more likely to die during a 5-year follow-up period than the general population, 5.0 fold more likely to die than those with RA alone, and 2.4 fold more likely to die than those with bronchiectasis alone (Awinson et al., 1997). Despite this association with higher mortality, it is reported that the presence of bronchiectasis is not correlated with the severity of RA (Manjinatha et al., 2010). Bronchiectasis associated with RA can precede the development of arthritis, but may also occur during the course of the disease (Gorman et al., 2002). A relatively recent study reported that the most frequent HRCT finding in RA patients was bronchiectasis, which was observed in 41.3% of patients, with clear differences detected in early (diagnosed within 1 year; 33.8%) and longstanding RA patients (duration >3 years; 49.2%) (Mori et al., 2008). An association has also been suggested between connective tissue disorder and susceptibility to NTM (Guide & Holland,

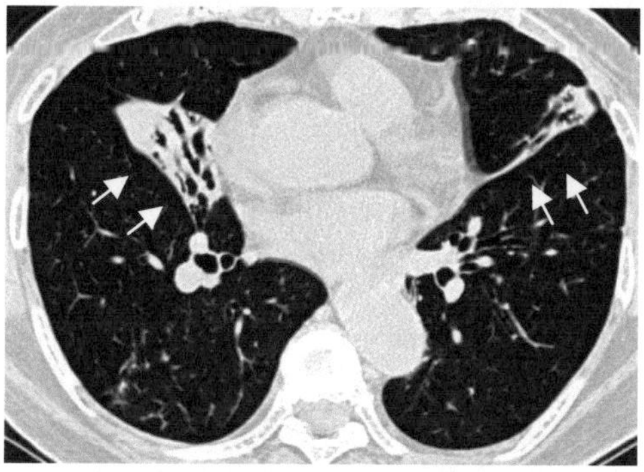

Fig. 3. HRCT image of the lungs of a 72-year-old woman suffering from RA for five years (stage 3, class 2). No NTM were detected in several analysed sputum cultures. The level of anti-GPL core IgA antibodies was negative (0.26 IU/l). Bronchiectasis was seen in the right middle lobe and lingula with infiltration (arrows).

2002). Among RA patients, NTM is more common in women >50 years of age (Gabriel, 2001; Griffith et al., 2007). According to United States Food and Drug Administration (FDA) MedWatch database, among patients with NTM disease receiving TNF-α blockers, the median age was 62 years, 65% were female, and the majority had RA. Notably, NTM infections were associated with all available TNF-α blockers, and MAC species were most commonly implicated as the infecting agents (Winthrop et al., 2009).

3. A new diagnostic tool for MAC-PD using an EIA kit detecting anti-GPL core antigen IgA antibodies

GPLs are the major cell-surface antigens of slowly growing mycobacteria, such as MAC, whereas *M. kansasii* and *M. tuberculosis* complex, and bacilli Calmette-Guerin (BCG) do not have GPLs in their cell walls (Brennan & Nikaido, 1995). The chemical structure of GPL consists of a common GPL core, with the different oligossacharide (polar GPL) moieties linked at the Thr substituent of the core. There are 31 distinct GPL serotypes, of which the complete structures of 14 have been identified (Aspinall et al., 1995; Brennan & Nikaido, 1995; Fujiwara et al., 2007; Kitada et al., 2005). Kitada et al. (2008) established an EIA kit for the serological diagnosis of MAC-PD that is based on the levels of serum IgA antibody to the GPL core. On examination of the MAC-specific IgG, IgA, and IgM immunoglobulin subclasses, the best results were obtained by the measurement of IgA, with a sensitivity of 92.5% and specificity of 95.1% for the GPL core. The serological testing of GPL core antibody levels could accurately differentiate MAC-PD from pulmonary TB, *M. kansasii*-PD, MAC colonization/contamination, and healthy subjects (Kitada et al., 2008). Furthermore, the GPL core-based EIA for diagnosing MAC disease is not affected by prior vaccination with BCG, because GPLs are not present in *M. tuberculosis* complexes (Brennan & Nikaido, 1995). Kitada et al. (2008) also reported that the levels of GPL core antibody, as measured by the developed EIA kit, in fibrocavitary disease and the nodular bronchiectasis-type of MAC-PD were significantly higher in the latter, although higher seropositivity was detected in fibrocavitary disease patients. Using the developed EIA kit, 15.8% false-negative determinations were made for patients with MAC-PD. Kitada et al. (2008) proposed several possible explanations for the false-negative results: (1) recently diagnosed disease; (2) change of GPL core antigenicity after chemotherapy; or (3) diversity of immune responses to GPL core in individual patients, potentially related to human leukocyte antigen genes.

In recent years, the number of case reports of NTM-PD disease among patients using TNF-α blockers has increased (Maimon et al., 2007; van Ingen et al., 2007; Winthrop et al., 2008). According to recent analysis of NTM infections associated with TNF-α blockers, of 105 confirmed or probable cases, most involved women (65%) and the median age was 63 years (range 20-90 years). Among these cases, *M. avium* was the most common etiologic organism identified (49%), followed by rapidly growing mycobacteria (19%) and *M. marinum* (8%) (Winthrop et al., 2009). As previously described, the diagnosis of MAC-PD is often challenging. Furthermore, bronchiectasis and NTM infection, predominantly MAC, often coexist (Griffith et al., 2007), and it is difficult to distinguish airway involvements due to bronchiectasis or bronchiolitis from those of MAC-PD on chest radiographs or HRCT. Moreover, before initiating TNF-α blockers, further pulmonary testing with sputum is indicated to rule out active NTM disease (van Ingen et al., 2008). However, as sputum cultures are not sufficiently sensitive for the diagnosis of NTM-PD, more invasive methods, such as bronchoalveolar lavage and biopsy, may be required to assess NTM infection (Huang et al., 1999).

Unlike bronchoscopy, the EIA kit developed by Kitada et al. (2008) is a rapid (results within a few hours) and noninvasive assay with high sensitivity and specificity for diagnosing MAC-PD. Therefore, we investigated the usefulness of anti-GPL core IgA antibodies in the diagnosis of MAC-PD in RA patients. Sixty-three RA patients were enrolled: 17 with MAC-PD, including 3 with positive cultures of NTM isolates other than MAC, 16 with pulmonary abnormalities characteristic of NTM, such as bronchiectasis, on CT but undetected in sputum culture, and 30 control subjects with normal chest CT and no respiratory symptoms. The mean levels of antibodies in patients with MAC-PD, abnormal chest CT without NTM, and controls were 1.08 ± 1.42, 0.04 ± 0.09, and 0.09 ± 0.12 IU/l, respectively, representing a significantly higher titer of EIA antibody in the MAC-PD group than that in the abnormal chest CT without NTM group (p=0.02). Furthermore, the serum antibody levels were significantly higher in the patients with MAC-PD than those with abnormal chest CT without NTM when compared to controls (p=0.02). With the cutoff points set at 0.7 IU/l, the sensitivity and specificity of the GPL core IgA antibody between MAC-PD and control RA patients were 43% and 100%, respectively. Using receiver operating characteristic analysis for MAC-PD and control patients, the area under the curve of anti-GPL core IgA antibody titers was significant large (p<0.005). GPL core antigen is also useful for the rapid and less invasive serodiagnosis of MAC-PD in RA patients. Representative HRCT images of the lungs of a 32-year-old woman with RA (stage 4, class 2) suffering from sinusitis and respiratory symptoms, including phlegm and cough, are presented in Fig. 4. *M. avium* was detected in the patient's sputum culture despite treatment with ethambutol and high-dose clarithromycin. The level of anti-GPL core IgA antibodies in this patient was correspondingly positive (0.88 IU/l; cutoff value, 0.7 IU/l) (Watanabe et al., 2011). Kitada et al. (2007, 2005) described that the effects of treatment on the EIA titers were limited because anti-GPL core IgA antibody levels did not change with failure of chemotherapy, and there was no conversion to seronegative from seropositive status. However, on monitoring of the patient shown in Fig. 4, we observed that the EIA titer declined gradually and became seronegative after antimycobacterial treatment (Watanabe et al., 2011).

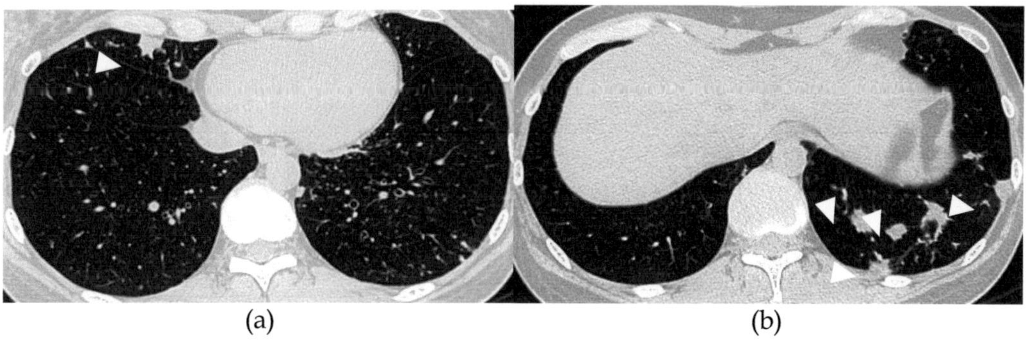

Fig. 4. HRCT images of the lungs of a 32-year-old woman with RA (stage 4, class 2) who had been suffering from sinusitis and respiratory symptoms. *M. avium* was detected in the patient's sputum culture despite of antimycobaterial treatment. Multiple nodules (arrowheads) were seen in the right middle and left lower lobes ((a) and (b)). Centrilobular tree-in-bud opacities with slight bronchiectasis were seen in the left lower lobe (a). EIA results were positive for the level of anti-GPL core IgA antibodies (0.88 IU/l).

4. Conclusion

NTM infection is one of the most important adverse events in RA patients, particularly those receiving TNF-α blockers, as infections can lead to severe or even fatal disease. NTM are associated with several types of illness, including pulmonary manifestations, with bronchiectasis representing the most frequent pulmonary involvement in RA patients. However, RA bronchiectasis is not easily distinguishable from bronchiectasis caused by NTM on HRCT, and the diagnosis of NTM-PD is often difficult due to contamination by ubiquitous environmental NTM isolates. Therefore, less invasive examination methods, in place of bronchoscopy, are needed for the diagnosis of NTM-PD. MAC is the most common pathogen of NTM-PD patients receiving TNF-α blockers. A newly developed EIA method for detecting the GPL core antigen IgA antibodies of MAC was shown to be highly specific, rapid, and have low invasiveness; thus, the EIA kit may be useful as an additional tool for the diagnosis of MAC-PD in RA patients. Although more examinations are needed to evaluate the clinical effectiveness of the EIA kit, it may be useful not only as a diagnostic tool, but also for monitoring the treatment of MAC-PD in RA patients receiving TNF-α blockers. The EIA kit may aid in the determination to restart TNF-α blockers in patients with severe RA and MAC-PD.

5. References

Akira M, Sakatani M, Hara H. (1999). Thin-section CT findings in rheumatoid arthritis-associated lung disease: CT patterns and their courses. *J Comput Assist Tomogr,* 23, 941-948.

Albelda SM, Kern JA, Marinelli DL, Miller WT. (1985). Expanding spectrum of pulmonary disease caused by nontuberculous mycobacteria. *Radiology,* 157, 289-296.

Anaya JM, Diethelm L, Ortiz LA, Gutierrez M, Citera G, Welsh RA, Espinoza LR. (1995). Pulmonary involvement in rheumatoid arthritis. *Semin Arthritis Rheum,* 24, 242-254.

Arend SM, van Soolingen D, Ottenhoff TH. (2009). Diagnosis and treatment of lung infection with nontuberculous mycobacteria. *Curr Opin Pulm Med,* 15, 201-208.

Arend SM, Breedveld FC, van Dissel JT. (2003). TNF-alpha blockade and tuberculosis: better look before you leap. *Neth J Med,* 61, 111-119.

Aspinall GO, Chatterjee D, Brennan PJ. (1995). The variable surface glycolipids of mycobacteria: structures, synthesis of epitopes, and biological properties. *Adv Carbohydr Chem Biochem,* 51, 169-242.

Barker AF. (2002). Bronchiectasis. *N Engl J Med,* 346, 1383-1393.

Bean AG, Roach DR, Briscoe H, France MP, Korner H, Sedgwick JD, Britton WJ. (1999). Structural deficiencies in granuloma formation in TNF gene-targeted mice underlie the heightened susceptibility to aerosol Mycobacterium tuberculosis infection, which is not compensated for by lymphotoxin. *J Immunol,* 162, 3504-3511.

Beglinger C, Dudler J, Mottet C, Nicod L, Seibold F, Villiger PM, Zellweger JP. (2007). Screening for tuberculosis infection before the initiation of an anti-TNF-alpha therapy. *Swiss Med Wkly,* 137, 620-622.

Belknap R, Reves R, Burman W. Immune reconstitution to Mycobacterium tuberculosis after discontinuing infliximab. (2005). *Int J Tuberc Lung Dis,* 9, 1057-1058.

Boulman N, Rozenbaum M, Slobodin G, Rosner I. (2006) Mycobacterium fortuitum infection complicating infliximab therapy in rheumatoid arthritis. *Clin Exp Rheumatol,* 24, 723.

Brennan PJ, Nikaido H. (1995). The envelope of mycobacteria. *Annu Rev Biochem,* 64, 29-63.

Bryckaert M, Fontenay M, Lioté F, Bellucci S, Carriou R, Tobelem G. (1994). Increased mitogenic activity of scleroderma serum: inhibitory effect of human recombinant interferon-gamma. *Ann Rheum Dis,* 53, 776-779.

Cappelluti E, Fraire AE, Schaefer OP. (2003). A case of ""hot tub lung"" due to Mycobacterium avium complex in an immunocompetent host. *Arch Intern Med,* 14, 163, 845-848.

Carmona L, Gómez-Reino JJ, Rodr íguez-Valverde V, Montero D, Pascual-Gómez E, Mola EM, Carreño L, Figueroa M; BIOBADASER Group. (2005) Effectiveness of recommendations to prevent reactivation of latent tuberculosis infection in patients treated with tumor necrosis factor antagonists. *Arthritis Rheum,* 52, 1766-1772.

Centers for Disease Control and Prevention (CDC). (2004). Tuberculosis associated with blocking agents against tumor necrosis factor-alpha--California, 2002-2003. *MMWR Morb Mortal Wkly Rep,* 53, 683-686.

Chalermskulrat W, Gilbey JG, Donohue JF. (2002). Nontuberculous mycobacteria in women, young and old. *Clin Chest Med,* 23, 675-686.

Chan ED, Kaminska AM, Gill W, Chmura K, Feldman NE, Bai X, Floyd CM, Fulton KE, Huitt GA, Strand MJ, Iseman MD, Shapiro L. (2007). Alpha-1-antitrypsin (AAT) anomalies are associated with lung disease due to rapidly growing mycobacteria and AAT inhibits Mycobacterium abscessus infection of macrophages. *Scand J Infect Dis,* 39, 690-696.

Christensen EE, Dietz GW, Ahn CH, Chapman JS, Murry RC, Anderson J, Hurst GA. (1981). Initial roentgenographic manifestations of pulmonary Mycobacterium tuberculosis, M kansasii, and M intracellularis infections. *Chest,* 80, 132-136.

Cook JL. (2010). Nontuberculous mycobacteria: opportunistic environmental pathogens for predisposed hosts. *Br Med Bull,* 96, 45-59.

Corbett EL, Churchyard GJ, Clayton T, Herselman P, Williams B, Hayes R, Mulder D, De Cock KM. (1999). Risk factors for pulmonary mycobacterial disease in South African gold miners. A case-control study. *Am J Respir Crit Care Med,* 159, 94-99.

Cortet B, Flipo RM, Rémy-Jardin M, Coquerelle P, Duquesnoy B, Rémy J, Delcambre B. (1995). Use of high resolution computed tomography of the lungs in patients with rheumatoid arthritis. *Ann Rheum Dis,* 54, 815-819.

Crum NF, Lederman ER, Wallace MR. (2005). Infections associated with tumor necrosis factor-alpha antagonists. *Medicine (Baltimore),* 84, 291-302.

Daley CL, Griffith DE. (2002). Pulmonary disease caused by rapidly growing mycobacteria. *Clin Chest Med,* 23, 623-632.

Dhillon SS, Watanakunakorn C. (2000). Lady Windermere syndrome: middle lobe bronchiectasis and Mycobacterium avium complex infection due to voluntary cough suppression. *Clin Infect Dis,* 30, 572-575.

Ehlers S. (2005). Tumor necrosis factor and its blockade in granulomatous infections: differential modes of action of infliximab and etanercept? Clin Infect Dis, 41, S199-203.

Ehlers S, Benini J, Kutsch S, Endres R, Rietschel ET, Pfeffer K. (1999). Fatal granuloma necrosis without exacerbated mycobacterial growth in tumor necrosis factor receptor p55 gene-deficient mice intravenously infected with Mycobacterium avium. *Infect Immun,* 67, 3571-3579.

Ellis SM, Hansell DM. (2002). Imaging of Non-tuberculous (Atypical) Mycobacterial Pulmonary Infection. *Clin Radiol,* 57, 661-669.

Embil J, Warren P, Yakrus M, Stark R, Corne S, Forrest D, Hershfield E. (1997). lmonary illness associated with exposure to Mycobacterium-avium complex in hot tub water. Hypersensitivity pneumonitis or infection? *Chest,* 111, 813-816

Ergin A, Hascelik G. (2004). Non tuberculous mycobacteria (NTM) in patients with underlying diseases: results obtained by using polymerase chain reaction-restriction enzyme analysis between 1997-2002. *New Microbiol,* 27, 49-53.

Falkinham JO 3rd. (2002). Nontuberculous mycobacteria in the environment. *Clin Chest Med,* 23, 529-551.

Falkinham JO 3rd. (1996) Epidemiology of infection by nontuberculous mycobacteria. *Clin Microbiol Rev,* 9, 177-215.

Field SK, Cowie RL. (2006). Lung disease due to the more common nontuberculous mycobacteria. *Chest,* 129, 1653-1672.

Fowler SJ, French J, Screaton NJ, Foweraker J, Condliffe A, Haworth CS, Exley AR, Bilton D. (2006). Nontuberculous mycobacteria in bronchiectasis: Prevalence and patient characteristics. *Eur Respir J,* 28, 1204-1210.

Fujiwara N, Nakata N, Maeda S, Naka T, Doe M, Yano I, Kobayashi K. (2007). Structural characterization of a specific glycopeptidolipid containing a novel N-acyl-deoxy sugar from mycobacterium intracellulare serotype 7 and genetic analysis of its glycosylation pathway. *J Bacteriol,* 189, 1099-1108.

Gabriel SE. (2001). The epidemiology of rheumatoid arthritis. *Rheum Dis Clin North Am,* 27, 269-281.

Garcia Vidal C, Rodríguez Fernández S, Martínez Lacasa J, Salavert M, Vidal R, Rodríguez Carballeira M, Garau J. (2005). Paradoxical response to antituberculous therapy in infliximab-treated patients with disseminated tuberculosis. *Clin Infect Dis,* 40, 756-759.

Gardam MA, Keystone EC, Menzies R, Manners S, Skamene E, Long R, Vinh DC. (2003). Anti-tumour necrosis factor agents and tuberculosis risk: mechanisms of action and clinical management. *Lancet Infect Dis,* 3, 148-155.

Gauhar UA, Gaffo AL, Alarcón GS. (2007). Pulmonary manifestations of rheumatoid arthritis. *Semin Respir Crit Care Med,* 28, 430-440.

Glassroth J. (2008). Pulmonary disease due to nontuberculous mycobacteria. *Chest,* 133, 243-251.

Goo JM, Im JG. (2002). CT of tuberculosis and nontuberculous mycobacterial infections. *Radiol Clin North Am,* 40, 73-87.

Gorman JD, Sack KE, Davis JC Jr. (2002) Treatment of ankylosing spondylitis by inhibition of tumor necrosis factor alpha. *Engl J Med,* 346, 1349-1356.

Griffith DE, (2010). Nontuberculous mycobacterial lung disease. *Curr Opin Infect Dis,* 23, 185-190.

Griffith DE, Aksamit T, Brown-Elliott BA, Catanzaro A, Daley C, Gordin F, Holland SM, Horsburgh R, Huitt G, Iademarco MF, Iseman M, Olivier K, Ruoss S, von Reyn CF,

Wallace RJ Jr, Winthrop K; ATS Mycobacterial Diseases Subcommittee; American Thoracic Society; Infectious Disease Society of America. (2007). An official ATS/IDSA statement: diagnosis, treatment, and prevention of nontuberculous mycobacterial diseases. *Am J Respir Crit Care Med,* 2007, 175, 367-416.

Griffith DE, Brown-Elliott BA, Langsjoen B, Zhang Y, Pan X, Girard W, Nelson K, Caccitolo J, Alvarez J, Shepherd S, Wilson R, Graviss EA, Wallace RJ Jr. (2006). Clinical and molecular analysis of macrolide resistance in Mycobacterium avium complex lung disease. *Am J Respir Crit Care Med,* 174, 928-934.

Griffith DE, Girard WM, Wallace RJ Jr. (1993) Clinical features of pulmonary disease caused by rapidly growing mycobacteria. An analysis of 154 patients. *Am Rev Respir Dis,* 147, 1271-1278.

Gubler JG, Salfinger M, von Graevenitz A. (1992). Pseudoepidemic of nontuberculous mycobacteria due to a contaminated bronchoscope cleaning machine. Report of an outbreak and review of the literature. *Chest,* 101, 1245-1249.

Guide SV, Holland SM. (2002). Host susceptibility factors in mycobacterial infection. Genetics and body morphotype. Infect Dis Clin North Am, 16, 163-186.

Han D, Lee KS, Koh WJ, Yi CA, Kim TS, Kwon OJ. (2003). Radiographic and CT findings of nontuberculous mycobacterial pulmonary infection caused by Mycobacterium abscessus. *Am J Roentgenol,* 181, 513-7.

Hartman TE, Swensen SJ, Williams DE. (1993). Mycobacterium avium-intracellulare complex: evaluation with CT. *Radiology,* 187, 23-26.

Hassan WU, Keaney NP, Holland CD, Kelly CA. (1995). High resolution computed tomography of the lung in lifelong non-smoking patients with rheumatoid arthritis. *Ann Rheum Dis,* 54, 308-310.

Haverkamp MH, van Dissel JT, Holland SM. (2006). Human host genetic factors in nontuberculous mycobacterial infection: lessons from single gene disorders affecting innate and adaptive immunity and lessons from molecular defects in interferon-gamma-dependent signaling. *Microbes Infect,* 8, 1157-1166.

Haverkort F; Australian Mycobacterium Reference Laboratory Network; Special Interest Group in Mycobacteria within the Australian Society for Microbiology. (2003). National atypical mycobacteria survey, 2000. *Commun Dis Intell,* 27, 180-189.

Hillarby MC, McMahon MJ, Grennan DM, Cooper RG, Clarkson RW, Davies EJ, Sanders PA, Chattopadhyay C, Swinson D. (1993) HLA associations in subjects with rheumatoid arthritis and bronchiectasis but not with other pulmonary complications of rheumatoid disease. *Br J Rheumatol,* 32, 794-797.

Hollings NP, Wells AU, Wilson R, Hansell DM. (2002). Comparative appearances of non-tuberculous mycobacteria species: a CT study. *Eur Radiol,* 12, 2211-2217.

Huang JH, Kao PN, Adi V, Ruoss SJ. (1999). Mycobacterium avium-intracellulare pulmonary infection in HIV-negative patients without preexisting lung disease: diagnostic and management limitations. *Chest,* 115, 1033-1040.

Inderlied CB, Kemper CA, Bermudez LE. (1993). The Mycobacterium avium complex. *Clin Microbiol Rev,* 6, 266-310.

Iseman MD, Buschman DL, Ackerson LM. (1991). Pectus excavatum and scoliosis. Thoracic anomalies associated with pulmonary disease caused by Mycobacterium avium complex. *Am Rev Respir Dis,* 144, 914-916.

Jacobs M, Togbe D, Fremond C, Samarina A, Allie N, Botha T, Carlos D, Parida SK, Grivennikov S, Nedospasov S, Monteiro A, Le Bert M, Quesniaux V, Ryffel B. (2007).Tumor necrosis factor is critical to control tuberculosis infection. *Microbes Infect,* 9, 623-628.

Jarzembowski JA, Young MB. (2008). Nontuberculous mycobacterial infections. *Arch Pathol Lab Med,* 132, 1333-1341.

Jenkins PA, Campbell IA, Banks J, Gelder CM, Prescott RJ, Smith AP. (2008). Clarithromycin vs ciprofloxacin as adjuncts to rifampicin and ethambutol in treating opportunist mycobacterial lung diseases and an assessment of Mycobacterium vaccae immunotherapy. *Thorax,* 63, 627-34.

Kahana LM, Kay JM, Yakrus MA, Waserman S. (1997). Mycobacterium avium complex infection in an immunocompetent young adult related to hot tub exposure. *Chest,* 111, 242-245.

Keane J, Bresnihan B. (2008). Tuberculosis reactivation during immunosuppressive therapy in rheumatic diseases: diagnostic and therapeutic strategies. *Curr Opin Rheumatol,* 20, 443-449.

Keane J, Gershon S, Wise RP, Mirabile-Levens E, Kasznica J, Schwieterman WD, Siegel JN, Braun MM. (2001). Tuberculosis associated with infliximab, a tumor necrosis factor alpha-neutralizing agent. *N Engl J Med,* 345, 1098-1104.

Keane J. (2005). TNF-blocking agents and tuberculosis: new drugs illuminate an old topic. *Rheumatology (Oxford),* 44, 714-720.

Khoor A, Leslie KO, Tazelaar HD, Helmers RA, Colby TV. (2001). Diffuse pulmonary disease caused by nontuberculous mycobacteria in immunocompetent people (hot tub lung). *Am J Clin Pathol,* 115, 755-762.

Kim TS, Koh WJ, Han J, Chung MJ, Lee JH, Lee KS, Kwon OJ. (2005). Hypothesis on the evolution of cavitary lesions in nontuberculous mycobacterial pulmonary infection: thin-section CT and histopathologic correlation. *Am J Roentgenol,* 184, 1247-1252.

Kindler V, Sappino AP, Grau GE, Piguet PF, Vassalli P. (1989). The inducing role of tumor necrosis factor in the development of bactericidal granulomas during BCG infection. *Cell,* 56, 731-740.

Kitada S, Kobayashi K, Ichiyama S, Takakura S, Sakatani M, Suzuki K, Takashima T, Nagai T, Sakurabayashi I, Ito M, Maekura R; MAC Serodiagnosis Study Group. (2008). Serodiagnosis of Mycobacterium avium-complex pulmonary disease using an enzyme immunoassay kit. *Am J Respir Crit Care Med,* 177, 793-797.

Kitada S, Maekura R, Toyoshima N, Naka T, Fujiwara N, Kobayashi M, Yano I, Ito M, Kobayashi K. (2005). Use of glycopeptidolipid core antigen for serodiagnosis of mycobacterium avium complex pulmonary disease in immunocompetent patients. *Clin Diagn Lab Immunol,* 12, 44-51.

Koh WJ, Kwon OJ. (2005) Mycobacterium avium complex lung disease and panhypopituitarism. *Mayo Clin Proc,* 80, 961-962.

Koh WJ, Lee KS, Kwon OJ, Jeong YJ, Kwak SH, Kim TS. (2005). Bilateral bronchiectasis and bronchiolitis at thin-section CT: diagnostic implications in nontuberculous mycobacterial pulmonary infection. *Radiology,* 235, 282-288.

Kubo K, Yamazaki Y, Hachiya T, Hayasaka M, Honda T, Hasegawa M, Sone S. (1998). Mycobacterium avium-intracellulare pulmonary infection in patients without known predisposing lung disease. *Lung,* 176, 381-391.

Ledingham J, Wilkinson C, Deighton C. (2005). British Thoracic Society (BTS) recommendations for assessing risk and managing tuberculosis in patients due to start anti-TNF-{alpha} treatments. *Rheumatology (Oxford)*, 44, 1205-1206.

Lubberts E. (2008). IL-17/Th17 targeting: on the road to prevent chronic destructive arthritis? *Cytokine*, 41, 84-91

Lynch DA, Simone PM, Fox MA, Bucher BL, Heinig MJ. (1995). CT features of pulmonary Mycobacterium avium complex infection. *J Comput Assist Tomogr*, 19, 353-360.

Maimon N, Brunton J, Chan AK, Marras TK. (2007). Fatal pulmonary Mycobacterium xenopi in a patient with rheumatoid arthritis receiving etanercept. Thorax, 62, 739-740.

Manjunatha YC, Seith A, Kandpal H, Das CJ. (2010). Rheumatoid arthritis: spectrum of computed tomographic findings in pulmonary diseases. *Curr Probl Diagn Radiol*, 39, 235-46.

Marie I, Heliot P, Roussel F, Hervé F, Muir JF, Levesque H. (2005). Fatal Mycobacterium peregrinum pneumonia in refractory polymyositis treated with infliximab. *Rheumatology (Oxford)*, 44, 1201-1202.

Martín-Casabona N, Bahrmand AR, Bennedsen J, Thomsen VO, Curcio M, Fauville-Dufaux M, Feldman K, Havelkova M, Katila ML, Köksalan K, Pereira MF, Rodrigues F, Pfyffer GE, Portaels F, Urgell JR, Rüsch-Gerdes S, Tortoli E, Vincent V, Watt B; Spanish Group for Non-Tuberculosis Mycobacteria. (2004). Non-tuberculous mycobacteria: patterns of isolation. A multi-country retrospective survey. *Int J Tuberc Lung Dis*, 8,1186-1193.

Maugein J, Dailloux M, Carbonnelle B, Vincent V, Grosset J; French Mycobacteria Study Group. (2005). Sentinel-site surveillance of Mycobacterium avium complex pulmonary disease. *Eur Respir J*, 26, 1092-1096.

McGrath EE, Blades Z, McCabe J, Jarry H, Anderson PB. (2010). Nontuberculous mycobacteria and the lung: from suspicion to treatment. *Lung*, 188, 269-282.

McInnes IB, Liew FY. (2005). Cytokine networks--towards new therapies for rheumatoid arthritis. *Nat Clin Pract Rheumatol*, 1, 31-39.

Mdluli K, Swanson J, Fischer E, Lee RE, Barry CE 3rd. (1998). Mechanisms involved in the intrinsic isoniazid resistance of Mycobacterium avium. *Mol Microbiol*, 27, 1223-1233.

Moore EH. (1993). Atypical mycobacterial infection in the lung: CT appearance. *Radiology*,187, 777 782.

Mori S, Cho I, Koga Y, Sugimoto M. (2008). Comparison of pulmonary abnormalities on high-resolution computed tomography in patients with early versus longstanding rheumatoid arthritis. *J Rheumatol*, 35, 1513-1521.

Morita H, Usami I, Torii M, Nakamura A, Kato T, Kutsuna T, Niwa T, Katou K, Itoh M. Isolation of nontuberculous mycobacteria from patients with pneumoconiosis. (2005). *J Infect Chemother*, 11, 89-92.

Morrissey BM. (2007). Pathogenesis of bronchiectasis. *Clin Chest Med*, 28, 289-296.

Mufti AH, Toye BW, Mckendry RR, Angel JB. (2005) Mycobacterium abscessus infection after use of tumor necrosis factor alpha inhibitor therapy: case report and review of infectious complications associated with tumor necrosis factor alpha inhibitor use. *Diagn Microbiol Infect Dis*, 53, 233-238.

Mutlu GM, Mutlu EA, Bellmeyer A, Rubinstein I. (2006). Pulmonary adverse events of anti-tumor necrosis factor-alpha antibody therapy. *Am J Med*, 119, 639-646.

Obayashi Y, Fujita J, Suemitsu I, Kamei T, Nii M, Takahara J. (1999). Successive follow-up of chest computed tomography in patients with Mycobacterium avium-intracellulare complex. *Respir Med,* 93, 11-15.

Okubo H, Iwamoto M, Yoshio T, Okazaki H, Kato T, Bandoh M, Minota S. (2005). Rapidly aggravated Mycobacterium avium infection in a patient with rheumatoid arthritis treated with infliximab. *Mod Rheumatol,* 15, 62-64.

Okumura M, Iwai K, Ogata H, Ueyama M, Kubota M, Aoki M, Kokuto H, Tadokoro E, Uchiyama T, Saotome M, Yoshiyama T, Yoshimori K, Yoshida N, Azuma A, Kudoh S. (2008). Clinical factors on cavitary and nodular bronchiectatic types in pulmonary Mycobacterium avium complex disease. *Intern Med,* 47, 1465-1472.

Olivier KN. (1998). Nontuberculous mycobacterial pulmonary disease. *Curr Opin Pulm Med,* 4, 148-53.

Perez T, Remy-Jardin M, Cortet B. (1998). Airways involvement in rheumatoid arthritis: clinical, functional, and HRCT findings. *Am J Respir Crit Care Med,* 157, 1658-1665.

Pfeffer K, Matsuyama T, Kündig TM, Wakeham A, Kishihara K, Shahinian A, Wiegmann K, Ohashi PS, Krönke M, Mak TW. (1993). Mice deficient for the 55 kd tumor necrosis factor receptor are resistant to endotoxic shock, yet succumb to L. monocytogenes infection. *Cell,* 73, 457-467.

Piersimoni C, Scarparo C. (2008) Pulmonary infections associated with non-tuberculous mycobacteria in immunocompetent patients. *Lancet Infect Dis,* 8, 323-334.

Primack SL, Logan PM, Hartman TE, Lee KS, Müller NL. (1995). Pulmonary tuberculosis and Mycobacterium avium-intracellulare: a comparison of CT findings. *Radiology,* 194, 413-417.

Prince DS, Peterson DD, Steiner RM, Gottlieb JE, Scott R, Israel HL, Figueroa WG, Fish JE. (1989). Infection with Mycobacterium avium complex in patients without predisposing conditions. *N Engl J Med,* 321, 863-868.

Reich JM, Johnson RE. (1992). Mycobacterium avium complex pulmonary disease presenting as an isolated lingular or middle lobe pattern. The Lady Windermere syndrome. *Chest,* 101, 1605-1609.

Reich JM, Johnson RE. (1991). Mycobacterium avium complex pulmonary disease. Incidence, presentation, and response to therapy in a community setting. *Am Rev Respir Dis,* 143, 1381-1385.

Remy-Jardin M, Remy J, Cortet B, Mauri F, Delcambre B. (1994). Lung changes in rheumatoid arthritis: CT findings. *Radiology,* 193, 375-382.

Saag KG, Teng GG, Patkar NM, Anuntiyo J, Finney C, Curtis JR, Paulus HE, Mudano A, Pisu M, Elkins-Melton M, Outman R, Allison JJ, Suarez Almazor M, Bridges SL Jr, Chatham WW, Hochberg M, MacLean C, Mikuls T, Moreland LW, O'Dell J, Turkiewicz AM, Furst DE; American College of Rheumatology. (2008). American College of Rheumatology 2008 recommendations for the use of nonbiologic and biologic disease-modifying antirheumatic drugs in rheumatoid arthritis. *Arthritis Rheum,* 59, 762-784.

Salliot C, Dougados M, Gossec L. (2009). Risk of serious infections during rituximab, abatacept and anakinra treatments for rheumatoid arthritis: meta-analyses of randomised placebo-controlled trials. *Ann Rheum Dis,* 68, 25-32.

Salvana EM, Cooper GS, Salata RA. (2007). Mycobacterium other than tuberculosis (MOTT) infection: an emerging disease in infliximab-treated patients. J Infect, 55, 484-7.

Shadick NA, Fanta CH, Weinblatt ME, O'Donnell W, Coblyn JS. (1994). Bronchiectasis. A late feature of severe rheumatoid arthritis. *Medicine (Baltimore)*, 73, 161-170.

Shelburne SA 3rd, Hamill RJ. (2003). The immune reconstitution inflammatory syndrome. *AIDS Rev*, 5, 67-79.

Sonnenberg P, Murray J, Glynn JR, Thomas RG, Godfrey-Faussett P, Shearer S. (2000).Risk factors for pulmonary disease due to culture-positive M. tuberculosis or nontuberculous mycobacteria in South African gold miners. Eur Respir J, 15, 291-296.

Stewart MW, Alvarez S, Ginsburg WW, Shetty R, McLain WC, Sleater JP. (2006). Visual recovery following Mycobacterium chelonae endophthalmitis. *Ocul Immunol Inflamm*, 14, 181-183.

Stout JE. (2006). Evaluation and management of patients with pulmonary nontuberculous mycobacterial infections. Expert Rev Anti Infect Ther, 4, 981-993.

Sugita Y, Ishii N, Katsuno M, Yamada R, Nakajima H. (2000). Familial cluster of cutaneous Mycobacterium avium infection resulting from use of a circulating, constantly heated bath water system. *Br J Dermatol*, 142, 789-793.

Swensen SJ, Hartman TE, Williams DE. (1994) Computed tomographic diagnosis of Mycobacterium avium-intracellulare complex in patients with bronchiectasis. *Chest*, 105, 49-52.

Swinson DR, Symmons D, Suresh U, Jones M, Booth J. (1997). Decreased survival in patients with co-existent rheumatoid arthritis and bronchiectasis. *Br J Rheumatol*, 36, 689-691.

Taiwo B, Glassroth J. (2010). Nontuberculous mycobacterial lung diseases. *Infect Dis Clin North Am*, 24, 769-789.

Tanaka D, Niwatsukino H, Oyama T, Nakajo M. (2001). Progressing features of atypical mycobacterial infection in the lung on conventional and high resolution CT (HRCT) images. *Radiat Med*, 19, 237-245.

Tanaka E, Amitani R, Niimi A, Suzuki K, Murayama T, Kuze F. (1997) Yield of computed tomography and bronchoscopy for the diagnosis of Mycobacterium avium complex pulmonary disease. *Am J Respir Crit Care Med*, 155, 2041-2046.

Tanaka N, Kim JS, Newell JD, Brown KK, Cool CD, Meehan R, Emoto T, Matsumoto T, Lynch DA. (2004). Rheumatoid arthritis-related lung diseases: CT findings. *Radiology*, 232, 81-91

Teo SK, Lo KL. (1992). Nontuberculous mycobacterial disease of the lungs in Singapore. *Singapore Med J*, 33, 464-466.

Thomsen VO, Andersen AB, Miörner H. (2002). Incidence and clinical significance of non-tuberculous mycobacteria isolated from clinical specimens during a 2-y nationwide survey. *Scand J Infect Dis*, 34, 648-653.

Tortoli E. (2009). Clinical manifestations of nontuberculous mycobacteria infections. *Clin Microbiol Infect*, 15, 906-910.

Tortoli E. (2006). The new mycobacteria: an update. *FEMS Immunol Med Microbiol*, 48, 159-178.

Turesson C, O'Fallon WM, Crowson CS, Gabriel SE, Matteson EL. (2003). Extra-articular disease manifestations in rheumatoid arthritis: incidence trends and risk factors over 46 years. *Ann Rheum Dis*, 62, 722-727.

van Ingen J, Boeree MJ, Dekhuijzen PN, van Soolingen D. (2008). Mycobacterial disease in patients with rheumatic disease. *Nat Clin Pract Rheumatol,* 4, 649-656.

van Ingen J, Boeree M, Janssen M, Ullmann E, de Lange W, de Haas P, Dekhuijzen R, van Soolingen D. (2007). Pulmonary Mycobacterium szulgai infection and treatment in a patient receiving anti-tumor necrosis factor therapy. *Nat Clin Pract Rheumatol,* 3, 414-419.

Wallis RS. (2005). Reconsidering adjuvant immunotherapy for tuberculosis. *Clin Infect Dis,* 41, 201-208.

Wallis RS, Broder M, Wong J, Beenhouwer D. (2004). Granulomatous infections due to tumor necrosis factor blockade: correction. *Clin Infect Dis,* 39, 1254-1255.

Wallis RS, Broder MS, Wong JY, Hanson ME, Beenhouwer DO. (2004) Granulomatous infectious diseases associated with tumor necrosis factor antagonists. *Clin Infect Dis,* 38, 1261-1265.

Watanabe M, Banno S, Sasaki K, Naniwa T, Hayami Y, Ueda R. (2011).Serodiagnosis of Mycobacterium avium-complex pulmonary disease with an enzyme immunoassay kit that detects anti-glycopeptidolipid core antigen IgA antibodies in patients with rheumatoid arthritis. *Mod Rheumatol,* 21, 144-149.

Wickremasinghe M, Ozerovitch LJ, Davies G, Wodehouse T, Chadwick MV, Abdallah S, Shah P, Wilson R. (2005). Non-tuberculous mycobacteria in patients with bronchiectasis. *Thorax,* 60, 1045-1051.

Winthrop KL, Chang E, Yamashita S, Iademarco MF, LoBue PA. (2009) Nontuberculous mycobacteria infections and anti-tumor necrosis factor-alpha therapy. *Emerg Infect Dis,* 15, 1556-1561.

Winthrop KL, Yamashita S, Beekmann SE, Polgreen PM; Infectious Diseases Society of America Emerging Infections Network. (2008). Mycobacterial and other serious infections in patients receiving anti-tumor necrosis factor and other newly approved biologic therapies: case finding through the Emerging Infections Network. *Clin Infect Dis,* 46, 1738-1740.

Wittram C, Weisbrod GL. (2002) Mycobacterium avium complex lung disease in immunocompetent patients: radiography-CT correlation. *Br J Radiol,* 75, 340-344.

Witty LA, Tapson VF, Piantadosi CA. (1994) Isolation of mycobacteria in patients with pulmonary alveolar proteinosis. *Medicine (Baltimore),* 73, 103-109.

Woodring JH, Vandiviere HM, Melvin IG, Dillon ML. (1987). Roentgenographic features of pulmonary disease caused by atypical mycobacteria. *South Med J,* 80, 1488-1497.

Yim K, Nazeer SH, Kiska D, Rose FB, Brown D, Cynamon MH. (2004). Recurrent Mycobacterium xenopi infection in a patient with rheumatoid arthritis receiving etanercept. *Scand J Infect Dis,* 36, 150-154.

Increased Mortality Rate in Rheumatoid Arthritis Patients with Neurological Symptoms or Signs Secondary to Cervical Spine Subluxations – Reduced Mortality if Postoperative Ankylosis is Achieved

Albert C. Paus[1], Harald Steen[1], Petter Mowinckel[2],
Jo Røislien[3] and Jens Teigland[1]
[1]*Orthopaedic Department, Oslo University Hospital, Oslo,*
[2]*Department of Paediatrics, Division Woman and Child, Oslo University Hospital, Oslo,*
[3]*Department of Biostatistics, Institute of Basic Medical Sciences, University of Oslo,*
Norway

1. Introduction

Patients in Norway with rheumatoid arthritis (RA) and involvement of the cervical column with subluxations during the years 1974-1999 were routinely referred to the Rheumasurgical Department of Oslo Sanitetsforening's Rheumatism Hospital in Oslo (OSR) for critical evaluation, treatment and follow-up. The patients were recruited from a large and widely dispersed area of the country.

The primary aim of the current study was to assess the mortality rate of operated patients with cervical neurological symptoms or signs in this cohort and compare the results with RA patients operated during the same period for cervical involvement without relevant neurology. Secondarily we wanted to disclose important factors affecting the mortality rate in operated RA patients with neurology. The results for the total RA population with cervical subluxations (n=532) treated during the same 25 year period (217 operated and 315 non-operated) have been published previously (Paus et al., 2008).

2. Material and methods

2.1 Patients

All patients referred with RA and neurological symptoms or signs related to involvement of the cervical column, were consecutively included from 1974 in the present prospective cohort study. Patients with other differential diagnoses, e.g. spondyl-arthritis, were excluded. After the end-point on December 31st 1999, all medical journals of included patients were revisited.

During this period 75 patients with RA and cervical spine subluxations with cervical radiculopathy, myelopathy or paresthesia were operated on in our department. There were 54 females (72%) and 21 males (28%) with a mean age at the first visit of 60 (SD, 11.9) years.

The RA diagnosis had been made at the mean age of 41 (SD, 13.7) years. By the end-point date, 51 (68%) patients had died at a mean age of 69 (SD, 9.3) years (Table 1).

	Operated with Neurology	Operated without Neurology	Total
Total number	75	142	217
Female/male	54/21	99/43	153/64
Age at RA diagnosis	41 (13.7)	39 (14.1)	40 (13.9)
Age at first visit	60 (11.9)	56 (12.3)	57 (12.3)
Age at operation	61 (11.5)	58 (12.0)	59 (11.9)
Follow-up period (years)	6.7 (5.5)	9.8 (5.8)	8.5 (5.9)
No of dead patients (%)	51 (68)	93 (65)	144 (66)
Age at death	69 (9.3)	69 (11.0)	69 (10.5)

Table 1. Various Data of Operated RA Patients with Cervical Subluxation with and without Neurological Symptoms or Signs. Mean Values with Standard Deviations (SD)

The total number of patients with RA and cervical problems operated in the neck during the same period was 217 patients, i.e. 142 patients without relevant, specific neurology.

The follow-up period after surgery till death or to Dec 31st 1999 for all the operated patients (n=217) was mean 8.5 (SD, 5.9) years, for those with relevant neurology (n=75) mean 6.7 (SD, 5.5) years and for those without (n=142) mean 9.8 (SD, 5.8) years. Fifty one (68%) of the patients with relevant neurology, and 93 (65%) of the patients without, died during the follow-up.

The defined selection criteriae for surgical intervention were existing or increasing atlantoaxial or subaxial subluxations above certain limits. The patients had cervical symptoms (e.g paresthesia) or neurological signs (e.g loss of sensibility, paresis or increased reflexes) from radiculopathy or myelopathy in addition to unspecific local pain not responding to conservative treatment. The neurological findings were paresthesia in 35 patients, paresis in 32, acute radiating pain in the arm(s) in 15, hyperreflexia in 14 and difficulties with urinary control in 8 patients. The localisation was in the upper extremity in 63 (84%), in the lower limb in 41 patients (55%) and in both extremity levels in 29 (39%) patients.

The aims of the operations were to remove or reduce neurological symptoms and signs with pain, stabilize the cervical spine to prevent further subluxations both horizontally and vertically, and to prevent future neurological involvement.

The medical treatment for the patients' RA was continued by the referring rheumatologist.

Operative methods changed over time, and different techniques were used with or without decompression of the spinal canal, depending on the type of cervical instability. Initially, atlantoaxial (AA) fusion would also include additional fusion to the occiput (Brattstrom & Granholm, 1976) but later AA fusion included spondylodesis of atlas and axis only. The applied methods consisted of fixation of occiput to atlas and axis in 12 patients (16%; two combined with laminectomy), fixation of atlas to axis only in 37 patients (49%; 5 of these in combination with laminectomy), 18 patients (24%) had a posterior fusion further down the cervical spine (16 of these combined with laminectomy), and 8 had laminectomy only (Table 2). The need for laminectomy was significantly ($p<0.001$) higher in the cohort with cervical neurology (31/75) than in the cohort of patients without (5/142).

	All	Alive	Dead
Number	75	24 (32)	51 (68)
Operated with arthrodesis	67 (89)	18 (75)	49 (96)
Arthrodesis Occiput - C1 - C2	12 (16)	4 (17)	8 (16)
Arthrodesis C1 – C2	37 (49)	8 (33)	29 (57)
Arthrodesis below C1 – C2	18 (24)	6 (25)	12 (24)
Laminectomy	31 (41)	11 (46)	20 (39)
Postoperative ankylosis	51 (76)	18 (100)	33 (67)
Reoperation refixation	3 (4)	1 (6)	2 (4)
Reoperation cement removal	1 (1)	0	1 (2)
Release nervus occipitalis major	2 (3)	0	2 (4)

Table 2. Operated RA Patients with Cervical Subluxation and relevant Neurology. Levels of Fixation, Frequency of Laminectomy and Postoperative Results with Complications and Reoperations. Distribution among Alive and Dead during the Follow-up Period. Absolute Numbers (percentages)

2.2 Radiology

The diagnosis of instability was made from conventional lateral radiographs of the cervical spine in maximum extension and maximum flexion (Karhu et al., 2005; Kauppi & Neva, 1998; Kwek et al., 1998). Functional radiographs were often combined with plain tomography, and later during the study period with computer tomography (CT) or magnetic resonance imaging (MRI).

Radiographs were scored according to Teigland et al (1990) measuring both the anterior subluxation (AS) of atlas relative to axis and the vertical settling (VS) of atlas on axis measured as the so called 'AC distance'. In addition all posterior subluxations (PS) and subaxial subluxations (SS) were registered. The radiographs were not calibrated directly for distance measurements, but all examinations were taken in the same laboratory with the same equipment and with a standard distance and positioning of the head and neck relative to the film during exposures. The numbers and mean values of cervical spine subluxations for the various subgroups of patients are presented in Table 3. Bony ankylosis was evaluated by examination of ordinary 2-plane cervical radiographs.

2.3 Statistical analysis

Values are presented as absolute numbers N (proportions) or mean (SD). Student's t-test and chi square test were used for testing group differences for continuous and categorical variables, respectively. Cox Proportional Hazard regression analysis was used to identify possible predictors for survival. As reference point for the time-to-event analyses we used the time at operation. Martingale residuals were used to assess the validity of the models. As the assumption of proportionality of the hazard rates was violated, an interaction term between the indicator for cervical neurology and the time variable 'years survival following operation' was included in the final model.

All P-values equal to or below 0.05 were considered statistically significant. Statistical analyses were performed with SPSS software, version 12.0 (SPSS Inc., Chicago), R (R Foundation for Statistical Computing, http://www.R-project.org) and Statistical Analysis System (SAS version 9.1.3; Cary, North Carolina, USA).

	Total N	AS (mm)	VS (mm)	SS N (%)
All	217	10.7 (3.6)	19.7 (7.0)	25 (12)
Alive	73	10.9 (3.4)	21.2 (5.9)	7 (10)
Dead	144	10.5 (4.0)	18.8 (7.5)	18 (13)
Operated with neurology	75	9.4 (4.5)	18.2 (8.3)	23 (31)
Alive	24	9.6 (4.6)	20.6 (7.6)	7 (29)
Dead	51	9.3 (5.2)	16.9 (8.6)	16 (31)
Operated without neurology	142	11.2 (2.9)	21.1 (5.3)	2 (1)
Alive	49	11.5 (2.4)	21.7 (4.3)	0
Dead	93	11.1 (3.1)	20.7 (5.9)	2 (2)

AS - Anterior subluxation
VS - Vertical settling
SS - Subaxial subluxation(s)

Table 3. Cervical Spine Subluxations in Operated RA Patients with and without Neurological Symptoms or signs. Distribution among Alive and Dead during the Follow-up Period. Total Numbers, Mean values with Standard Deviations (SD)

3. Results

In the group of patients with neurological signs or symptoms 66 patients (88%) had per definition (Teigland et al., 1990) a pathological AS of more than 2 mm, with an average of 10.7 (SD, 3.8) mm, and 40 patients (53%) had an AS of more than 10 mm, with an average of 13.2 (SD, 2.0) mm. In 24 patients (32%) the VS was 25 mm or less (normal values 30 mm or more), with 9 patients (12%) having an impaction between 5 and 9 mm, and 15 patients (20%) an impaction of 10 mm or more. In 23 patients (31%) SS was found in the cervical column, in 10 patients at 1 level, 6 patients at 2 levels, 2 patients at 3 levels, and in 5 patients at 4 levels. The levels were C2/C3 in 10 cases, C3/C4 in 15 cases, C4/C5 in 13 cases and C5/C6 in 10 cases. There was a significantly ($p<0.001$) higher incidence of SS in the group of patients

	Operated with Neurology N (%)	Operated without Neurology N (%)	*P*
Moderate AS 3 – 10 mm	26 (35)	32 (22)	0.055
Severe AS > 10 mm	40 (53)	107 (73)	0.001
Moderate VS 21 – 25 mm	9 (12)	13 (9)	0.13
Severe VS ≤20 mm	15 (20)	14 (10)	0.04
SS at one level	10 (13)	2 (1)	< 0.001
SS at two or more levels	13 (17)	0 (0)	< 0.001

AS - Anterior subluxation
VS - Vertical settling
SS - Subaxial subluxation(s)

Table 4. Operated RA Patients with Cervical Subluxation with (N=75) and without (N=142) Neurological Symptoms or signs. Severity of Dislocations Distributed between the two Groups with Statistical Differences. Absolute Numbers (percentages)

with cervical neurological symptoms or signs. In the group of patients operated without relevant neurology there were only 2 patients with SS. The incidence of severe VS was higher in the group of patients with relevant neurology (p=0.04). Interestingly, severe AS was significantly higher in the group of patients without relevant neurology (p=0.001) (Table 4).
The survival rate of the studied cohort with neurological symptoms or signs was significantly reduced (p<0.001) when compared to the cohort of RA patients without relevant neurology operated for involvement of the cervical column (Figure 1).

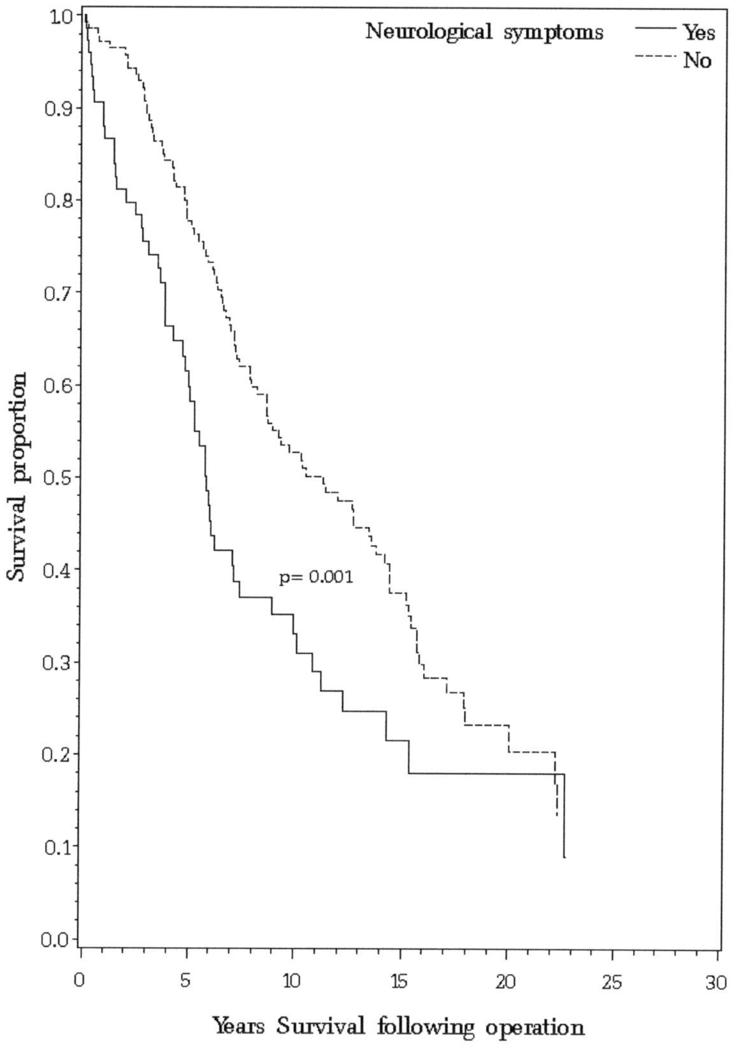

Fig. 1. Survival for operated RA patients with and without preoperative cervical neurological symptoms and signs.

The presence of a significant interaction term (p=0.015) indicates that the hazard for death changes over time postoperatively for the group with cervical neurological findings. The hazard ratio for this group compared with the group without relevant neurology starts at 2.69 for the first time period following operation decreasing to 2.47 at about 6 years postoperatively, indicating that the postoperative hazard ratio is different for the group with relevant neurology than for the group without. The older the patient is at operation, the hazard for death increases with 6% for each year of age (p<0.001), and the patients with relevant neurology have a 169% increased hazard each year (p=0.001). We also calculated that males have a 40% higher annual risk, but this difference was not statistically significant (p=0.07) (Table 5).

	HR	95% CI	*P*
Age at operation	1.06	1.04 - 1.08	< 0.001
Neurology as indication for operation	2.69	1.48 - 4.88	0.001
Time of follow-up	0.92	0.85 - 0.99	0.03
Gender	1.40	0.97 - 2.00	0.07

HR indicates Cox proportional hazard ratio; CI=95% Confidence interval

Table 5. Cox Proportional Hazard Ratio Regression for Survival in Operated Patients with and without Neurological Symptoms or signs.

Postoperatively 7 (9%) of the patients experienced residual neurological symptoms or signs. None of these were alive at the end of the study, indicating a poor prognosis for patients with residual cervical neurology after surgery (p=0.015).

In 4 patients (5%) reoperation was performed: rearthrodesis in 3 patients, fistula with removal of cement in 1. Additional operation with local superficial release of the greater occipital nerve was necessary in 2 patients (Table 2)

Among those still alive at the end of the follow-up 18 patients had had an arthrodesis performed, and all of these developed bony ankylosis. In the group of patients that died during the follow-up period 49 had had an arthrodesis performed, but only 33 achieved bony ankylosis which is a significantly poorer result (p=0.004).

Only 3 of the patients without neurological symptoms or signs before the operation developed relevant neurology during the follow-up period.

4. Discussion

RA is an independent risk factor for increased mortality (Hakoda et al., 2005; Sihvonen et al., 2004). When the cervical spine is involved this risk is increased (Paus et al., 2008; Riise et al., 2001; Shen et al., 2004). In the RA population the estimates of the number of patients with cervical involvement varies from 12% (Naranjo et al., 2004) to 57% (Neva et al., 2006).

Cervical spinal disorders should be diagnosed early and treated actively to prevent severe and potentially fatal complications (Neva et al., 2006). Early surgery corrects AS and prevents further instability (Grob et al., 1999; Hamilton et al., 2001; McRorie et al., 1996). Early surgery may also reduce mortality (Grob, 2000; Paus et al., 2008; Tanaka et al., 2005). Posterior fusion reduces pain and may improve neurological symptoms or signs (Eyres et al., 1998; Matsunaga et al., 2003) as well as preventing progression of existing neural lesions without undue risk for the patient (Kim & Hilibrand, 2005; Santavirta et al., 1988).

When cervical neurological symptoms or signs have developed, the literature agrees that there is indication for operative treatment (Kim & Hilibrand, 2005). In addition to reducing pain, neurological recovery is more consistent with lower grade of preoperative myelopathy (Monsey, 1997). An autopsy study suggests that paralysis may be due to both mechanical neural compression and vascular impairment (Delamarter & Bohlman, 1994).

It is claimed that patients with no clear radiographic evidence of fusion following occipitocervical instrumentation seemed to do just as well as those who have obvious fusion (Moskovich et al., 2000). In our total series of patients (Paus et al., 2008) we came to the same conclusion. However, when we consider the most severely affected patients (i.e. those with neurological symptoms or signs as in the present study), we find a significant better prognosis if ankylosis is achieved. To obtain a higher proportion of bony ankylosis we have changed operative method from Brattstrøm and Granholm (1976) to transarticular screws (Claybrooks et al., 2007; Cornefjord et al., 2003; Haid, Jr. et al., 2001; Henriques et al., 2000; Praveen & Regis, 2005) after this study.

In our minds, based on the present findings, patients with relevant neurology are late for operation, their prognosis being worse, and we advise that operative treatment is initiated prior to the development of neurological symptoms or signs. We disagree with the routine of conservative treatment until neurological complications develop. Residual neurological deficit following operation also resulted in a reduced prognosis in the present study, indicating that delayed treatment may be hazardous.

The high incidence of neurological involvement in patients with SS is well described in the literature (Moskovich et al., 2000; Stirrat & Fyfe, 1993), and we find that this group of patients has a worse prognosis. Our conclusions regarding these patients are more cautious as the operative procedure is more elaborate and carries a higher risk of morbidity, but despite this these patients may benefit from operation prior to the development of neurological complications.

VS can be stopped by AA fixation (Grob, 2000) and patients with neurological symptoms or signs have a significantly more serious settling. In patients with VS, early fixation may reduce the danger of developing neurological complications.

AS is the most frequently occurring dislocation in the spinal neck with an increasing number with increasing severity in both operated groups. However, severe AS is significantly more frequent in the non-neurological group, while SS and VS are over-represented in the group with relevant neurology. This suggests a weak association between degree of AS per se and neurological phenomena. In the non-neurological group, the majority of patients are operated related to severe AS. As neurological symptoms or signs with indication for surgery may develop before severe AS occurs in patients with SS and VS, this may explain the reduced number with severe AS in the group with relevant neurological findings.

5. Conclusion

Development of neurological symptoms or signs in RA patients with cervical subluxations significantly increases the mortality rate. It is therefore important to diagnose these patients early and if possible operate prior to the development of neurological complications. Early surgical intervention will reduce the patients' local symptoms as well as the danger of developing neurological complications which most likely will decrease their life-time expectancy.

6. References

Brattstrom, H. & Granholm, L. (1976). Atlanto-axial fusion in rheumatoid arthritis. A new method of fixation with wire and bone cement. *Acta Orthop.Scand.*, Vol. 47, No. 6, pp. 619-628.

Claybrooks, R., Kayanja, M., Milks, R., & Benzel, E. (2007). Atlantoaxial fusion: a biomechanical analysis of two C1-C2 fusion techniques. *The Spine Journal*, Vol. 7, No. 6, pp. 682-688.

Cornefjord, M., Henriques, T., Alemany, M., & Olerud, C. (2003). Posterior atlanto-axial fusion with the Olerud Cervical Fixation System for odontoid fractures and C1-C2 instability in rheumatoid arthritis. *European Spine Journal*, Vol. 12, No. 1, p. 91.

Delamarter, R. B. & Bohlman, H. H. (1994). Postmortem osseous and neuropathologic analysis of the rheumatoid cervical spine. *Spine*, Vol. 19, No. 20, pp. 2267-2274.

Eyres, K. S., Gray, D. H., & Robertson, P. (1998). Posterior surgical treatment for the rheumatoid cervical spine. *Br.J.Rheumatol.*, Vol. 37, No. 7, pp. 756-759.

Grob, D. (2000). Atlantoaxial immobilization in rheumatoid arthritis: a prophylactic procedure? *Eur.Spine J.*, Vol. 9, No. 5, pp. 404-409.

Grob, D., Schutz, U., & Plotz, G. (1999). Occipitocervical fusion in patients with rheumatoid arthritis. *Clin.Orthop.Relat Res.*, No. 366, pp. 46-53.

Haid, R. W., Jr., Subach, B. R., McLaughlin, M. R., Rodts, G. E., Jr., & Wahlig, J. B., Jr. (2001). C1-C2 transarticular screw fixation for atlantoaxial instability: a 6-year experience. *Neurosurgery*, Vol. 49, No. 1, pp. 65-68.

Hakoda, M., Oiwa, H., Kasagi, F., Masunari, N., Yamada, M., Suzuki, G. et al. (2005). Mortality of rheumatoid arthritis in Japan: a longitudinal cohort study. *Ann.Rheum.Dis.*, Vol. 64, No. 10, pp. 1451-1455.

Hamilton, J. D., Johnston, R. A., Madhok, R., & Capell, H. A. (2001). Factors predictive of subsequent deterioration in rheumatoid cervical myelopathy. *Rheumatology*, Vol. 40, No. 7, pp. 811-815.

Henriques, T. M., Cunningham, B. W. M., Olerud, C. M., Shimamoto, N. M., Lee, G. A. M., Larsson, S. M. et al. (2000). Biomechanical Comparison of Five Different Atlantoaxial Posterior Fixation Techniques. *Spine*, Vol. 25, No. 22, pp. 2877-2883.

Karhu, J. O., Parkkola, R. K., & Koskinen, S. K. (2005). Evaluation of flexion/extension of the upper cervical spine in patients with rheumatoid arthritis: an MRI study with a dedicated positioning device compared to conventional radiographs. *Acta Radiol.*, Vol. 46, No. 1, pp. 55-66.

Kauppi, M. & Neva, M. H. (1998). Sensitivity of lateral view cervical spine radiographs taken in the neutral position in atlantoaxial subluxation in rheumatic diseases. *Clin.Rheumatol.*, Vol. 17, No. 6, pp. 511-514.

Kim, D. H. & Hilibrand, A. S. (2005). Rheumatoid arthritis in the cervical spine. *J.Am.Acad.Orthop.Surg.*, Vol. 13, No. 7, pp. 463-474.

Kwek, T. K., Lew, T. W., & Thoo, F. L. (1998). The role of preoperative cervical spine X-rays in rheumatoid arthritis. *Anaesth.Intensive Care,* Vol. 26, No. 6, pp. 636-641.

Matsunaga, S., Sakou, T., Onishi, T., Hayashi, K., Taketomi, E., Sunahara, N. et al. (2003). Prognosis of patients with upper cervical lesions caused by rheumatoid arthritis: comparison of occipitocervical fusion between C1 laminectomy and nonsurgical management. *Spine,* Vol. 28, No. 14, pp. 1581-1587.

McRorie, E. R., McLoughlin, P., Russell, T., Beggs, I., Nuki, G., & Hurst, N. P. (1996). Cervical spine surgery in patients with rheumatoid arthritis: an appraisal. *Ann.Rheum.Dis.,* Vol. 55, No. 2, pp. 99-104.

Monsey, R. D. (1997). Rheumatoid Arthritis of the Cervical Spine. *J.Am.Acad.Orthop.Surg.,* Vol. 5, No. 5, pp. 240-248.

Moskovich, R., Crockard, H. A., Shott, S., & Ransford, A. O. (2000). Occipitocervical stabilization for myelopathy in patients with rheumatoid arthritis. Implications of not bone-grafting. *J.Bone Joint Surg.Am.,* Vol. 82, No. 3, pp. 349-365.

Naranjo, A., Carmona, L., Gavrila, D., Balsa, A., Belmonte, M. A., Tena, X. et al. (2004). Prevalence and associated factors of anterior atlantoaxial luxation in a nation-wide sample of rheumatoid arthritis patients. *Clin.Exp.Rheumatol.,* Vol. 22, No. 4, pp. 427-432.

Neva, M. H., Hakkinen, A., Makinen, H., Hannonen, P., Kauppi, M., & Sokka, T. (2006). High prevalence of asymptomatic cervical spine subluxation in patients with rheumatoid arthritis waiting for orthopaedic surgery. *Ann.Rheum.Dis.,* Vol. 65, No. 7, pp. 884-888.

Paus, A. C., Steen, H., Roislien, J., Mowinckel, P., & Teigland, J. (2008). High mortality rate in rheumatoid arthritis with subluxation of the cervical spine: a cohort study of operated and nonoperated patients. *Spine,* Vol. 33, No. 21, pp. 2278-2283.

Praveen, M. & Regis, H. (2005). Atlantoaxial fixation: Overview of all techniques. *Neurology India,* Vol. 53, No. 4, p. 408.

Riise, T., Jacobsen, B. K., & Gran, J. T. (2001). High mortality in patients with rheumatoid arthritis and atlantoaxial subluxation. *J.Rheumatol.,* Vol. 28, No. 11, pp. 2425-2429.

Santavirta, S., Slatis, P., Kankaanpaa, U., Sandelin, J., & Laasonen, E. (1988). Treatment of the cervical spine in rheumatoid arthritis. *J.Bone Joint Surg.Am.,* Vol. 70, No. 5, pp. 658-667.

Shen, F. H., Samartzis, D., Jenis, L. G., & An, H. S. (2004). Rheumatoid arthritis: evaluation and surgical management of the cervical spine. *Spine J.,* Vol. 4, No. 6, pp. 689-700.

Sihvonen, S., Korpela, M., Laippala, P., Mustonen, J., & Pasternack, A. (2004). Death rates and causes of death in patients with rheumatoid arthritis: a population-based study. *Scand.J.Rheumatol.,* Vol. 33, No. 4, pp. 221-227.

Stirrat, A. N. & Fyfe, I. S. (1993). Surgery of the rheumatoid cervical spine. Correlation of the pathology and prognosis. *Clin.Orthop.Relat Res.,* No. 293, pp. 135-143.

Tanaka, N., Sakahashi, H., Hirose, K., Ishima, T., Takahashi, H., & Ishii, S. (2005). Results after 24 years of prophylactic surgery for rheumatoid atlantoaxial subluxation. *J.Bone Joint Surg.Br.,* Vol. 87, No. 7, pp. 955-958.

Teigland, J., Ostensen, H., & Gudmundsen, T. E. (1990). Radiographic measurements of occipito-atlanto-axial dislocation in rheumatoid arthritis. *Scand.J.Rheumatol.,* Vol. 19, No. 2, pp. 105-114.

16

Surgical Considerations of Rheumatoid Disease Involving the Craniocervical Junction and Atlantoaxial Vertebrae

T.M. Murphy, L. McEvoy and C. Bolger
Beaumont Hospital, Dublin, Ireland

1. Introduction

Rheumatoid arthritis is a progressive systemic erosive inflammatory polyarthropathy causing symptoms both as a result of disease progression, (Zikow et al 2005, Gorter et al 2010, Klarenbeek at al 2010), and as result of medical management of the disease process itself (Haugeberg et al 2003). It affects synovial joints in 1% of the world's population (Matteson 2003) , with more than 50% of those affected experiencing involvement of the cervical spine (Cabot & Becker 1978, Yurube et al 2011, Garcia- Arias et al 2011) It is characterised by an erosive synovitis, causing destruction of the articular joint surfaces, joint capsules and supporting ligaments for the joints. The atlantoaxial joint is the most commonly affected (Dreyer et al 1999). Though the disease process can cause horrendous morphological change to the cervical joints, with concomitant changes to joint function and stability, neurological dysfunction is surprisingly uncommon. The importance of regular neurological assessment and rapid intervention lie in the rapid progression to disability with the onset of neurological deficits (Rana 1989), allied with a significantly increased mortality rate (Mikulowski et al 1975, Paus et al 2008).

Great strides in the development and evolution of spine surgery techniques and instrumentation have been made treating individuals with cervical and craniocervical junction dysfunction. The complexities encountered when approaching the craniocervical junction of a severe rheumatoid neck, and the anatomical variability of the neural and vascular structures that may be iatrogenically breached (Bruneau 2006) mandate the use of image guidance techniques and/or conductivity detection devices (Kelleher et al 2006) to limit intraoperative risk (Kotani et al 2003, Aryon et al 2008).

The vertebrae of the region most commonly affected by rheumatoid degenerative disease, namely the craniocervical junction and the atlantoaxial joints, have a very complex anatomical relationship with traversing nerves, vessels, and of course the spinal cord (Oliveira et al 1985), and an appreciation of the structure and function of the components of these joints (including how degenerative changes alter the kinematics and structural integrity) is integral to safe surgery in the region.

The most common causes for surgical review of the cervical spine of rheumatoid patients include basilar invagination, atlantoaxial instability and subaxial subluxation (Boden et al 1993). Despite an improvement in spine surgical techniques and technology, rheumatoid disease of the cervical spine remains a challenging opponent for the modern day spine surgeon. The challenge lies in both the poor general medical condition of most rheumatoid patients with cervical spine dysfunction (Skues & Welchew 1993), and the bone destruction and ligamentous laxity that make instrumentation difficult in all but the most specialists of practices. A predilection for developing post-operative infections also contributes to an understandable wariness on the part of non-specialist neurosurgical/orthopaedic surgeons of embarking on major instrumentation without having ready access to the necessary back-up should complications arise (Lidgran 1973, Grennan et al 2001).

2. Epidemiology of upper cervical spine involvement in rheumatoid disease

Rheumatoid arthritis has a mean age of onset at 50 years old. The first documented case of rheumatoid involvement of the cervical spine was reported by Garrod, who noted clinical evidence of rheumatoid disease in the cervical spines of 36% of his 500 rheumatoid patients. It is a ubiquitous condition, and has a male: female incidence ratio of 1:3. Initiation of combination drug therapy of disease-modifying-agents (e.g. sulfasalazine, methotrexate, hydroxychloroquine, prednisolone) at an early stage in the disease process, before extensive cervical or systemic damage has been caused, has been shown to retard the development of upper cervical subluxations (Neva et al 2000). It has been estimated that cervical involvement occurs in over 60% of rheumatoid cases (Dickman et al 1997), with atlantoaxial subluxation occurring in almost 70% of these cases (Boden et al 1993). Whilst basilar invagination and cranial settling are less commonly seen, the associated neurological deficits can be dire, with wide ranges of associated neurological deficits are reported (Zeidman & Ducker 1994), resulting in an estimated cost per case to the taxpayer of over €9500 per annum in late cases (Westhovens et al 2005). Initiation of combination drug therapy of disease-modifying-agents (e.g. sulfasalazine, methotrexate, hydroxychloroquine, prednisolone) at an early stage in the disease process, before extensive cervical or systemic damage has been caused, has been shown to retard the development of upper cervical subluxations (Neva et al 2000).

3. Cellular / molecular factors

Analysis of synovial tissue specimens taken from affected knee joints reveals a typical finding of 2 distinct cell types: Type A cells contain Golgi complexes and resemble macrophages, whose function is predominately one of phagocytosis, and Type B cells contain a proper nucleus and rough endoplasmic reticulum, whose function is mainly protein synthesis (Rooney et al 1988). The histological analysis of affected tissue in the cervical spine demonstrates that the histopathological process of late rheumatoid progression may be different compared with that of the joints of the appendicular skeleton (O'Brien et al 2002). Analysis of chronic rheumatoid disease in the craniocervical junction reveals ligamentous and bony destruction allied with a replacement of rheumatoid synovium of atlantoaxial and subaxial joints with fibrous tissue. Gross mechanical instability at the heavy-weight-bearing craniocervical junction and atlantoaxial joints is caused by bony destruction and replacement of ligamentous structures, as opposed to the acute rheumatoid inflammatory processes commonly seen in appendicular joints. Craniocervical junction chronic rheumatoid arthritis may be considered to be a progressive mechanical disabling process, as opposed to the metabolically active prevalent in other locations.

4. Radiological assessment of the rheumatoid craniocervical junction and atlantoaxial joint

The most commonly used radiological screening tool in nonspecialist units are x-rays of the cervical spine in maximum flexion and extension. However, many cases of subluxation will only reveal themselves on maximum pain-free flexion and extension views.

Computed tomography (CT) is vital when considering which surgical approach to use when fusing posteriorly with a rod and screw fixation. Anomalies such as anomalous courses of vertebral arteries, the presence of arcuate foramina, a small pars interarticularis of C2, or a small lateral mass of C1 can all be appreciated on review of 3D-reconstruction of contiguous axial images stretching from the inion to C4, with added benefit of being suitable for use also for neuronavigation-aided screw placement (Mayer 2005). Soft tissue windowing allows evaluation of pannus. CT is also the ideal imaging modality for evaluation of rotatory subluxations (Rahimi et al 2003).

Magneitic resonance imaging (MRI) is of particular use when reviewing patients with multilevel rheumatoid involvement or in evaluating cases of cranial settling. When compared with CT, MRI is more accurate in evaluating soft-tissue and pannus. It does however have serious limitations when attempting to evaluate bony anatomy. We have performed dynamic flexion MRIs in the past as suggested by some authors, but haven't found it to be of significantly more use than conventional static MRI (Reijnierse et al 2000) in the majority of cases. It may be suitable for a small number of cases where stability or compression is in doubt. In cases being considered for surgical intervention we advocate x-rays, CT, and MR imaging.

No matter which modality is presented to the clinician, he/she must be aware of the various radiographic measurements used when determining cranial settling and atlantoaxial subluxation. However, these measurements are now largely of academic interest, having been replaced in day to day practice by the direct visualisation of the anatomical structures with MRI. Projection of the odontoid peg tip above McRae's Line is considered abnormal, as is projection of the odontoid peg tip more than 3mm past Chamberlain's line. A Ranawat's distance of less than 13mm is also suggestive of cranial settling (Smoker 1994). Whilst the anterior atlantodental interval has been shown to be of great use when assessing non-rheumatoid patients for the presence or absence of spinal cord compression, rheumatoid cases are quite different. In this group of patients the pannus surrounding the odontoid peg can be quite large, and use of the anterior atlantodental interval may in fact underestimate the amount of spinal cord compression. An atlantodental interval of greater than 10mm suggests an incompetent transverse ligament (Dickman et al 1996). The transverse ligament may be lax, as in rheumatoid patients, or may be breached as is more commonly seen in trauma cases (Dickman. et al 1991). The posterior atlantodental interval has been shown to be a greater predictor of space available for cord, and of severity of neurological dysfunction (Boden et al 1993). Posterior atlantodental intervals of 14mm or more are considered to be the lower limit of normal (Oda, et al 1995). Post-operative radiographic images should be interpreted in the setting of such radiographic and craniometric measurements.

The ease of use and ready availability of MRI scanning to directly visualise the neural elements has largely superseded these measurements.

5. Upper cervical spine anatomy as it applies to screw placement and kinematics in rheumatoid patients

An in-depth knowledge of the unique anatomy in the region of the craniocervical junction and the atlantoaxial joint is mandatory when assessing neck pain or myelopathy of rheumatoid patients, and especially when considering surgical fixation of the region. The thirty two synovial lined joints of the cervical spine make this region of the body especially susceptible to becoming floridly symptomatic in individuals affected by rheumatoid arthritis. The occipitocervical and atlantoaxial motion segments have different biomechanical properties conferred on them through their bony and ligamentous relationships respectively.

5.1 Occipital bone

The occipital bone extends from the clivus anteriorly to the lambdoid suture posteriorly, it's embryologic origins being four primary cartilaginous centres laid down in the chondrocranium around the foramen magnum, and a fifth membranous element (Shaprio & Robinson 1976). The superior nuchal line serves as a rough guide for the location of the transverse sinus, and the inion, found in the midline along this line, approximates the torcula herophili. The insertion of the semispinalis capitis may be the most accurate landmark for the confluence of the sinuses (Martin et al 2010). Awareness of the presence of these venous structures lurking beneath the surface of the occipital bone is paramount when placing occipital screws to avoid poor screw purchase and a devastating egress of blood if screw removal is attempted (Roberts et al 1998). The occipital bone is thickest in the midline, with the raised osseous keel being an ideal place to position screws of high pull-out-strength, compared with the thinner more inconsistent lateral portions. Safe regions for locating screws close to the occipital keel are 2cm off the midline at the nuchal line, with an 8mm occipital bone depth being usual, this "safe-zone", however, decreases in width from the midline as one approaches the opisthion (Ebraheim et al 1996). The greater occipital nerve of Arnold is found 15mm off the midline, the importance of preservation through a strict subperiosteal surgical approach lying in posterior scalp numbness or neuralgia should the nerve be damaged (Vital et al 1989).

The occipital condyles, which function as skull-base weight-bearing facets, angle medially and inferiorly at average angles of 55 and 117.5 degrees when viewed from behind (Konig et al 2005). These shape of these condyles positioned on either side of the foramen magnum allow the skull articulate with the cervical spine, whilst the angles prevent excessive axial rotation at the craniocervical junction (Noble & Smoker 1996).

5.2 Atlas

The atlas has its origins in the fourth occipital and first cervical sclerotomes. It is unique among vertebrae in not having a body, is formed from three ossification sites: the anterior arch or centrum, and two neural arches which fuse in later life to become a unified posterior arch, thereby completing the osseous ring which surrounds the spino-medullary junction (Kim et al 2007). An appreciation that this ring is incomplete in up to 5% of patients is important if one is to avoid causing a durotomy or spinal cord injury when approaching the craniocervical junction posteriorly(Torriani & Lourenco 2002, Denaro et al 2010).

The ring of the atlas consists approximately of one-fifth anterior arch, two-fifths posterior arch, with the remaining two-fifths being contributed by the lateral masses (Gray 1918). The longus colli muscles and the anterior longitudinal ligament, which contribute to anterolateral flexion and resistance to hyperextension of the cervical spine respectively, are attached to the anterior tubercle found in the midline on the anterior arch. Two important membranes also arise from this portion of the atlas: the anterior atlantooccipital membrane connecting the atlas to the occipital bone, and the anterior atlantoaxial ligament extending from the atlas to the axis immediately inferior. The anterior atlantal arch is usually directly opposed to the odontoid peg of the axis. The lateral masses of the atlas have a mean width of 15mm (Dong et al 2003), providing both an adequate avenue for potential instrumentation by the spine surgeon, and allowing support of the weight of the head. Atlantal lateral masses have both a superior articular facet and an inferior articular facet. These true synovial joints allow articulation with the occipital condyles and the axis respectively. The atlantooccipital joints orientation at caudal angles of 129 degrees from lateral to medial limits the rotation possible, compared with the atlantoaxial joint with a cranially biased angulation of between 130-135 degrees, where much greater rotation is possible (Konig et al 2005). A posterior tubercle is found in the midline posteriorly providing attachment for the rectus capitis and the ligamentum nuchae. The posterior atlantooccipital membrane extends from the superior border of the posterior arch of the atlas, to the anterior surface of the rim of the foramen magnum (Fitzgerald at al 2002).

5.3 Axis

The axis is formed from five ossification centres: one in the body, one in each vertebral arch, and two in the odontoid process (Lustrin et al 2003) . It acts as a pivot around which the atlas rotates; the odontoid peg which rises perpendicularly from its body, allowing this unique functionality. The pars interarticularis is found directly adjoining the lateral mass-laminar junction. Successful placement of C2-pars screws mandates appreciation of the borders of this continuous bony area by the operating surgeon. The atlantoaxial joint is

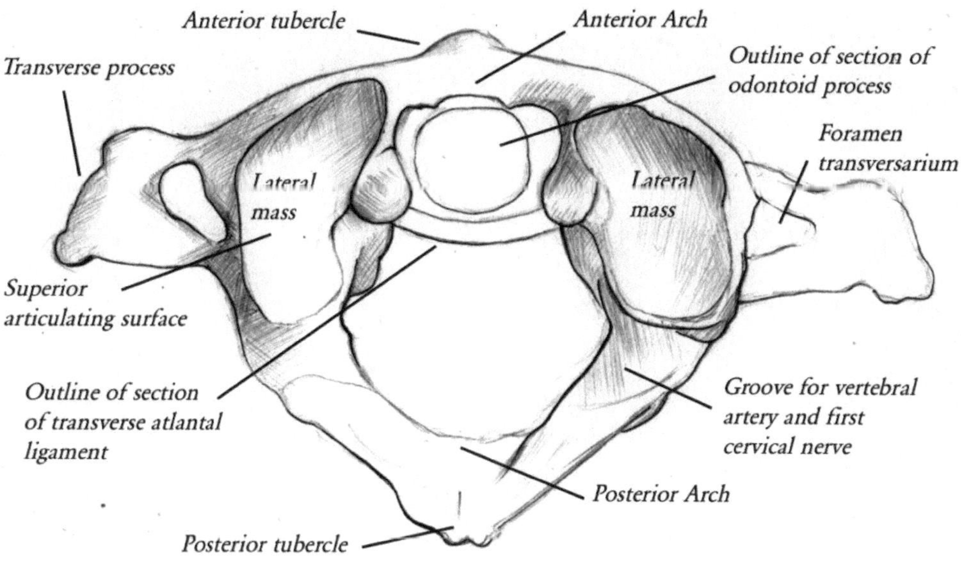

Fig. 1. The Atlas with the odontoid process being restrained by the transverse atlantal ligament.

usually angled 35 degrees oblique in the coronal plane, thereby allowing a consistently safe trajectory stretching from the caudal aspect of the lamina of the axis, through the pars interarticularis of the axis into the atlantoaxial joint, finishing in the lateral mass of the atlas. Pre-operative confirmation of the course of the vertebral artery prior to undertaking any such screw placement will be stressed later in the chapter.

5.4 The vertebral artery

The vertebral artery ascends rostrally through the foramina tranversaria from C6 to C2. Prior to entering the foramen at C2 the artery passes under the pars of C2 where it is vulnerable to injury from placement of C2 OR C1/C2 screws, The vertebral artery exits the superior aspect of the axis, and then passes laterally, to pass through the C2 foramen The vessel at this stage courses posteromedially over the superior aspect of the atlas, where it is vulnerable to injury from overly aggressive dissection by an inexperienced surgeon, before piercing the dura close to the midline and coursing cephalad to the foramen magnum. The left vertebral artery is deemed dominant in 35% of patients, whereas the right side is dominant in 23%. Equivalent vertebral arteries are present in 41% of cases (Menendez & Wright 2007, Tokuda et al 1985). . Particularly in rheumatoid patients the vertebral artery groove is variable in diameter and may encroach sufficiently on the C2 pars to render safe placement of C2 screws impossible.

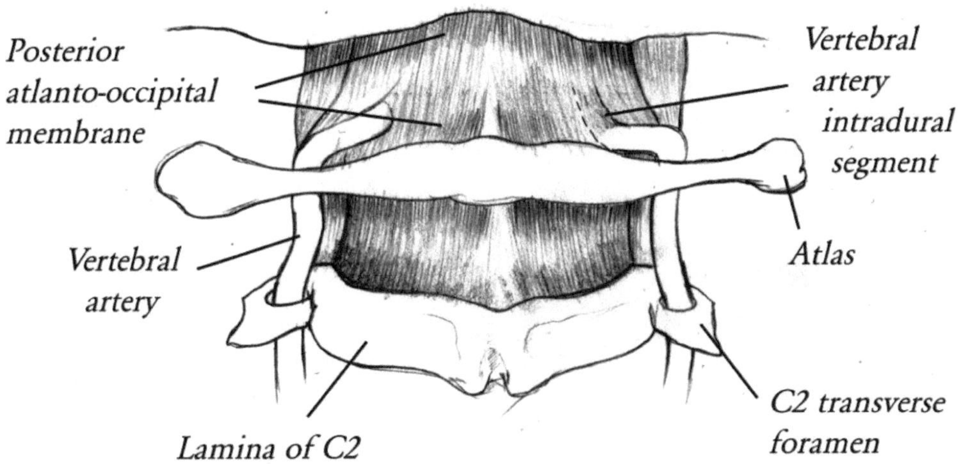

Fig. 2. The anatomy of the vertebral artery during its course from the C3 transverse process to its entry into the spinal dural canal at the level of C1

5.5 Ligaments

The osseous structures described in detail above articulate with each other through synovial joints, muscles, ligaments, and membranes. The slowly destructive process of rheumatoid arthritis is wrought on all of these, but it's effects on the regions ligaments are probably the most important of all. A thorough understanding of the role that ligaments play in providing both flexibility & stability to the upper cervical spine is of vital importance when considering whether a patient would benefit from internal fixation, and also when deciding on the optimum approach to be used. The ligaments of the craniovertebral junction may be broadly divided into an extrinsic group consisting of fibroelastic membranes, the ligamentum flavum between the atlas and axis, and the ligamentum nuchae, and the intrinsic group which consists of the tectorial membrane, the accessory atlantoaxial ligament, the cruciate ligament, the odontoid apical and alar ligaments, and the anterior atlanto-occipital membrane. Our discussion will focus primarily on the intrinsic group due to their importance in appreciating instability in cases of rheumatoid arthritis.

The apical ligament is found in the midline between the anterior atlanto-occipital membrane, has a triangular shape and extends from the tip of the odontoid peg to the anterior most lip of the foramen magnum (Tubbs et al 2000). Though reported to be absent in up to 20% of cadaveric case series, its absence or laxity is not thought to be of functional or structural significance if such abnormality occurs in isolation. The Ligament of Barkow (Tubbs et al 2010) present in 92% of studied cases inserts anterior to the alar ligaments and is often adhered to the anterior atlantooccipital membrane. Its primary function is thought to be in resisting extension of the atlantooccipital joint, acting synergistically to achieve this with the anterior atlantooccipital membrane.

The cruciform ligament is composed of both a longitudinal part (running from upper surface of the clivus to the posterior surface of the body of the axis) and a transverse part (running between the medial sides of the lateral masses of the atlas) arching behind the odontoid peg (Debernardi et al 2011). It's thickness of 2.5mm accounts for its reputation as the strongest ligament in the entire spine (failure strength of 350N), and is composed almost exclusively of collagen fibres arranged in a special lattice arrangement (Miyamoto et al, 2004, Dvorak et al 1988). This ligament functions as the major stabiliser of the atlas, tightly constraining the odontoid peg against the ring of the atlas, thus allowing axial rotation and lateral bending of the C1/C2 junction, whilst restricting flexion. When reviewing trauma radiographs or sagittal MRIs if an increase in the anterior atlantodental space above 3mm is noted, or reduction of the posterior atlantodental distance below 13mm, the clinician must assume that the transverse ligament is not intact.

A pair of alar V-shaped ligaments run from the upper one-third of the dens, where the origin is quite narrow, laterally to insert more broadly on the lateral masses of C1 & the occiput. The mainly horizontal alignment of the collagen fibres and their failure strength at about 200N allow them to restrict axial rotation in the craniocervical junction. The left alar ligament restricts axial rotation to the right, and vice-versa. The tensile strength of the alar ligaments account for the forced coupled rotation of the axis during lateral rotation.

The importance of the great strength of these ligaments is clear when one considers that an intact dorsal ring of the atlas is not required for stability. Instead an intact ventral ring of atlas and intact transverse and alar ligaments suffice for stability at the atlantoaxial junction.

The tectorial membrane is a cranial extension of the posterior longitudinal ligament running from the axis body to the basilar groove of the occipital bone. The central portion of the membrane merges with the dura mater, whilst the lateral portions merge with Arnold's ligaments (Tubbs 2007). A higher proportion of elastic fibres compared with other previously discussed ligaments account for its lack of tensile strength & its minimal contribution toward the stability of the craniocervical junction.

The accessory atlantoaxial ligament runs from the lateral mass of the atlas to the dorsal aspect of the body of the axis and to the occiput. Differences remain in the literature regarding whether this ligament is a part of or separate to Arnold's ligament (Tubbs 2004, Brolin & Halldin 2004). It is thought to play an important role in restricting craniocervical rotation.

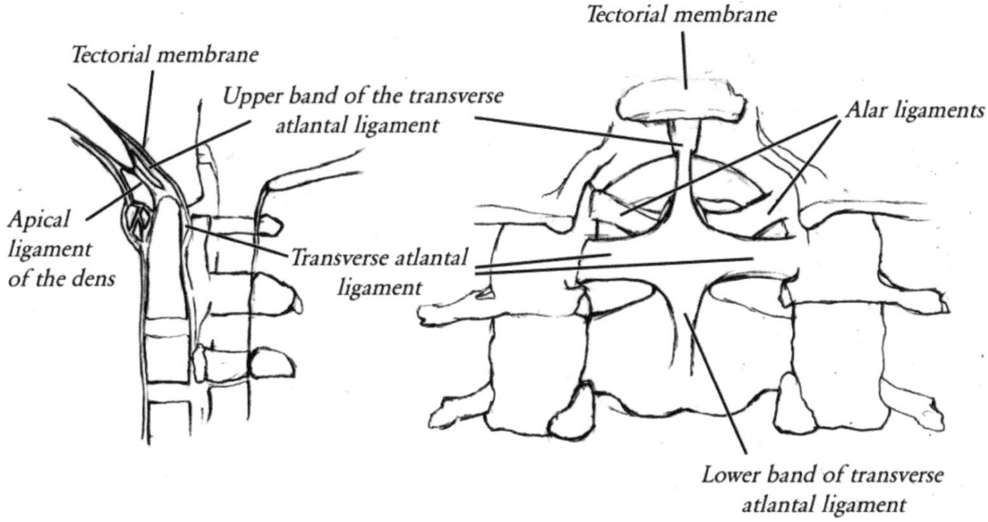

Fig. 3. (a) and (b): The ligaments of the craniocervical junction

(a) Sagittal view showing the posterior longitudinal ligament continuing rostrally as the tectorial membrane
(b) View of the cruciate ligament and alar ligaments, the main stabilisers of the craniocervical junction

5.6 Nerves & their role in causing pain assoc with RA

The greater occipital nerve is the name by which the medial branch of the dorsal primary ramus of the second cervical spinal nerve is better known by. It arises between the atlas and axis, passing between the inferior oblique and semispinalis capitis muscles, through the trapezius muscle, before innervating the posterior scalp. The lesser occipital nerve innervates the lateral scalp posterior to the ear, and is composed of fibres from both the second and third cervical nerves. Occipital neuralgia refers to sharp, shooting pain arising at back of the head or upper neck, and spreading either to the top of the skull, or to the temple region. It may be present bilaterally, and arises usually in rheumatoid patients due to atlantoaxial subluxation or to C2 nerve root impingement by thickened ligaments. Published series have reported incidence rates as high as 30% in rheumatoid patients (Conroy et al 2010). C1 lateral mass screws have been reported as being an iatrogenic cause of such a syndrome also, and needs to be considered in the post-operative period (Conroy et al 2010). The use of nerve stimulators have been associated with a mean reduction of 96% on the visual analogue score (Magown et al 2009), and are the treatment of choice in our institution (in the absence of atlantoaxial instability) post-successful diagnostic occipital nerve blocks.

6. Biomechanics of the upper cervical joints and the influence of rheumatoid changes on joint kinesiology

The atlantooccipital joint's main motion is one of flexion-extension of the head. Extension is limited by the tectorial membrane, and flexion is limited in turn by the dens meeting the foramen magnum lip. Lateral bending averages 4 degrees per side (one-sixth that possible in flexion-extension at the same joint), and is limited by the atlanto-condylar joint angulation and also by the alar ligaments (Panjabi et al 1988, Bogduk & Mercer 2000, Steinmetz et al 2010). The atlantoaxial joints on the other hand allow significant axial rotation due to the biconvex nature of the joint. Much less flexion is possible at the atlantoaxial joint compared to the occipitocervical joint due to the presence of the transverse ligament (Dvorak et al 1988), whilst extension is limited by the tectorial membrane and the atlantoaxial joint structure itself. Anterior sagittal translation of C1 on C2 is resisted by a combination of the transverse ligament, the alar and capsular ligaments, with the main resisting strength coming from the former (Dvorak et al 1987, Panjabi at al 1991). In the non-pathological state, adult anterior sagittal translation is limited to 3mm at most (Hung 2010).

Significant compromise of the integrity of the transverse ligament-odontoid peg unit is commonly seen in the rheumatoid arthritis patient. Enzymatic degradation causing erosion of the odontoid process have been shown to occur (Scutellario & Orzincolob 1988, Mancur & Williams 1995), a biomechanical process of osteolysis occurring at the odontoid peg base which also causes bony resorption. This phenomenon, consistent with Wolff's Law, occurs in rheumatoid patients due to transverse ligament laxity resulting in significant odontoid peg stress reduction and resultant localised osteopenia (Puttlitz et al 2000). This ligamentous laxity-odontoid osteopenia cycle results in the commonly seen atlantoaxial instability in rheumatoid patients. Puttlitzz's study (Puttlitz et al 2000) of a validated fully three-dimensional finite element model of rheumatoid development and progression also suggests a biomechanical mechanism underlying the resorption of lateral masses of rheumatoid atlases. An alteration in the contact force data, resulting in an unloading of the lateral aspects of the atlantoaxial and occipitoatlantal joints will result in localised resorption and osteopenia. The decreased articular joint force transmission is compensated to some extent at least by increased loading of the capsular ligaments, resulting over time in capsular ligamentous laxity through direct mechanical stretching of the capsule fibres. Much greater flexion-extension motion is allowed at an atlantoaxial joint with severe transverse ligamentous laxity, further eroding the lateral joint surfaces through joint range movement beyond the normal limits.

Whilst atlantoaxial ventral sagittal subluxation is a relatively early development in rheumatoid arthritis, cranial subluxation tends to occur at a much later stage (Slatis et al 1989). Ligamentous laxity can on its own result in ventral subluxation, whereas osseous destruction is required in addition to earlier ligamentous derangement, to cause cranial subluxation. A partial collapse of the atlantoaxial facet-joint complexes results in a cranial subluxation of the odontoid process into the foramen magnum. This process of progressive contact of the odontoid peg with the medulla is known as cranial settling when occurring as a result of rheumatoid disease (El-Khoury et al 1980). Identification of the onset of cranial settling is especially important, as it serves as a surrogate marker for patients prone to poorer outcome (Sherk 1978).

Lateral atlantoaxial subluxation occurs in 20% of cases of documented rheumatoid subluxation at the C1-C2 level (Lipson 1984), and is a clear indicator of asymmetric destruction of an atlantoaxial joint. Differing degrees of bone loss result in differing ranges of lateral subluxation. A limit of 2.5mm atlantal lateral subluxation is possible with 1mm loss of atlantal lateral mass or C2 articular surface subchondral bone, whereas if the bone loss depth increases more than 1mm, the lateral slippage can reach up to 5mm, being stopped at this limit only by the odontoid peg reaching the medial surface of the atlas lateral mass.

Posterior dislocation is found in less than 10% of cases of confirmed rheumatoid atlantoaxial dislocation (Lipson 1985). Destruction of the odontoid peg through a combination of previously described biomechanical and enzymatic means, results in the atlas subluxing posteriorly on the axis. The incidence of neurological deficit is very high due to the end position of the posterior arch of the atlas becoming wedged anterior to the spinous process of C2.

Rotatory dislocation is a less studied entity in the setting of rheumatoid disease. It is thought to occur in the setting of unilateral atlantoaxial joint destruction coinciding with severe transverse ligament laxity or destruction (Bouchaud & Liote. 2002).

It is rare when assessing a rheumatoid patient to find that the anatomical abnormality can be neatly pigeon-holed into one of the described entities. Far more commonly, patients will have subluxed in a number of axes and directions, a concept of importance when considering instrumenting such cases. As a rough rule of thumb, anterior atlantoaxial dislocation occurs first, followed by cranial settling, before subluxation of C3-C7 occurs in advanced cases (Paimela et al 1997).

7. Indications for surgical intervention

A common question posed at both rheumatology and spine conferences is whether rheumatoid disease of the cervical spine is a surgical entity or not. Most clinicians would agree that the answer to this lies in the precise neurological and radiological findings at time of presentation. The three principal agreed indications for surgical intervention in rheumatoid patients are spinal cord compression, debilitating pain, or significant dislocation on radiology imaging (King 1985, Bland 1990, Bouchaud & Liote 2002).

Spinal cord compression may be noted on either clinical or radiological examination as detailed previously in this chapter. It is indisputable that spinal cord compression visible on radiological examination, in a patient medically fit for anaesthesia and not bedbound, mandates urgent spinal cord decompression and arthrodesis in the presence of neurological deficit. Indeed some authors have stated that such spinal cord compression in patients with neurological deficits is the only indication for surgical decompression (Pellicci et al 1981).

Intractable pain secondary to compression of the greater occipital nerve or the exiting two most cranial nerve roots, or perhaps true neck pain caused by irritation and strain of the synovial joint capsules and joint ligaments, can become debilitating despite maximal medical management (Pellicci et al 1981). Decompression, stabilisation and fusion of the cervical spine is indicated in this group of patients also. We do, however, advise a thorough assessment by a pain specialist and psychologist before embarking on surgical intervention in such cases (Borghouts et al 1998, Edwards et al 2006).

The last, and in our view the most difficult group to gain universal agreement on, are those rheumatoid patients without significant signs or symptoms, but who do display significant subluxation on radiology imaging. Some authors have noted spontaneous radiological fusion occurring on serial follow up, but a significant proportion of these "auto-fused" patients will progress to displaying neurological deterioration. Though the timing of, and indications for, surgical intervention in such individuals remain controversial, many authors advocate decompression and arthrodesis, on the basis that the degree of neurological compromise often does not correlate with the degree of radiological subluxation (Rana et al 1973, Bland 1990, Oostveen et al 1999). Further, arthrodesis with the appropriate technique has been shown to prevent progression, particularly in relation to C1/C2 subluxation progressing to basilar invagination. Early intervention in these cases may obviate the need for later trans-oral decompression, a much more invasive procedure (Crockard et al 1986). Each case needs individual consideration both of the risks associated with surgical intervention, and also with the substantial risk of neurological compromise and mortality associated with conservative non-operative management (Sunchara et al 1997). Our practice advocates aggressive surgical management of such cases, in the belief that delaying intervention only places patients with impending neurological deficits at an unacceptably high risk of neurological compromise (Matsunaga et al 1976, Pellicci et al 1981, Casey et al 1996), whilst the patient's overall medical condition and mobility deteriorates, thereby raising the risk of inevitable surgical intervention.

Identification of asymptomatic patients likely to progress to neurological deterioration without arthrodesis relies on the experienced spine surgeon liaising with his rheumatology colleagues, and facilitating quick decompression and stabilisation should signs of early myelopathy become apparent. An atlantoaxial dental interval of greater than 10mm is certainly an indication for surgical intervention (Rana et al 1973), though intervals between the 5mm and 10mm need to be considered in the setting for the potential for progression to neurological dysfunction. Conventional trauma-based measurements cannot be extrapolated to rheumatoid patients, given that 5mm AADI is often seen in rheumatoid spines, as opposed to the 3mm limit of normal in unaffected adult individuals (Oda et al 1991, Shen et al 2004). We routinely favour the use of the posterior atlantodental interval as a more accurate screening mechanism for such patients, using a cut-off of 14mm as favoured by Boden et al, to stratify those at high risk of impending neural damage (Boden et al 1993). However, in our opinion, the overriding radiological measure is the presence of significant compromise on MRI imaging.

8. Peri-operative considerations in rheumatoid patients undergoing arthrodesis

A complete assessment of the patient by an internal medicine physician and an anaesthetist is vital prior to the patient undergoing general anaesthesia. Cardiological manifestations such as pericarditis, arrhymthmias, and valvular incompetence occur at much greater incidence in this cohort when compared with their peers (Conlon et al 1966, Del Rincón. et al 2001). Similarly rheumatoid patients have twice the mortality rate from pulmonary disease (Gonzolez-Juanatey et al 2003). We do routinely monitor these patients in a high dependency setting postoperatively, until they are stable enough to be transferred to a low dependency and rehabilitation setting. Anaemia is a common finding in patients with well established rheumatoid arthritis (Doyle et al 2000), though in our experience pre-operative transfusion is the exception as opposed to the rule. It is our practice to continue intravenous antibiotics for a period of 3 days post-operatively, with the initial dose being administered at time of induction, due these patients tendency to develop both early and late infections (Maury et al 1988, Wimmer et al 1998, Carpenter et al 1996).

A particularly difficult issue for surgeons to grapple with is the question of when to discontinue disease modifying drugs. Though a recent trial failed to show any significant difference (Grennan et al 2001),these medications had previously been shown to delay wound healing, a most undesirable complication in an already vulnerable group of patients (Abhilash et al 2002, Hamalainen et al 1984). Our practice is to discontinue such medications four weeks prior to surgery, having discussed the case with the patient's rheumatologist.

Such disease-modifying agents are recommenced after a period of 12 weeks to allow the maximum bony fusion to occur around the arthrodesis. The one exception in the disease modifying drug group is glucocorticoids. Rheumatoid patients have commonly been receiving oral glucocorticoids as a adjunct to other agents for a few decades by the time surgical intervention is recommended. By such a stage the hypothalamic-pituitary-adrenal has been completely suppressed, placing them at risk of an Addisonnian crisis if such medications are not administered. A large bolus of steroids is usually administered at the same time as that of antibiotics, with "stress-doses" continued for 3 days post-operatively. Due to the severity of the subluxation and deformity seen in the spines of these patients, along with accompanying cricoarytenoid and temporomandibular arthritis (Chen et al 2005, Paulsen 2000), the anaesthetists fibreoptically place the endotracheal tube whilst the patient remains awake.

9. Pre-operative traction

The practice in our unit for a number of years has been to initiate preoperative traction using an MRI compatible HALO ring (Oda et al 1991). This traction is then maintained during the surgical procedure to prevent the loss of valuable millimetres gained during the preceding days in traction, when the patient is being transferred to the operating table. Such millimetres may prove vital in cases of cranial settling and basilar invagination, in improving the degree of medullary compression. Should adequate reduction be possible with the traction, we proceed with a posterior-only decompression and fusion. Adequate and maintained reduction is successful in the majority of cases of rheumatoid atlantoaxial subluxation, as opposed to cases of basilar invagination with concurrent Chiari malformations (Caird & Bolger 2005). In cases of inadequate reduction, we believe our decision to proceed with an anterior odontoidectomy, and subsequent posterior stabilisation, is strengthened despite the slightly greater risks associated with such an approach. Placement of pre-operative tracheostomy and gastrostomy tubes facilitate healing of such anterior approach wounds, whilst allowing regular respiratory toilet and enhanced caloric intake, reducing risks of pneumonia or catabolism.

Rod and screw instrumentation is our favoured method of treating instability in the upper cervical spine. Techniques such as sublaminar wiring, loops or autologous grafting do not provide immediate stability, thereby mandating prolonged use of impractical HALO-vests or hard collars. A rapid return to mobilisation achievable through use of a variety of rod and screw arthrodises will optimise the chances of a full return to independent living in this vulnerable patient cohort.

The goal with all of the surgical techniques used to treat rheumatoid cervical disease is to restore or preserve neurologic function. The precise technique used by the surgeon to achieve this will depend both on the individual radiological findings and on surgeon preference.

10. C1C2 Transarticular screws

In cases of atlantoaxial subluxation, without evidence of cranial settling, we advocate stabilisation of the C1-C2 segment through the use of transarticular screws (Krauss et al 2010). Careful scrutiny of preoperative CT imaging will identify cases where such screw trajectories are dangerous or impossible, such as abnormal positioning of the transverse foraminae or aberrant vertebral artery (Ebraheim et al 1998, Golanki & Crockard 1999, Nagaria et al 2009). We routinely use stealth neuronavigation when planning screw trajectories to minimise the risk to both vertebral arteries and neural structures. In our experience myelopathic patients who have successful reduction and immobilisation of the C1C2 segment will not require laminar decompression. In cases of aberrant vertebral arteries we place a unilateral transarticular screw, with a lateral mass screw in C1 and a pars screw in C2 being placed on the "aberrant" side, if safe to do so, however, an aberrant vertebral artery can also preclude safe C2 pars screw insertion and we have not experienced any failures over a 15 year period with unilateral screw placement. Though some authors routinely reinforce their constructs with a Gallie or Brooks fusion, this has not been our practice. Successful placement of bilateral transarticular screws provides 38mm of fixation which more than adequately stabilises the segment (Yoshida et al 2006), without the added 5 - 7% risk of neurologic injury associated with wire constructs (Ebraheim et al 2000).

Having applied the Mayfield skull clamp either to the skull or to the halo ring itself if previously applied, an image intensifier is used to confirm correct alignment of the atlantoaxial joint and the subaxial cervical spine. A midline posterior incision from C1 arch to C2/C3 spinous interspace level is followed by a subperiosteal exposure of both atlas and axis, and of the occiput itself in cases of occipitocervical fusion. The posterior arches of C1 and C2 are exposed at C1 as far laterally as the medial border of the lateral mass and inferiorly as far as the C2/3 joint avoiding disruption of the joint itself. The destruction wrought by the rheumatoid inflammatory process on the normal anatomical landmarks of the atlas and axis makes placing C1-C2 screws without the use of neuronavigation hazardous at best, and foolhardy in some cases. The pars of C2 is exposed subperiostially as far as the C1/C2 joint remaining anterior to the traversing C2 root. Blunt dissection along the superior aspect of the C2 lamina allows the operator to appreciate the medial aspect of the C2 pedicle. Successful identification of the C2 pedicle and the pars as it extends superiorly toward the C1-C2 articulation, allows a safe entry into the C1-C2 joint. It is important in this area to maintain a subperiosteal approach with a sharp dissector to avoid venous haemorrhage. The joint may be entered, curetted and graft inserted directly. This step may be facilitated with the use of an operating microscope. It has been our practice to perform this additional step where the space between the articular surfaces of C1 and C2 allow it, particularly in those cases with incomplete reduction of C1 on C2. The approximate entry point for transarticular screw placement is 2mm lateral to the medial border of the C2-C3 facet joint. Stab incisions as per image guidance bilaterally allow the desired screw trajectory aiming toward the upper half of the C1 anterior tubercle. Use of neuronavigation to confirm screw trajectory minimises the danger of encountering either the vertebral artery (which may easily be damaged with a lateral or inferior trajectory (Geremia et al 1985) or the spinal cord. The vertebral artery is most at risk from a trajectory that is too low rather than one that is too lateral. This is especially important in cases when incomplete reduction of C1 and C2 has been achieved where an anterior target above the tubercle of C1 should be chosen. In these cases the choice of the anterior tubercle of C1 as a target causes a low trajectory through C2 with the risk of cortical perforation inferiorly. If this is kept in mind, incomplete reduction of C1 on C2 does not preclude C1/C2 transarticular screw fixation. An image-guided drill-guide is passed percutaneously to the posterior arch of C2, and aligned with the planned entry point on the neuronavigation. A guide K-wire is drilled into C2 using the drill-guide, and using lateral fluoroscopy to identify the trajectory to C1 through the C1-C2 joint toward the anterior tubercle of C1. Self-taping screws are passed over the K-wire, which is then safely removed. In cases of incomplete reduction, lag screws (partially threaded screws) may be used to improve the reduction.

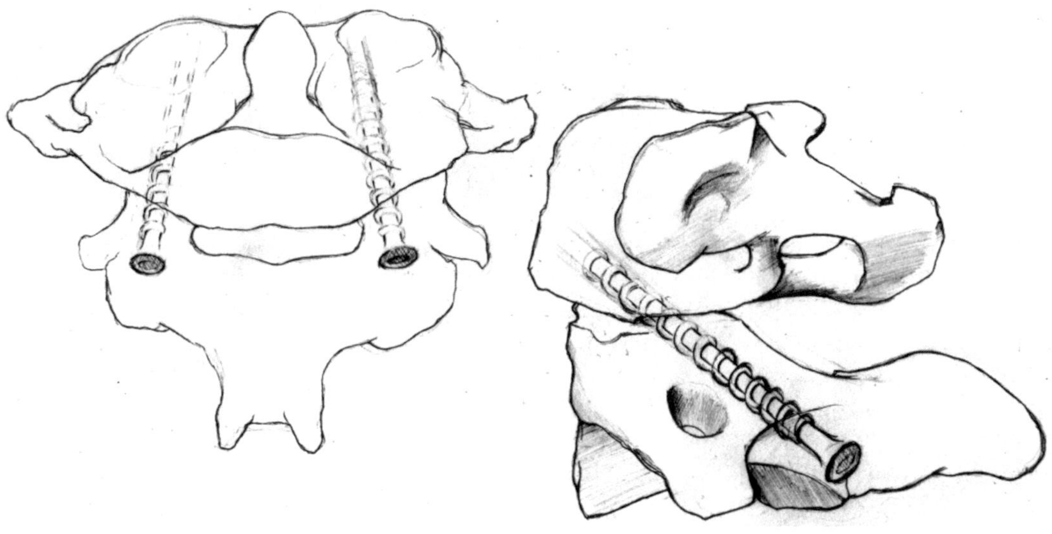

Fig. 4. Trajectory of transarticular screws aiming toward the upper anterior.

Given that up to one-fifth of patients will not be suitable for bilateral safe placement of C1/C2 transarticular screws due to abnormal vertebral artery position (Wright & Lauryssen 1998), all available technologies to reduce the risk of potentially catastrophic vascular injury must be made available to the operating surgeon. The first clinical series involving the use of image guidance in C1/C2 transarticular screws demonstrated no neurovascular injuries in a series of 84 screws (38 bilateral and 8 unilateral) performed in 46 patients with atlantoaxial instability due to rheumatoid arthritis (Paramore et al 1996). Preoperative planning using the contiguous axial images allowed careful planning of the screw trajectory; keeping in mind the position of the intraosseous portion of the vertebral arteries, the diameter of the pars interarticularis and the quality of bone in the axis.
Independent review of postoperative radiographs by consultant radiologists confirmed good screw position in all instances. In 8 cases pre-operative assessment demonstrated a pars diameter which precluded the safe placement of a C2 pars screw, so alternative posterior stabilisation methods were undertaken on the reduced pars diameter side. Such is the biomechanical strength of a properly placed transarticular screw, however, that both in our own practice and those of other authors excellent results have been achieved with a unilateral transarticular screw and Philadelphia collar (Wigfield & Bolger 2001).

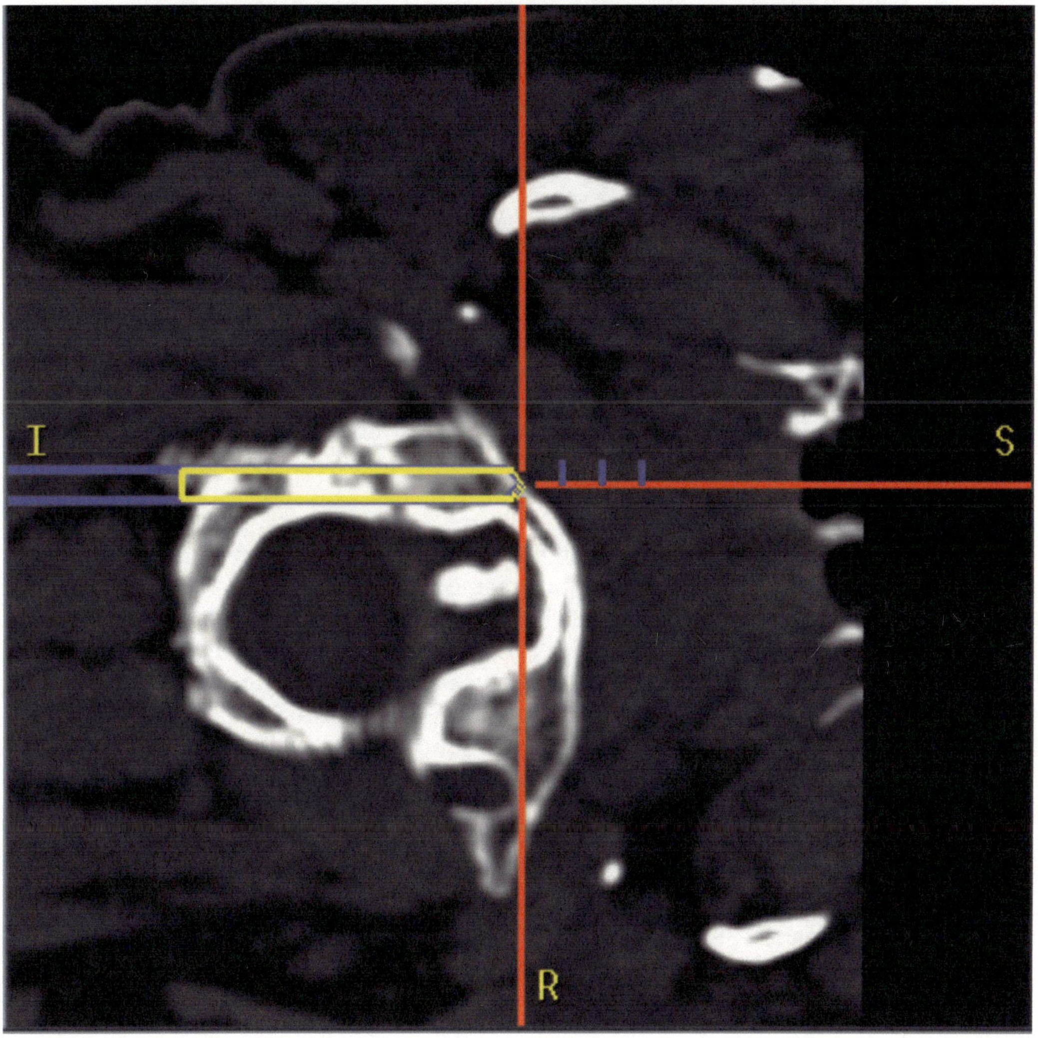

Fig. 5. Neuronavigation trajectory planning of a C1 screw

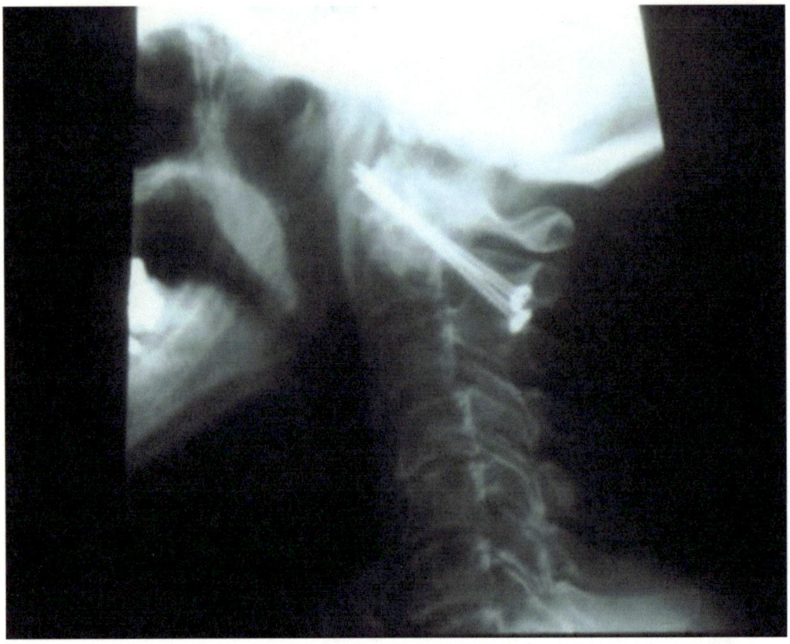

Fig. 6. Lateral radiograph demonstrating bilateral C1C2 transarticular screw placement

11. Occipital-cervical fusion

The occipitocervical junction (consisting of the occipitoatlantoaxial complex) is a multi-joint complex of 4 synovial joints. An important biomechanical nuance to be overcome when fusing this joint complex is the sharp angle between the occiput and the upper cervical spine readily appreciable on lateral x-rays or MRI sagittal views. This sharp angle makes access to the joints quite challenging in rheumatoid patients and also contributes, along with the 5kg weight of the head, to a large moment arm necessitating the most rigid of constructs. Unfortunately fusion and immobilisation of this junction will eliminate up to 50% of the normal range of motion of the head and neck. Our main indication for such "drastic" reduction in mobility in rheumatoid patients is in cases with a large ventral pannus causing cord compression.

The most common complications, other than infection and persistent neck pain, are fixation of the patient's head in an excessively flexed or extended position, thereby increasing the risk of falls in an already vulnerable and sometimes unsteady patient cohort. Our practice of placing these patients pre-operatively in a HALO-brace will accomplish the dual goals of checking whether the ventral compression is relieved on distraction (through visualisation of CSF anterior to the cord on MRI), and will allow the physiotherapists to check patient safety on mobilising.

Though historically the cervical fixation was achieved with interspinous wiring or lateral mass wiring in combination with preformed rods such as the Ransford loop, our practice is to use lateral mass or transarticular screws, with off-set connectors if necessary as the bony anatomy is commonly distorted in rheumatoid patients. These more modern techniques have demonstrated higher fusion rates (Shad et al 2002, Kelleher et al 2008) and lower pseudoarthrosis rates (Abumi et al 1999) when compared to their wire-based predecessors.

Surgeons now have a choice of 2 types of occipital fusion systems. The older "Grob-style" plating system utilises the thick keel-like midline portion of the occipital bone, with the inverted Y-shaped plate being fixed to the occipital midline through a set of predetermined screw positions. The greater thickness of the bone in this location increases the pull-out resistance. We favour such plating systems where the occipital bone is intact. Our practice, however, involves treating patients who have commonly undergone previous suboccipital decompression, with loss of this midline portion of occipital bone. In such cases we more commonly utilise an "all-in-one" cervical rods with integrated occipital plates which are secured to the previously placed lateral mass/transarticular screws with locking cap screws. This construct allows the use of bicortical polyaxial screws of differing length, and also allows the surgeon to vary the screw position and trajectory. This 2-plate occipital fixation provides more rotational stability than the mid-line only Grob-plate occipital fixation. A variation on this solution is the use of modular plate rod constructs allowing a further degree of surgical screw-placement freedom.

No clear biomechanical data exists regarding where the caudal-most screw fixation point ought to be placed. Our practice is to have at least 3 solid lateral mass screws or a transarticular screw and 2 lateral mass screw fixation points on each side of the subaxial spine to. The published literature does not give any guidance on which patients may be treated with constructs that end at the axis, and which patients require subaxial stabilisation as part of an occipitocervical fusion. Martin et al's (2010a) cadaveric study suggested that occipital plate and transarticular screw constructs restricted motion equally well whether or

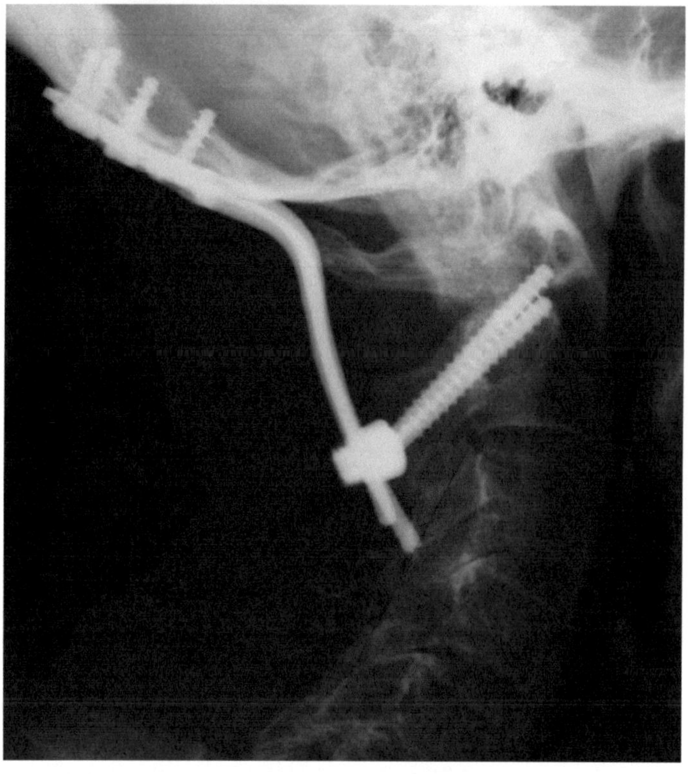

Fig. 7. Occipitocervical fusion utilising transarticular screw fixation of the axis

not subaxial fixation were included as part of the construct. Criticisms such as the female-only nature of the cadaveric specimens and the use of non-contiguous subaxial fixation points have been robustly refuted by the authors as being of limited clinical relevance.

Nowhere in spine surgery is the concept of ultimate mechanical fatigue and subsequent failure of greater importance than at the occipitocervical junction. The large moment arm generated with an adult head and the steep angles required in excessively lordotic porotic rheumatoid cervical spine account for these high failure figures. We use a combination of the autologous bone-chippings on the decorticated bone surfaces, and osteoconductive and osteoinductive bone void-fillers superimposed on our construct to maximise the chance of securing bony fusion. Osseous fusion is necessary for ultimate success of this procedure, as in its absence metal fatigue and subsequent catastrophic construct failure is virtually guaranteed. Rigid internal fixation at time of surgery obviates the need for use of post-operative HALO-bracing, though a custom-fitted Miami-J collar beneath the patient's chin will prevent premature excessive neck flexion and screw pull-out. Careful adherence to a professionally devised and supervised nutrition programme is also part of any follow-up

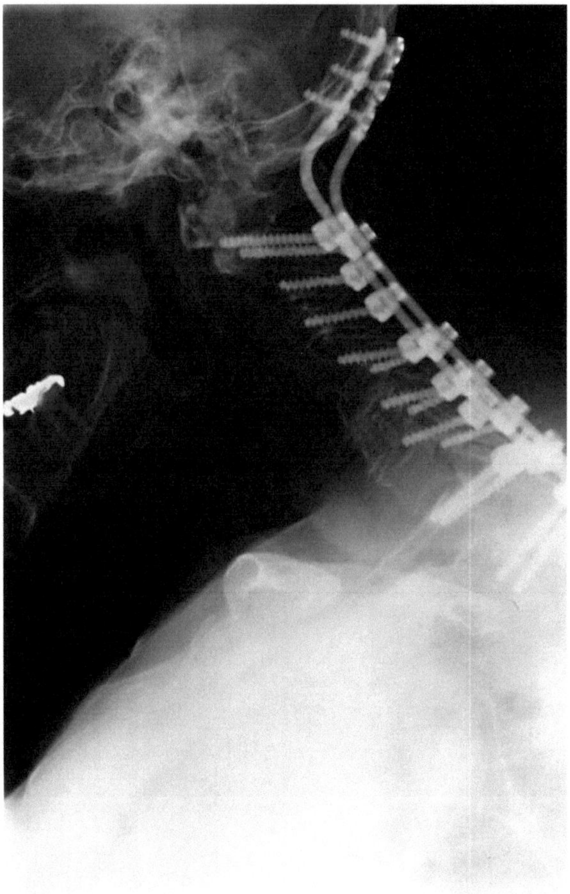

Fig. 8. Occipitocervical fusion using a transarticular screw fixation of the C1C2 complex, and lateral mass fixation of C3-C7. The construct was extended into the upper thoracic levels. Note that single screws were only possible at the C3 and C4 levels

schedule after such fusions to enhance healing rates. Despite poor bone quality we have not encountered any incidents of screw pull-out or construct-failure in our published series of rheumatoid cervical fusions (Heller et al 1991).

12. C1 Lateral mass screw placement

Though we prefer to use C1/C2 transarticular screws, anatomical or surgical circumstances pertaining to this challenging patient cohort occasionally mandate the use of C1 lateral mass screws. C1 lateral mass screws are technically demanding, but we do use them regularly in cases of rheumatoid C1-2 fusions. These may be inserted in cases in which transarticular screws are contraindicated because of anatomic constraints. Such cases include patients with anomalous vertebral arteries, though in such cases it is essential to show on 3D CT that placement of a C2 pars screw is possible. Seventeen (18%) of 94 patients had a high-riding transverse foramen on at least one side of the axis that would prohibit the placement of conventional C1/C2 transarticular screws (Mummaneni & Haid 2005, Nagaria et al 2009). C1 lateral mass screw-rod constructs are preferred over conventional atlantoaxial transarticular screws by certain authors due to a variety of factors (Paramore et al 1996, Currian & Yaszemski 2004). The C1 lateral mass screws can be inserted before reduction of the atlantoaxial joints, thereby enabling the surgeon to use the screws as method of achieving a reduction. The screws do not violate the C1-2 joints, and therefore they can be used for temporary immobilization in trauma patients; however this is not a consideration in the rheumatoid patient. C1 lateral mass screws can also be used when the C1 arch is deficient. The presence of an arcuate foramen (ponticulus posticus) in the atlas, seen in up to 18% of cases, through which the vertebral artery and first cervical nerve traverse, precludes the use of this technique (Gunnarsson et al 2007).

Beginning the passage of C1 lateral mass screw can be quite a challenge due to the almost constant presence of a venous plexus at the insertion site caudal to the posterior lateral arch of the atlas. We use a combination of Surgicel and thrombin glue to achieve haemostasis, and a slightly more rostral entry point, on the posterior lateral arch itself using a pneumatic drill to drill away the undersurface of the posterior lateral arch. Using such an entry point, in conjunction with neuronavigation, allows one to avoid the vertebral artery and spinal cord, whilst also avoiding the worst of the bleeding from the venous plexus. Such an approach is possible in over 85% of cases (Huang & Glaser 2003). The internal carotid artery and hypoglossal nerve lie over the anterior aspect of the lateral mass of the atlas and are at risk from bicortical C1 lateral mass screws. Some authors have advocated use of unicortical C1 lateral mass screws in order to avoid such potential complications. Such opinions are supported by biomechanical data showing greater pull-out strength of both unicortical and bicortical C1 lateral mass screws compared with subaxial lateral mass screws. Our practice however is to aim for bicortical purchase, given the absence of adequate comparative data for rheumatoid patients, and the greater risk of screw pullout due to the tendency of the underlying rheumatoid disease to cause osteoporosis of the vertebrae (Wordsworth et al 1984, Lee et al 2006).

13. Anterior approaches

The most common indication historically for anterior approach to the craniocervical junction in rheumatoid patients was to perform a transoral odontoidectomy in cases of brainstem deformity caused by a fixed kyphotic deformity. Recent authors have published their series demonstrating that such an approach is not necessary if pre-operative traction is successful in reducing the kyphosis, given that the pannus causing the deformity resolves after a posterior immobilisation procedure (Martin M. et al 2010, Nagaria et al 2009). We reserve odontoidectomy for such cases of failed reduction with traction, concentrating on eliminating the medullary kink through resection of the odontoid itself, the body of C2 and a portion of the clivus, if necessary. Our practice is to confirm adequate medullary decompression with a post-operative MRI, before proceeding to a posterior stabilisation as a second procedure. Rheumatoid patients unfortunately are often unsuitable for this transoral approach to such ventral pathologies, due to an inability to open their mouths the required minimum of 2.5cm, or perhaps due to a fixed flexion deformity of their unstable cervical spine precluding adequate surgical access. Advantages of this approach include the presence of pannus usually being within 1.5cm of the midline (Grob et al 1997). The preparatory work and initial steps involving adequate neck extension in traction, use of Crockard transoral retractors to minimise swelling of tongue and lips, along with the midline posterior pharyngeal incision are described elsewhere (Fessler & Sekhar 2006). We often use a posterior pharyngeal flap allowing for greater exposure and less mucosal trauma from retraction.

A few salient anatomical points related specifically to removal of the rheumatoid pannus are warranted however. Direct incision over the tubercle of the atlas is vital as a first step to avoid straying off the midline, and placing neighbouring neural and vascular structures at significant risk. Once the anterior arch of C1 is removed, we dissect laterally to fully identify the borders of the Peg prior to beginning removal. In this way anatomical awareness is maintained throughout the procedure. Many authors advocate separating the peg inferiorly and delivering the upper end by pulling the, disarticulated, inferior end out, towards the surgeon. However we think that this practice is potentially dangerous with the tendency for the superior end of the peg to be displaced posteriorly into the medullary tissue during the manoeuvre. Our practice is to directly expose the upper end of the peg so it may be immobilised prior to any extraction manoeuvre.

Other authors stress the importance of closing the pharyngeal structures in 2 layers (Crockard et al 1986). We have found this almost impossible to achieve, due to the poor quality of the mucosa in these patients, particularly after prolonger retraction. We have routinely closed the posterior pharyngeal mucosa in a single layer without complication.

14. Subaxial instability & lateral mass screws

Inclusion of subaxial points of fixation as part of an occipitocervical or atlantoaxial fusion may be required depending on the individual case. Post-operative follow-up is of the utmost importance in rheumatoid patients. Nowhere is this demonstrated more readily than in severe rheumatoid patients who have undergone craniocervical fusions involving only the atlas and axis. Such constructs whilst immobilising the spine at the upper motion segments, will accentuate the stresses experienced in the subaxial levels, and accelerated adjacent level breakdown may be seen (Smith et al. 1972). The ligamentous laxity so commonly seen in these patients, allied to uncovertebral joint synovitis, further promotes a rapid degenerative process. Due to this tendency we advocate extending the level of fusion to the upper thoracic spine. Our practice is to extend the construct to T2 at least if we encounter a cervical spine that has undergone significant degenerative change; should the subaxial spine be relatively intact, and the subluxation be confined to the atlantoaxial joint, then we advocate simply performing a single level fusion. Avoiding including the very heavy skull and inferior subaxial levels will accomplish the dual goals of eliminating atlantoaxial subluxation, whilst also avoiding the creation of a very large moment arm about the fusion endpoint. If fixation to the skull is necessary we may extend the subaxial fixation as far as C4, but any longer fixation mandates extension of the fixation to T2. An intermediate level of fixation will produce a large moment arm with almost certain failure of the construct at its lower end. Our own series of 37 consecutive rheumatoid patients, with a minimum follow-up of 7 years post transarticular screw placement for atlantoaxial subluxation, demonstrated a 90% success rate in relief of neck pain and occipital neuralgia symptoms (Nagaria et al 2009). In our case series we defined "success" as at least a 50% reduction in the VAS. Both the Myelopathy Disability Indices and the Ranawat myelopathy score showed significant postoperative improvement. Bony fusion and stability was noted in 97% of cases on follow-up CT imaging and flexion/extension radiograph views of the C1/C2 motion segment.

Though described initially by Roy-Camille slightly more than thirty years ago (Nagaria et al 2009), lateral mass screws have been the posterior fixation method of choice for the majority of spine surgeons for the past 20 years. Lateral mass fixation has the advantage over wiring or laminar screw techniques in that it may be used in conjunction with laminectomies or laminoplasties. A disadvantage is the proximity of the vertebral artery, the exiting spinal nerve root, and indeed the cord itself. In the original description, Roy Camille proposed an entry point in the middle of the lateral mass, and a drill/screw trajectory 10 degrees lateral from the parasagittal plane. In an average patient, a screw length of 14-16mm will achieve the bicortical purchase so important in these commonly osteoporotic patients. A number of variations on the concept, involving slightly different entry points and trajectories have been described, but the end-results are biomechanically broadly similar (McKibbin 1979, Xu et al 1998), and all techniques have at their core an emphasis on placing the screw trajectory away from the nerve root and vertebral artery.

The Magerl technique describes the entry point as being 1mm medial to the centre of the lateral mass, and then angling the drill 20 degrees cephalad and 30 lateral trajectory. The vertebral artery usually lies anterior to the longitudinal depression or valley found in all cervical vertebrae between the laminae and lateral masses. Placing your entry point medial to the centre point of the lateral mass will lessen the risk of encountering the vertebral artery and nerve roots, whilst also maximising your screw length, thereby increasing the overall stability of your construct. Further variations of this original technique include the Anderson technique with entry point also 1mm medial to the mid-point and trajectory 10 degrees lateral in a rostrocaudal plane parallel to the facet joint.

Our lateral mass screw placement and trajectory is slightly different to these previously described techniques, with our focus being on achieving the longest possible bicortical screw placement through the lateral mass, whilst avoiding the nerve root or vertebral artery. To this end, we make our entry point at least 3 mm medial to the lateral mass midpoint, commonly along the lamina-lateral mass junction "valley", and then steeply angle laterally and caudally at angles of 30 degrees and 45 degrees respectively. Resting the drill guide on the spinous process of the inferior vertebra is a reasonable rule-of-thumb for the required trajectory (Varrey et al 2004), though in deformed rheumatoid patients especially this rule may not be completely reliable. In our experience it is often necessary to remove the tops of the spinous processes to achieve the required "back-and-out" drill slant. Previous biomechanical studies have shown the more laterally divergent screws of the Magerl technique to have greater pull-out strength compared with the 10 degree Roy-Camille screw (Chin et al 2006), and we believe that our own variation on this with increased screw length at least partly accounts for our success in achieving fusion despite significant comorbidities (Heller et al 1991).

Inclusion of the C7 lateral mass may be required in a minority of cases. In such instances the surgeon's task is eased somewhat by the absence of the vertebral artery from the vertebral foramen, but it must be borne in mind that the C7 lateral mass is the smallest of all in the cervical spine. For this reason placement of a C7 pedicle screw with a 30 degree medial and perpendicular rostrocaudal trajectory is our usual practice. Should the occiput be included in such constructs however we advocate inclusion of at least T1 and T2 in the construct due to the dangers (screw pull-out and kyphosis) of stopping such a large moment arm at a transition junction. Careful review of 3D CT cervical spine pre-operatively will allow the surgeon to gauge pedicle size, and also recognise any aberrant vertebral artery anatomy.

15. Use of PediGuard™

Misplacement and breach of pedicle cortex occurs in approximately 20% of attempted screw placements. Given the much softer consistency of rheumatoid bones, and the importance of avoidance of creating any false tracts down narrow pedicles, it is of utmost importance to ensure that each "screw placement counts". A screw which breaches the pedicle will not be able to contribute its required resistance to flexion, extension or torque forces, and so will significantly weaken the entire construct, perhaps even placing the patient at risk of

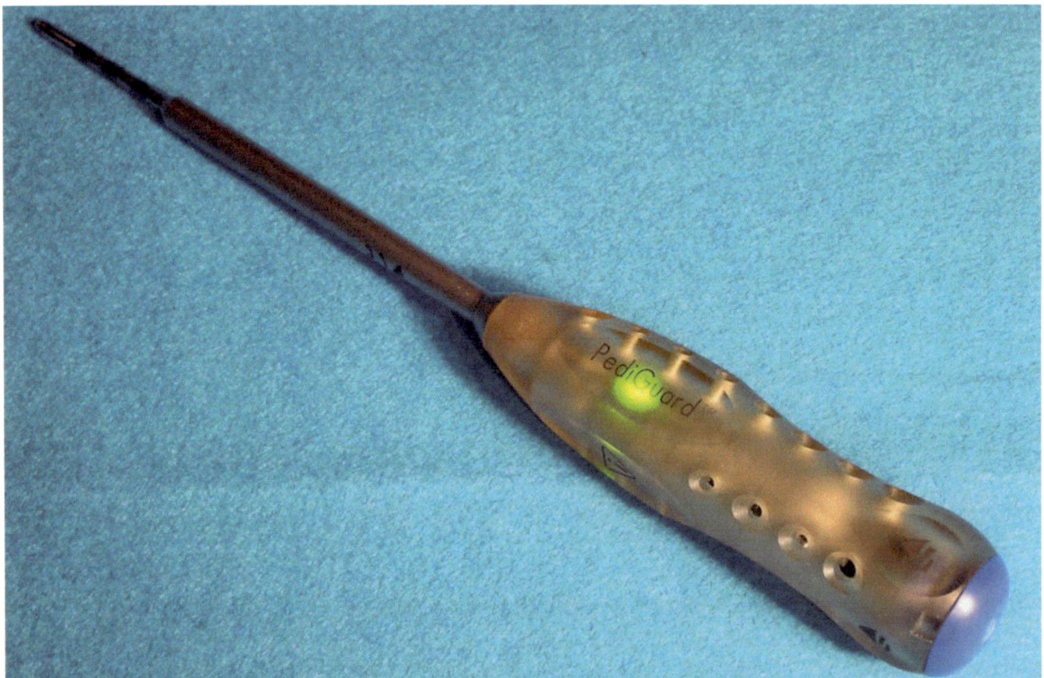

Fig. 9. PediGuard™ Picture

developing a significant neurological morbidity. Our practice when placing pedicle screws in such patients is to utilise the Pediguard™, a device which doubles both as a hand-held awl and which also detects changes in electrical conductance at the device tip. Variation of conductivity occurs when passing between different media, such as exiting the osseous pedicle into surrounding soft-tissue, as occurs during an iatrogenic pedicle perforation. Our series demonstrated a sensitivity of >98% in detecting breaches, more than twice the rate reported by surgeons performing the same surgeries (Bolger et al 2007, Anzhsn 2011).

16. Conclusion

Rheumatoid arthritis affecting the craniovertebral junction and subaxial cervical spine remains a challenging surgical entity despite recent technological advances. Such cases need a pre-operative assessment by a multi-disciplinary team to ensure adequate medical optimisation prior to such invasive procedures, thereby limiting the risk of post-procedure medical deterioration. Symptomatic instability may require instrumentation, and success in such cases depends on the specialist knowledge of the unique altered bone morphology and the plethora of traversing neural and vascular structures. An appreciation of the biomechanical forces which instrumented constructs in this area experience is mandatory if a safe solid pain-free end-result is to be achieved.

17. References

Abhilash J. et al (2002) Influence of steroids and methotrexate on wound complications after elective rheumatoid hand and wrist surgery. *Journal Hand Surgery 27(3), 449 – 455.*

Abumi K. et al (1999) Posterior occipitocervical reconstruction using cervical pedicle screws and plate-rod systems. *Spine 24(14), 1425 – 1434.*

Agarwal A. (1992) Recurrence of cervical spine instability in rheumatoid arthritis following previous fusion: can disease progression be prevented by early surgery? *The Journal Of Rheumatology. 19(9), 1364 – 1370.*

Anzhsn (2011) PediGuard™ Available from: http://www.euroscan.org.uk/technologies/technology/view/1643

Aryon H.E. et al (2008) Stabilization of the atlantoaxial complex via C-1 lateral mass and C-2 pedicle screw fixation in a multicenter clinical experience in 102 patients: modification of the Harms and Goel techniques. *Journal of Neurosurgery: Spine - 8(3), 222-22.*

Assalt K.M. et al (2001) Outcome of cervical spine surgery in patients with rheumatoid arthritis. *Annals of the Rheumatic Diseases 60 (5), 448 – 452.*

Baer A. (1990) The pathogenesis of anemia in rheumatoid arthritis: A clinical and laboratory analysis. *Seminars in Arthritis & Rheumatism 19(4), 209 – 223.*

Bland J.H. (1990) Rheumatoid subluxation of the cervical spine. *The Journal Of Rheumatology 17(2), 134 – 137.*

Boden S. et al (1993) Rheumatoid arthritis of the cervical spine. A long-term analysis with predictors of paralysis and recovery. *Journal of Bone and Joint Surgery 75(9), 1282 – 1297.*

Bogduk N. & Mercer S. (2000) Biomechanics of the cervical spine. I: Normal kinematics. *Clinical Biomechanics 13(9), 633 – 648.*

Bolger C. et al (2007) Electrical conductivity measurement: a new technique to detect iatrogenic initial pedicle perforation. *European Spine Journal 16(11), 1919 – 1924.*

Borghouts J. et al (1998) The clinical course and prognostic factors of non-specific neck pain: a systematic review. *Pain 77(1), 1 – 13.*

Bouchaud C. & Liote F. (2002) Cervical spine involvement in rheumatoid arthritis. A Review. *Joint Bone Spine 69(2), 141 – 154.*

Brolin K. & Halldin P. (2004) Development of a finite element model of the upper cervical spine and a parameter study of ligament characteristics. *Spine 29(4), 376 – 385.*

Bruneau M. (2006) Anatomical Variations of the V2 Segment of the Vertebral Artery. *Neurosurgery 59(1), 20 – 24.*

Cabot A & Becker A. (1978) The Cervical Spine in Rheumatoid Arthritis. *Clinical Orthopaedics and Related Research 131, 130-140.*

Caird J. & Bolger C. (2005) Preoperative cervical traction in cases of cranial settling with halo ring and Mayfield skull clamp. *British Journal of Neurosurgery 19(6), 488 – 489.*

Carle R.S. et al (2006) Perioperative Management of Medications Used in the Treatment of Rheumatoid Arthritis. *Hospital Special Surgery Journal 2(2), 141 – 147.*

Carpenter et al (1996) Postoperative joint infections in rheumatoid arthritis patients on methotrexate therapy. *Orthopedics 19(3), 207 – 210.*

Casey A. et al (1996) Surgery on the rheumatoid cervical spine for the non-ambulant myelopathic patient—too much, too late? *The Lancet 347(9007), 1004 – 1007.*

Chen J.J et al (2005) Cricoarytenoid Rheumatoid Arthritis: An Important Consideration in Aggressive Lesions of the Larynx. *American Journal of Neuroradiology 26, 970 – 972.*

Chin K.R. et al (2006) Use of spinous processes to determine drill trajectory during placement of lateral mass screws: a cadaveric analysis. *Journal of Spinal Disorders and Techniques 19(1), 18 – 21.*

Conlon P.W. et al (1966) Rheumatoid Arthritis of the Cervical Spine: An Analysis of 333 Cases. *Annals of the Rheumatoid Diseases.*

Conroy E. et al (2010) C1 lateral mass screw-induced occipital neuralgia: a report of two cases. *European Spine Journal 19(3), 474 – 476.*

Crockard HA et al (1986) Transoral decompression and posterior fusion for rheumatoid atlanto-axial subluxation. *Journal of Bone and Joint Surgery - British Volume,* Vol 68-B, Issue 3, 350-356.

Currian B. & Yaszemski M. (2004) The use of C1 lateral mass fixation in the cervical spine. *Current Opinion in Orthopaedics 15(3), 184 – 191.*

Debernardi A. et al (2011) The Craniovertebral Junction Area and the Role of the Ligaments and Membranes. *68(2),Neurosurgery 291 – 301.*

Del Rincón I. et al (2001) High incidence of cardiovascular events in a rheumatoid arthritis cohort not explained by traditional cardiac risk factors. *Arthritis & Rheumatism 44(12), 2737 – 2745.*

Denaro L et al [Ed] (2010) Pitfalls in Cervical Spine Surgery: Avoidance and Management of Complications. Springer Publications. ISBN 978-3-540-85019-9.

Dickman C.A. et al (1991) Magnetic resonance imaging of the transverse atlantal ligament for the evaluation of atlantoaxial instability. *Journal of Neurosurgery 75(2), 221-22.*

Dickman C.A. et al (1996) Injuries Involving the Transverse Atlantal Ligament: Classification and Treatment Guidelines Based upon Experience with 39 Injuries. *Neurosurgery 38(1), 44 – 50.*

Dickman C.A. et al (1997) Surgery of the craniovertebral junction. Thieme Publications ISBN 3-13-107181-8.

Dong Y. et al (2003) Quantitative Anatomy of the Lateral Mass of the Atlas. *Spine 28(9), 860 – 863.*

Doyle J.J et al (2000) Prevalence of Pulmonary Disorders in Patients with Newly Diagnosed: Rheumatoid Arthritis. *Clinical Rheumatology,19(3), 217 – 221.*

Dreyer S. et al (1999) Natural History of Rheumatoid Arthritis of the Cervical Spine. *Clinical Orthopaedics and Related Research 366, 98 – 106.*

Dvorak J. et al (1987) Functional Anatomy of the Alar Ligaments. *Spine 12(2), 183 – 189.*

Dvorak J. et al (1988) Biomechanics of the craniocervical region: The alar and transverse ligaments. *Journal of Orthopaedic Research, 6(3), 452 – 461.*

Ebraheim N. et al (1996) An Anatomic Study of the Thickness of the Occipital Bone: Implications for the occipitalcervical instrumentation. *Spine 21(15), 1725 – 1729.*

Ebraheim N. et al (1998) The Quantitative Anatomy of the Vertebral Artery Groove of the Atlas and Its Relation to the Posterior Atlantoaxial Approach. *Spine 23(3), 320 – 323.*

Ebraheim N. et al (2000) The optimal transarticular C1-2 screw length and the location of the hypoglossal nerve. *Surgical Neurology 53(3), 208 – 210.*

Edwards R.R. et al (2006) Catastrophizing and pain in arthritis, fibromyalgia, and other rheumatic diseases. *Arthritis Care & Research 55(2), 325 – 332.*

El-Khoury G.Y. et al (1980) Cranial settling in rheumatoid arthritis. *Radiology 137, 637 – 642.*

Fessler R.G. & Sekhar L. [ed] (2006) Atlas of Neurosurgical Techniques: Spine and Peripheral Nerves. Thieme Publications ISBN: 9783131275318.

Fitzgerald R.H. at al (2002) Orthopaedics. Mosby Inc. ISBN 0-323-01318-X.

Garcia- Arias M. et al (2011) Complex Situations in Rheumatoid Arthritis. *Autoimmune Diseases* 27-44, DOI: 10.1007/978-0-85729-358-9_4

Geremia G.K. et al (1985) Complications of sublaminar wiring. *Surgical Neurology 23(6), 629 – 634.*

Golanki G. & Crockard A. (1999) Peroperative Determination of Safe Superior Transarticular Screw Trajectory Through the Lateral Mass. *Spine 24(14), 1477.*

Gonzolez - Juanatey et al (2003) Increased Prevalence of Severe Subclinical Atherosclerotic Findings in Long-Term Treated Rheumatoid Arthritis Patients Without Clinically Evident Atherosclerotic Disease. *Medicine 82(6), 407 – 413.*

Gord D. (1993) Principles of surgical treatment of the cervical spine in rheumatoid arthritis. European Spine journal, 2(4), 180 - 190

Gorter S.L. et al (2010) Extended report: Current evidence for the management of rheumatoid arthritis with glucocorticoids: a systematic literature review informing the EULAR recommendations for the management of rheumatoid arthritis. Annals of the Rheumatic Diseases 69: 1010 - 1014.

Gray, H. (1918) Anatomy of the Human Body http://www.bartleby.com/107/

Grennan D.M. et al (2001) Methotrexate and early postoperative complications in patients with rheumatoid arthritis undergoing elective orthopaedic surgery. *Annals of the Rheumatic Diseases 60 (3), 214 – 217.*

Grob D. et al (1997) Atlantoaxial Fusion and Retrodental Pannus in Rheumatoid Artritis. *Spine 22(14), 1580 – 1583.*

Grob D. et al. (1992) Biomechanical evaluation of four different posterior atlantoaxial fixation techniques. *Spine (Phila Pa 1976) 17(5), 480 – 490.*

Gunnarsson T. et al (2007) The Use of C1 Lateral Mass Screws in Complex Cervical Spine Surgery: Indications, Techniques, and Outcome in a Prospective Consecutive Series of 25 Cases. *Journal of Spinal Disorders & Techniques 20(4), 308 – 316.*

Hamalainen M. et al (1984) *Post-operative* wound infection in rheumatoid arthritis surgery. *Clinical Rheumatology 3(3), 329 – 335.*

Haugeberg G. et al (2003) Effects of rheumatoid arthritis on bone. *Current Opinion in Rheumatology 15(4) 469 – 475.*

Heller J.G. et al (1991) Anatomic comparison of the Roy-Camille and Magerl techniques for screw placement in the lower cervical spine. *Spine 16(10), S552 – 557.*

Huang M. & Glaser J. (2003) Complete Arcuate Foramen Precluding C1 Lateral Mass Screw Fixation in a Patient with Rheumatoid Arthritis: Case Report. *Iowa Ortho Journal 23, 96 – 99.*

Hung S.C. (2010) Revisiting Anterior Atlantoaxial Subluxation with Overlooked Information on MR Images. *American Journal of Neuroradiology 31(5), 838 – 843.*

Kelleher M.O. et al (2008) Lateral mass screw fixation of complex spine cases: a prospective clinical study. *British Journal of Neurosurgery 22(5), 663 – 668.*

Kim D.M. et al (2007) Surgery of the paediatric spine. Thieme Medical Publications. ISBN 978-3-13-141931-6.

King T.T. (1985) Rheumatoid subluxations of the cervical spine. *Annals of the Rheumatic Diseases, 44(12), 807 – 808.*

Klarenbeek N.B. et al (2010) Recent advances in the management of rheumatoid arthritis. *British Medical Journal,* 341 9642.

Konig S.A. et al (2005) Anatomical data on the craniocervical junction and their correlation with degenerative changes in 30 cadaveric specimens. *Journal of Neurosurgery: Spine 3(5), 379-385.*

Kotani Y. et al (2003) Improved accuracy of computer-assisted cervical pedicle screw insertion. *Journal of Neurosurgery: Spine 99(3), 257 – 263.*

Krauss W.E. et al (2010) Rheumatoid arthritis of the craniovertebral junction. *Neurosurgery 66(3), S83 – S85.*

Lee M. et al (2006) The Feasibility of Inserting Atlas Lateral Mass Screws via the Posterior Arch. *Spine 31(24), 2798 – 2801.*

Lidgran L. (1973) Orthopaedic Infections In Patients With Rheumatoid Arthritis. *Scandinavian Journal of Rheumatology 2(2), 92 – 96.*

Lipson S.J. (1984) Rheumatoid Arthritis of the Cervical Spine. *Clinical Orthopaedics and Related Research 182, 143 – 149.*

Lipson S.J. (1985) Cervical myelopathy and posterior atlanto-axial subluxation in patients with rheumatoid arthritis. *Journal of Bone and Joint Surgery 67(4), 593 – 597.*

Lustrin E.S. et al (2003) Paediatric Cervical Spine: Normal Anatomy, Variants, and Trauma. *Radiographics 23(3), 539 – 560.*

Magown P. et al (2009) Occipital Nerve Stimulation for Intractable Occipital Neuralgia: An Open Surgical Technique. *Clinical Neurosurgery 56, 119 – 124.*

Mancur C. & Williams H.J. (1995) Rheumatoid Arthritis: Status of Drug Therapies. *Physical Therapy 75(6), 511 – 525.*

Martin M. et al (2010a) Biomechanical Implications of Extending Occipitocervical Instrumentation to Include the Subaxial Spine. *Neurosurgery 66(6), 1148 – 1152.*

Martin M.D. et al (2010b) Anatomic and biomechanical considerations of the craniovertebral junction. *Neurosurgery 66(3S), 2 – 6.*

Matsunaga S. et al (1976) Prognosis of Patients With Upper Cervical Lesions Caused by Rheumatoid Arthritis: Comparison of Occipitocervical Fusion Between C1 Laminectomy and Nonsurgical Management. *Spine 28(4) 1581 – 1587.*

Matteson E. (2003) Cervical spine disease in rheumatoid arthritis: How common a finding? How uncommon a problem? *Arthritis & Rheumatism 48(7), 1775 – 1778.*

Maury C.P. et al 1988 Scientific Commons: Mechanism of anaemia in rheumatoid arthritis: demonstration of raised interleukin 1 beta concentrations in anaemic patients and of interleukin 1 mediated suppression of normal erythropoiesis and proliferation of human erythroleukaemia (HEL) cells in vitro. *Annuals of Rheumatic Diseases 47, 972 – 978.*

Mayer H.M. [Ed] (2005) Minimally invasive spine surgery 2nd Ed; Springer, New York – ISBN 3-540-21347-3.

McKibbin B. [Ed] (1979) Recent advances in orthopaedics 3. http://onlinelibrary.wiley.com/doi/10.1002/bjs.1800670531/abstract

Menendez J.A. & Wright N.M. (2007) Techniques of Posterior C1-C2 Stabilisation. *Neurosurgery 60(1S), S103 – S110.*

Mikulowski P. et al (1975) Sudden Death in Rheumatoid Arthritis with Atlanto-axial Dislocation. *Acta Medica Scandinavica 198 (1-6), 445 – 451.*

Miyamoto A. et al (2004) Traumatic Anterior Atlantoaxial Subluxation Occurring in a Professional Rugby Athlete: Case Report and Review of Literature Related to Atlantoaxial Injuries in Sports Activities. *Spine 29(3), 61 – 64.*

Mummaneni P.V. & Haid P.V. (2005) Transoral Odontoidectomy. *Neurosurgery 56(5), 1045 – 1950.*

Nagaria J. et al (2009) C1–C2 Transarticular Screw Fixation for Atlantoaxial Instability due to Rheumatoid Arthritis: A Seven-Year Analysis of Outcome. *Spine 34(26), 2880 – 2885.*

Neva M.M. et al (2000) Combination drug therapy retards the development rheumatoid atlantoaxial subluxations. *Arthritis & Rheumatism 43(11), 2397 – 2401.*

Noble E.R. & Smoker W.R.K. (1996) The forgotten condyle: the appearance, morphology, and classification of occipital condyle fractures. *American Journal of Neuroradiology 17(3), 507 – 513.*

O'Brien M. et al (2002) Histology of the Craniocervical Junction in Chronic Rheumatoid Arithritis: A clinicopathologic analysis of 33 operative cases. *Spine 27(20), 2245 – 2254.*

Oda T. et al (1991) Experimental Study of Atlas Injuries II: Relevance to Clinical Diagnosis and Treatment. *Spine 16(10) S466 – S473.*

Oda, T. et al (1995) Natural Course of Cervical Spine Lesions in Rheumatoid Arthritis. *Spine 20(10), 1128 – 1135.*

Oliveira E. et al (1985) Microsurgical anatomy of the region of the foramen magnum. *Surgical Neurology 24(3), 293 – 352.*

Oostveen J. et al (1999) Successful conservative treatment of rheumatoid subaxial subluxation resulting in improvement of myelopathy, reduction of subluxation, and stabilisation of the cervical spine. A report of two Cases. *Annals of the Rheumatic Diseases 58, 126 – 129.*

Paimela L. et al (1997) Progression of cervical spine changes in patients with early rheumatoid arthritis. *The Journal of Rheumatology 24(7), 1280 – 1284.*

Panjabi M. at al (1991) Effects of Alar ligament transection on upper cervical spine rotation. *Journal of Orthopaedic Research 9(4), 584 – 593.*

Panjabi M. et al (1988) Three-Dimensional Movements of the Upper Cervical Spine. *Spine 13(7), 726 – 730.*

Paramore C. et al (1996) The anatomical suitability of the C1–2 complex for transarticular screw fixation. *Journal of Neurosurgery 85(2), 221-224.*

Paulsen F.P. (2000) The Cricoarytenoid Joint Capsule and Its Relevance to Endotracheal Intubation. *Anesthesia & Analgesia 90(1), 180 – 185.*

Paus A.C. et al (2008) High Mortality Rate in Rheumatoid Arthritis With Subluxation of the Cervical Spine: A Cohort Study of Operated and Nonoperated Patients. Spine 33(21), 2278 - 2283.

Pellicci P.M. et al (1981) A prospective study of the progression of rheumatoid arthritis of the cervical spine. *Journal of Bone and Joint Surgery 63(3), 342 – 350.*

Puttlitz C. et al (2000) Biomechanical Rationale for the Pathology of Rheumatoid Arthritis in the Craniovertebral Junction. *Spine 25(13), 1607 – 1616.*

Rahimi S. et al (2003) Treatment of atlantoaxial instability in paediatric patients. *Neurosurgical Focus, 15(6); 1 – 4.*

Rana N. (1989) Natural History of Atlanto-Axial Subluxation in Rheumatoid Arthritis. *Spine 14(10), 1054 – 1056.*

Rana N.A. et al (1973) Atlanto-Axial Subluxation in Rheumatoid Arthritis. *Journal of Bone and Joint Surgery 55-B (3), 458 – 470.*

Reijnierse M. et al (2000) Are magnetic resonance flexion views useful in evaluating the cervical spine of patients with rheumatoid arthritis? *Skeletal Radiology 29(8), 85 – 89.*

Roberts D.A. et al (1998) Quantitative Anatomy of the Occiput and the Biomechanics of occipital screw fixation. *Spine 23(10), 1100 – 1107.*

Rooney M. et al (1988) Analysis of the histologic variation of synovitis in rheumatoid arthritis. *Arthritis & Rheumatism 31(8), 956 – 963.*

Rosher J.J & Cosh J.A (1978) Radiological study of cervical spine and hand in patients with rheumatoid arthritis of 15 years' duration: an assessment of the effects of corticosteroid treatment. *Annals of the Rheumatic Diseases 37 (6), 529 – 535.*

Scutellario P.N & Orzincolob C. (1988) Rheumatoid arthritis: sequences. *European Journal Radiology 27(1), S31 – S38.*

Shad A. et al (2002) Craniocervical fusion for rheumatoid arthritis: comparison of sublaminar wires and the lateral mass screw craniocervical fusion. *British Journal of Neurosurgery 16(5), 483 – 486.*

Shaprio R. & Robinson F. (1976) Embryogenesis of the human occipital bone. *American Journal of Roentgenology 126, 1063 – 1068.*

Shen F.H. et al (2004) Rheumatoid arthritis: evaluation and surgical management of the cervical spine. *Spine Journal 4(6), 389 – 700.*

Sherk H.H. (1978) Atlantoaxial instability and acquired basilar invagination in rheumatoid arthritis. *Orthop Clin North Am 9(4), 1053 – 1063.*

Skues M. & WElchew E. (1993) Anaesthesia and rheumatoid arthritis. *Anaesthesia 48 (11), 989 – 997.*

Slatis P. et al (1989) Cranial subluxation of the odontoid process in rheumatoid arthritis. *Journal of Bone and Joint Surgery 71(2), 189 – 195.*

Smoker W. (1994) Craniovertebral junction: normal anatomy, craniometry, and congenital anomalies. *Radiographics 14(2), 255 – 277.*

Song G. et al (1997) Unilateral posterior atlantoaxial transarticular screw fixation. *Journal Neurosurgery 87(6), 851 – 855.*

Steinmetz M.P. et al (2010) Craniovertebral junction: biomechanical considerations. *Neurosurgery 2010, 66(3), S7 – S12.*

Sunchara N. et al (1997) Clinical Course of Conservatively Managed Rheumatoid Arthritis Patients With Myelopathy. *Spine 22(22), 2603 – 2607.*

Tokuda K. et al (1985) Anomalous atlantoaxial portions of vertebral and posterior inferior cerebellar arteries. *Neuroradiology, 27(5), 410 – 413.*

Torriani M. & Lourenco J. (2002) Agenesis of the posterior arch of the atlas. *Revista do Hospital das Clínicas 57(2), 73 – 76.*

Tubbs R.S. (2004) The Accessory Atlantoaxial Ligament. *Neurosurgery 55(2), 400 – 404.*

Tubbs R.S. (2007) The tectorial membrane: anatomical, biomechanical and histological analysis. *Clinical Anatomy. 20(4), 382 – 386.*

Tubbs R.S. et al (2000) *The apical ligament: anatomy and functional significance. Journal of Neurosurgery: Spine, 92(2), 197-200.*

Tubbs R.S. et al (2010) Ligament of Barkow of the craniocervical junction: its anatomy and potential clinical and functional significance. *Journal Neurosurgical Spine12(6), 619 – 622.*

Varrey C. et al (2004) Biomechanical evaluation of cervical lateral mass fixation: a comparison of the Roy-Camille and Magerl screw techniques. *Journal of Neurosurgery: Spine 100(3), 268-276.*

Vital J. et al (1989) An anatomic and dynamic study of the greater occipital nerve (n. of Arnold). Applications to the treatment of Arnold's neuralgia. *Surgical & Radiologic Anatomy 11(3), 205 – 210.*

Westhovens R. et al (2005) Healthcare consumption and direct costs of rheumatoid arthritis in Belgium. *Clinical Rheumatology. 24(6), 615 – 619.*

Wigfield C. & Bolger C. (2001) A technique for frameless stereotaxy and placement of transarticular screws for atlanto-axial instability in rheumatoid arthritis. *European Spine Journal 10(3), 264 – 268.*

Wimmer C. et al (1998) Predisposing Factors for Infection in Spine Surgery: A Survey of 850 Spinal Procedures. *Journal of Spinal Disorders & Techniques 11(2), 124 – 128.*

Wordsworth B.P et al (1984) Metabolic Bone Disease Among In-Patients with Rheumatoid Arthritis. *Rheumatology 23(4), 251 – 257.*

Wright N. & Lauryssen C. (1998) Vertebral artery injury in C1–2 transarticular screw fixation: results of a survey of the AANS/CNS Section on Disorders of the Spine and Peripheral Nerves. *Journal of Neurosurgery 88(4), 634 – 640.*

Xu R. et al (1998) Modified Magerl technique of lateral mass screw placement in the lower cervical spine: an anatomic study. *Journal of Spinal Disorders and Techniques 11(3), 237 – 240.*

Yoshida M. et al (2006) Comparison of the Anatomical Risk for Vertebral Artery Injury Associated With the C2-Pedicle Screw and Atlantoaxial Transarticular Screw. *Spine 31 (15), E513 – E517.*

Yurube T. et al (2011) Progression of Cervical Spine Instabilities in Rheumatoid Arthritis: A Prospective Cohort Study of Outpatients over 5 Years. Spine 36(8), 647 - 653.

Zeidman S.M. & Ducker T.B. (1994) Rheumatoid arthritis. Neuroanatomy, compression, and grading of deficits. *Spine 19(20), 2259 – 2266.*

Zikow A. et al (2005) Radiological cervical spine involvement in patients with rheumatoid arthritis: a cross sectional study. *The Journal of Rheumatology 32(5) 801-806.*